FIFTH EDITION

OPHTHALMIC NURSING

FIFTH EDITION

OPHTHALMIC NURSING

Mary E. Shaw
University of Manchester, UK

Agnes Lee
Northampton General Hospital, UK

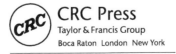

CRC Press
Taylor & Francis Group
Boca Raton London New York

CRC Press is an imprint of the
Taylor & Francis Group, an **informa** business

CRC Press
Taylor & Francis Group
6000 Broken Sound Parkway NW, Suite 300
Boca Raton, FL 33487-2742

Printed on acid-free paper
Version Date: 20160405

International Standard Book Number-13: 978-1-4822-4976-7 (Paperback)

This book contains information obtained from authentic and highly regarded sources. While all reasonable efforts have been made to publish reliable data and information, neither the author[s] nor the publisher can accept any legal responsibility or liability for any errors or omissions that may be made. The publishers wish to make clear that any views or opinions expressed in this book by individual editors, authors or contributors are personal to them and do not necessarily reflect the views/opinions of the publishers. The information or guidance contained in this book is intended for use by medical, scientific or health-care professionals and is provided strictly as a supplement to the medical or other professional's own judgement, their knowledge of the patient's medical history, relevant manufacturer's instructions and the appropriate best practice guidelines. Because of the rapid advances in medical science, any information or advice on dosages, procedures or diagnoses should be independently verified. The reader is strongly urged to consult the relevant national drug formulary and the drug companies' and device or material manufacturers' printed instructions, and their websites, before administering or utilizing any of the drugs, devices or materials mentioned in this book. This book does not indicate whether a particular treatment is appropriate or suitable for a particular individual. Ultimately it is the sole responsibility of the medical professional to make his or her own professional judgements, so as to advise and treat patients appropriately. The authors and publishers have also attempted to trace the copyright holders of all material reproduced in this publication and apologize to copyright holders if permission to publish in this form has not been obtained. If any copyright material has not been acknowledged please write and let us know so we may rectify in any future reprint.

Visit the Taylor & Francis Web site at
http://www.taylorandfrancis.com

and the CRC Press Web site at
http://www.crcpress.com

Contents

Contents

Foreword

There are few specialties within nursing and allied health where the patients are aged from preterm neonates to the very elderly, where those needing care may be suffering from trauma, acute illness, or chronic disease or may need support or rehabilitation.

The eye is the only organ whose inside can be examined without damaging the body to do so. Blood vessels and nerve tissue may be seen, working, inside the person. The organ of sight is incredibly complex and, because of this, it can malfunction in many different ways and these all have consequences for the individual experiencing the problem.

Ophthalmology then is a complex speciality within which nurses work as a vital part of the multidisciplinary team. The ophthalmic nurse must have a good working knowledge about ophthalmology in order to provide individualised and effective care for their patients. The focus of our care is a patient with an eye problem but many other body systems may be involved and good, evidence-based care involves a knowledge of neurology, diabetology, rheumatology, oncology and all the other problems which are part of eye disease.

This book, the fifth edition of the text, provides an overview for those just setting out in a role within ophthalmic nursing. It includes basic and comprehensible anatomy and physiology (which are the foundations for understanding how the eye functions and why and how problems occur) and relates this to the care and needs of the patient. The chapters have been updated and include new colour images and diagrams and the most recent National Institute for Health and Care Excellence (NICE) guidelines for glaucoma and age-related macular degeneration.

The inclusion of reflective activities in each chapter allows readers to apply their knowledge to the realities of the care setting and use this to evidence portfolios, revalidation and knowledge and skills for the future.

The phrase 'knowledge is power' was coined by Francis Bacon, scientist and philosopher, in 1597. It has been used many times since, and it is as true now as it ever was. This book provides nurses with the ability to acquire knowledge and to use it to enhance their power to care for patients with eye problems.

I hope it instils in 'new' ophthalmic nurses the beginnings of a passion for ophthalmology and the care of patients with eye problems which I and many of my ophthalmic nursing colleagues have developed during our careers.

Janet Marsden
Professor of Ophthalmology and Emergency Care
Manchester Metropolitan University

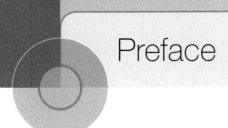

Preface

Since the publication of the fourth edition of this book, there have been many advances in the care and management of the ophthalmic patient. The role of the ophthalmic nurse has continued to expand, and as a result, other roles have developed. Assistant practitioners and other support worker roles have also developed in order to deliver timely, safe and effective care.

Some specialist ophthalmic nurses have completed prescribing courses as well as master's degrees and have become advanced nurses, functioning to a higher order of practice. Optometrists on the high street and in hospitals are increasingly responsible for managing the ocular health of the population, including managing glaucoma patients. Orthoptists are also expanding their roles to include the management of stable glaucoma patients.

This book continues to help and guide the practices of those caring for the ophthalmic patient. Once again in editing this edition, we have continued to build on the framework that has stood the test of time. Newer source materials have been included and are reflected in the chapters. References, further reading and websites have been updated to reflect current trends.

For the sake of ease and clarity, the nurse/carer is referred to as 'she' and the patient as 'he' with no discrimination intended.

Mary Shaw and Agnes Lee

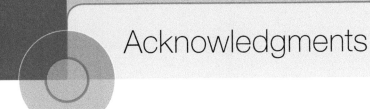

Acknowledgments

We would like to thank all of those who have been supportive to us as we undertook the re-working of this edition, especially our families and the publisher. We particularly wish to thank Debbie Morley, Specialist Nurse; Rita McLauchlan, Vitreo Retinal Nurse; John Cooper, Advanced Nursing Practitioner and Nigel Poole, Senior Fields Technician, for their contributions to chapters in this book. We would also like to thank the staff at the Manchester Royal Eye Hospital, including Louise Edwards and the Ophthalmic Imaging Department who provided images, and also staff at the University of Manchester, School of Nursing, Midwifery and Social Work.

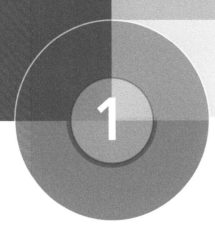

The ophthalmic patient

This chapter looks at the nature of the patients seen in ophthalmic or in primary care settings.

INTRODUCTION

The ophthalmic patient may be of any age and from any background. Ophthalmic conditions affect all age groups – ranging from a few days to more than 100 years old – although, in most ophthalmic settings, the majority of patients seen are elderly.

Infants and children will have parents or guardians who wish to be involved in their child's care. The infant or child whose parents or guardians are either unable or unwilling to become involved will need the extra care and attention of a nurse to reassure him in unfamiliar and possibly frightening surroundings.

The ophthalmic patient may have other diseases such as diabetes mellitus (type 1 or type 2), ankylosing spondylitis or arthritis, as these conditions have ocular manifestations. He may also suffer from unrelated diseases. Patients with co-morbidity can be challenging for the ophthalmic nurse who will have to make decisions about care and management based on need.

Many people with learning disabilities are known to have ocular problems, including visual impairment, refractive errors, squint, keratoconus, nystagmus, cataract and glaucoma. They face more problems than most members of society, including having difficulty accessing services when disease is detected, and few ophthalmic nurses have training specifically designed to meet the needs of these people.

The ophthalmic patient will arrive at the eye hospital or unit either as a referral to the outpatient department or as a casualty, where many are self-referred and may not be 'emergencies' as such. They will present with a variety of conditions, from a lump on the lid to sudden visual loss or severe ocular trauma. In addition, the ophthalmic patient may access care via walk-in centres, National Health Service (NHS) direct, the high street optometrist or GP services, including the practice nurse. The Darzi report (Department of Health 2008a) is driving the agenda for an increasing amount of care in the community, and the author insists that the care should be of a high quality. There is also an emphasis on patient well-being and preventive care.

Most people will be anxious on a first visit to a hospital or other healthcare setting. Even for the elderly but otherwise fit person, it might be his first experience of a hospital. Those arriving following trauma will be in varying degrees of shock depending on the nature and type of accident and they, and their relatives, may be very anxious. Something that seems fairly minor

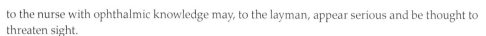

to the nurse with ophthalmic knowledge may, to the layman, appear serious and be thought to threaten sight.

Many people have a fear of their eyes being touched, making examination difficult. Some feel faint – or do faint – while certain procedures, such as removal of a foreign body, are being performed.

There are some old wives' tales about the eye. One of the most common is that the eye can be removed from the socket for examination and treatment, and be replaced afterwards. This kind of false information does not help the patient's frame of mind.

Each person will arrive at the hospital with his own individual personality and past experience to influence any attitude towards the eye condition. Some will be stoical, others extremely agitated. Those with chronic or recurrent eye conditions may become more accustomed to visiting the eye hospital. Most patients having ophthalmic surgery are outpatients, day cases or overnight-stay patients and not necessarily in a dedicated ophthalmic bed with ophthalmic trained staff to care for them. This means they have a very short time to adjust to the hospital setting and have little time to ask the questions that may be initially forgotten in the midst of all the activity. They may feel reluctant to express minor concerns when there appears to be little contact time with nurses.

The actual visual impairment experienced by the patient will vary with the eye condition. With many conditions there is no, or only slight, visual impairment and this may be temporary. Other conditions cause gross visual loss that may have occurred suddenly or gradually over the years. This visual loss may be untreatable and permanent, may be progressive, or sight may be restored. Some patients will have only one eye affected and others both eyes, probably to different degrees. Some will have blurred vision; some will only be able to make out movements. Others will be able to differentiate only between light and dark, or will see nothing at all. Some will have lost their central vision, others their peripheral vision. A number of patients will see better in bright light than dim light, and vice versa. Some degree of visual loss can be very upsetting to the patient and can prove to be a severe impairment to daily living. All patients experiencing severe visual loss will require practical and emotional help in coming to terms with their loss, regardless of the cause and the course it has taken.

REGISTRATION FOR THE SIGHT-IMPAIRED OR SEVERELY SIGHT-IMPAIRED

Research carried out by the Royal National Institute of Blind People (RNIB) (Bruce et al., 1991) suggested that there are three times more people eligible for registration as sight-impaired or severely sight-impaired than are in fact registered. There is no reason to suppose that this situation has changed. People are reluctant to take the final step as it can appear to be the giving up of any hope that treatment will help. This need not be the case, however: sight-impaired or severely sight-impaired registration can be a much more liberating experience for many as they realise, with help and support, that they can maximise their quality of life. Being registered blind or severely sight impaired *may* give access to a variety of benefits, including tax allowance, parking concession (blue badge) and a reduction in TV licence fee.

SEVERELY SIGHT IMPAIRED

The statutory definition for the purpose of registration as a blind person under the National Assistance Act 1948 is that the person 'is so blind as to be unable to perform any work for which eyesight is essential'. This refers to any form of employment, not only that which the patient formerly followed. It also only takes into account visual impairment, disregarding other bodily or mental infirmities. People with a visual acuity of less than 3/60 on the Snellen (1.0 LogMAR) chart, or with a visual acuity of 6/60 (1.0 LogMAR) but with a marked peripheral field defect, will be eligible for registration.

SIGHT IMPAIRED

There is no statutory definition of partial sight, although a person who does not qualify to be registered as blind but nevertheless is substantially visually impaired can be registered as partially sighted. Those people with 3/60–6/60 (1.0 LogMAR) vision and full peripheral field, those with vision up to 3/60 with moderate visual field contraction, opacities in the media, aphakia and those with 6/18 (10.5 [approximately] LogMAR) or better visual acuity but marked field loss can be included on this register.

Registering blind or partially sighted is a relatively easy process. The register is held by the local Social Services team. There are two forms of registration: Severely Sight Impaired (Blind) and Sight Impaired (Partially Sighted). It should be noted that access for help from social services is not dependent on being on the register.

An ophthalmologist must sign the registration form. To arrive at this point, the patient will have been referred to an ophthalmologist by his GP or optometrist.

The ophthalmologist will determine the patient's eligibility for being registered. It should be noted that registration is a voluntary process. Even if the form has been completed, Social Services will contact the patient and will ask him whether he wants to go onto the register, having explained the benefits of doing so.

In England and Wales the Certificate of Vision Impairment (CVI) is used. In Scotland it is form PP1, and in Northern Ireland form A655 is used (Department of Health, 2013).

ASSISTANCE AND REHABILITATION

The National Assistance Act 1948 directed all local authorities to compile a register of blind and partially sighted people residing in their area and to provide advice, guidance and services to enable them and their families to maintain their independence and to live as full a life as possible.

Registration is voluntary. People can choose to register but, if they do so, they can have their names removed from the register at any time should they wish. The local authority has the responsibility of reviewing the register regularly and updating the circumstances of the people on it. Local authorities must offer services to all those identified as visually impaired, whether they choose to register or not. However, registration is necessary to qualify for certain financial benefits and for help from the many voluntary organisations such as the National Library for the Blind. Registration is a good guide as to whether a person is coming to terms with his sight loss.

The social services department has the responsibility for registering people. Some social services departments have delegated this task to their local voluntary organisation that deals with the blind and partially sighted people within their area. The role of the social worker is that of counsellor, providing support and information about the services available. Such services include entitlement to benefits and referral to other statutory bodies involved with retraining, special needs education for those of school and college age, rehabilitation, employment, social, leisure and recreational activities and introduction to self-help groups.

VOLUNTARY ORGANISATIONS

A number of voluntary organisations work with the visually impaired and most local areas or counties have their own organisations, which were established to provide aids and social contact. Many local authorities have an arrangement with voluntary organisations to provide services to facilitate independent living, ranging from talking or tactile watches and clocks to alarms that sound when rained upon so that the washing can be brought in. Technological developments have resulted, for example, in equipment being available to enlarge print onto a computer screen, to convert the written word into Braille or to use voice synthesisers.

Local voluntary organisations are often centres of social contact for the visually impaired and their carers. Some voluntary organisations maintain contact through radio stations; Glasgow, for example, has a radio station dedicated entirely to people with visual impairment. Many self-help groups are supported by the voluntary sector; for example, glaucoma or macular disease support groups exist across the United Kingdom, with some being facilitated in hospital settings while others are supported in the community.

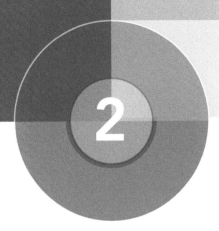

The ophthalmic nurse

This chapter explores the role of the nurse caring for the ophthalmic patient in a variety of settings.

INTRODUCTION

It is becoming increasingly common for ophthalmic patients to be cared for in environments other than specialist ophthalmic units. Primary care settings are the focus of many aspects of ophthalmic care, for example in walk-in centres where people attend with a variety of ailments for advice, treatment or referral. In addition, some high street optometrists have expanded the range of conditions they diagnose and manage.

The nurse with overall responsibility for the care of the ophthalmic patient should ideally hold a first degree and a specialist ophthalmic qualification. In addition, programmes to prepare others to care for the ophthalmic patient are available at national vocational qualification (NVQ) level 2 or 3. All must have gained applied knowledge and skills while practising clinically. Within the wider workforce planning agenda, other clinical roles are being developed such as assistant practitioners and surgical care practitioners.

Ophthalmic nurses will naturally be continuing to expand their practice to include, for example, nurse consent, pre-operative assessment, sub-Tenon's local anaesthesia and diagnosis and management of ocular emergencies (including telephone triage). As specialist or advanced practitioners, ophthalmic nurses will also care for and manage groups of patients linked to ophthalmic subspecialities: stable glaucoma patients, or those involving minor surgical oculoplastic procedures, cataracts, corneal conditions, uveitis or ophthalmic emergencies. With any of these expanded roles, the ophthalmic nurse must always be mindful of her professional accountability (Nursing and Midwifery Council 2015).

The ophthalmic nurse must naturally possess all the qualities required of a nurse working in any speciality or environment. Some characteristics, however, are more important to a nurse specialising in the diseases and conditions of the eye. The eye is very delicate and sensitive, and most of the patients the nurse will attend to will have varying degrees of anxiety about their eye and pain or discomfort in or around the eye. In order to allay any fears the patient may have about his eyes being touched, the ophthalmic nurse must be extremely gentle with her hands and in her manner. The nurse should be aware of her position and work on the patient's right-hand side when dealing with the right eye and vice versa with the left.

The eye is small, and there is not much room for manoeuvre around it when performing manual nursing procedures. The nurse therefore needs to be manually dexterous, and she also needs to have the best possible vision when performing nursing procedures. There is no place for vanity when dealing with the ophthalmic patient – wearing glasses for close work, should these be required, is essential.

As ophthalmic patients can be from any age group, the nurse needs to be familiar with the special requirements of all ages – those of the very young and the old in particular. However, it is recognised that specialist paediatric nurses should, as a matter of course, care for children. The difficulty here is that there are very few paediatric nurses with an ophthalmic qualification.

The nurse must be thoughtful in her approach to the visually impaired person. She must use a variety of interpersonal skills to their best advantage, including touching as appropriate to indicate presence or to show concern, introducing herself, indicating when she is leaving, and never shouting. There is a great temptation to assume that a person who is visually impaired is also hard of hearing.

The nurse must always bear in mind that there is an individual human being behind the eyes that are being treated, and each patient should be cared for as a whole, unique person.

ASSESSMENT OF PATIENTS

Ophthalmic patients receive treatment as outpatients, day cases and in primary care settings. If hospitalised, they tend to spend a minimum of time actually in hospital. Today's ophthalmic nurse has a limited amount of time in which to get to know the patient and be able to assess his needs and therefore must employ clear, succinct assessment skills in order to carry out an effective assessment. Many aspects of patient assessment are by necessity delegated to other carers in the team. For example, a clinical support worker may measure visual acuity, take blood samples or record an electrocardiogram (ECG), and a technician may perform biometry.

Patient assessment remains one of the most important interactions that nurses will have with their patients, and in order to do this thoroughly and efficiently, excellent communication skills are required. The ophthalmic nurse must therefore use verbal and non-verbal skills appropriately. Open-ended questions yield more information than closed questions. For example, asking a patient, 'Are you managing to put your drops in alright?' is likely to result in a simple yes or no reply, but had they been asked, 'How often do you miss putting in your drops?', they are in effect being given opportunity to admit to missing drops or having difficulty. An appropriate tone and pitch of voice should be employed. The ophthalmic nurse must be aware of the effects of eye contact, facial expression, posture, gestures and touch on the patients, remembering that non-verbal communication apart from touch may not always be immediately appropriate to the visually impaired. However, if the ophthalmic nurse does not utilise her non-verbal communication skills, it could affect her own attitude and behaviour, and the patient or the carer could in turn pick this up. It is also useful to integrate counselling skills such as the use of active listening, silence, attention and paraphrasing, in order to gain additional understanding of the patient's needs. The ophthalmic nurse also needs to be very observant. The importance of clear and concise record-keeping cannot be overemphasised.

PATIENT INFORMATION AND TEACHING

It is well recognised by nurses that giving information about procedures, for example, relieves anxiety and aids recovery. Not only do patients and carers need to know what is wrong with them and how they will be managed medically or surgically; the majority will also want to know why they are having that particular treatment. Patients and carers have ready access to Internet resources and frequently will have downloaded information about their condition and treatment options. The ophthalmic nurse needs to be aware of this and should be in a position to advise the patient as to the accuracy and reasonableness of information obtained from these resources. Many hospitals and clinics place patient information on their own Web pages as well as have such information available on a range of electronic media. Having an understanding of the rationale behind treatment will aid compliance and will enable the patient to be actively involved in his own care. Patients and carers need information at all stages of management. Patients do benefit from effective pre-operative teaching programmes.

Care systems are based on efficient multidisciplinary team working. Nurses alongside other allied health professionals, such as orthoptists and optometrists, also provide ophthalmic services and are considered key to the provision of quality services and the empowerment of the patient (Department of Health 2008b).

Voluntary sector organisations, for example Henshaw's Society for Blind People (HSBP), Macular Society, the International Glaucoma Association (IGA) and the Royal National Institute of Blind People (RNIB), continue to have a major role in ophthalmic care, and many outpatient departments have resident representatives to assist patients in coming to terms with their lives as people with visual impairment. Nurses are well placed to provide patients with sufficient information about their conditions and treatments. The ophthalmic nurse must, therefore, be in possession of sound knowledge in order to impart accurate information. She also needs time and the ability to use communication skills, mentioned above, appropriately. The nurse needs to assess how much information the patient needs, and in what depth, as well as whether to use lay or professional terminology. The ophthalmic nurse needs to be able to impart information to all age groups. As many of the patients are elderly, she needs a special understanding of the needs of this group of individuals. Although the senses are often reduced due to the ageing process, this does not mean that the elderly cannot learn about their health needs. Visually impaired elderly people with a hearing loss are a challenge to the ophthalmic nurse, especially as loss of both of these senses may cause them some confusion.

In addition to providing information on the various conditions and their treatment, the nurse needs to instruct the patient or carer in practical skills that need to be carried out at home or while at work, such as instilling drops, lid hygiene or inserting conformer shells. The patient or carer will need time to practise these skills following instruction from the nurse. It is vital that the nurse assesses their competence, which needs to be satisfactory if compliance is to be achieved. Many reasons exist as to why patients fail to adhere to their treatment plan, including poor understanding of the diagnosis, the chronic nature of the condition, forgetfulness, lack of motivation, physical problems such as rheumatoid arthritis of the hands or neck, side effects of the drops, frequency of drop instillation and multiple pharmacotherapy. Non-compliance may be as high as 95%, if one takes into account late instillation or missed doses. Physical problems such as hand tremor and weakness or arthritis may be overcome by the use of devices to help in the delivery of drops.

Teaching is another area that has been affected by the shortened contact time between nurse and patient. The actual organisation of when and where to carry out teaching is often difficult. Verbal information and instruction must be backed up with the written word – and both must be clear, unambiguous and appropriate for the individual. Written information includes the provision of leaflets in other languages, according to the community served. The patient's visual acuity and other aspects of vision must be taken into account when using such materials to ensure that the individual can indeed see them adequately. In addition, materials should be available on request in a format that the person with the disability can access readily, for example Braille or tape recordings. As mentioned, many hospitals and clinics now place patient information on the Internet. Some centres make use of having a DVD available to be viewed while the patient waits to see the clinician or as part of an individual teaching session. Others have created websites that patients can access at their leisure. In addition, some specialist centres are using patient group education as a means of enhancing the patient's knowledge and understanding of the condition and treatment.

The patient's need for information and the nurse's role to give it are vitally important and, in order to save unnecessary repetition in the following text, it will be assumed under each eye condition that this is carried out.

Above all, the ophthalmic nurse needs to be a knowledgeable, competent practitioner who instils confidence in the patients with whom she has contact.

PROFESSIONAL ISSUES

Ophthalmic nurses must be research-aware and should be encouraged to become involved in clinical research studies and clinical audit. While there is an increasing body of ophthalmic nursing research, much of what ophthalmic nurses do is not research based.

Health professionals are being encouraged to reflect on their practice and the ophthalmic nurse is no exception. Reflection allows time for nurses to ponder on their practice and discover ways to improve their performance. Reflection is encouraged as it goes some way to filling the theory/practice gap in nursing. Nurses have continued to expand their roles in response to the changing demands of the service, and are increasingly undertaking roles previously carried out by doctors. Some duties previously performed by ophthalmic nurses are now within the domain of assistant practitioners and clinical support workers. They too must have the required underpinning knowledge.

Ophthalmic nurses have a key role to play in health education and health promotion. This includes informing people of how to avoid accidents in the home or work setting and screening for diseases such as open-angle glaucoma.

Ophthalmic nurses have a prime responsibility for the quality of care they deliver, regardless of the setting. The ophthalmic nurse should use a quality framework to audit her practice and to make comparisons with practices outside her own unit/place of work.

THE NURSE IN THE OUTPATIENT DEPARTMENT

The outpatient department is the portal into the hospital or unit for the majority of patients attending with eye conditions and may be the only department they visit. It is therefore important that the nurse working there should be a good advertisement for the whole hospital or unit.

Standards exist to ensure that non-urgent patients do not have to wait longer than 18 weeks from referral to commencement of treatment and that urgent cases, such as cancer suspects, are seen within 2 weeks of GP referral (Comber 2015).

McBride (2000, 2002) has suggested that ophthalmic outpatient facilities fail to meet the needs of the patient with low vision and, while much has been done to improve on this situation, some work is still required. Nurses have a major role to play in ensuring that the environment and systems work for this category of patients and that they come up to a good standard. Low vision awareness training is one way to redress the situation, as is the introduction of initiatives such as 'the productive department' or 'the productive ward' (Department of Health 2008b).

Outpatient departments are always busy and, while great progress has been made in ensuring shorter waits for appointments (including booked appointments), there seems to be no answer to the problem of waiting time in the clinic itself. A number of methods for alleviating the frustrations and boredom experienced due to the waiting are available to the nurse running the clinic. She can inform the patient approximately how long the wait will be and give an explanation for any delay, if possible. This may help avoid tempers becoming frayed. It is also useful to have a snack bar to which patients and relatives may be directed, where they can while away the time and prevent hypoglycaemic episodes in the diabetic patient. It is also important to advise patients about how the clinic works so that they can understand, for example, that a patient returning from a test or investigation is not jumping the queue but rather is completing his consultation.

Some outpatient departments have involved other allied health professionals in the management of certain clinical cases. Optometrist-led glaucoma services are one such example. Other initiatives involve patients being seen in primary care settings.

All patients visiting the outpatient department have their visual acuity recorded, this usually being the responsibility of the nurse. Other nursing procedures may include

- Performing lacrimal sac washouts
- Performing epilation of lashes
- Taking conjunctival swabs
- Removing sutures
- Removing/inserting/cleaning contact lenses
- Instilling drops/ointment
- Removing/inserting ocular prostheses
- Testing for dry eyes using tear strips
- Applying eye pad and bandaging
- Recording blood pressure, as hypertension can be associated with retinopathies and central artery and vein occlusions; needs to be recorded if the patient is to undergo surgery, and for general screening
- Testing urine and/or blood glucose monitoring to ensure that the patient is not diabetic, as diabetes can cause various ophthalmic conditions, and for general screening
- Performing minor surgery and investigations carried out in the outpatient department; must become familiar with the procedures and instruments necessary to perform operations and tests under local anaesthetic, such as
  - Incision and curettage of chalazion
  - Lid surgery
  - Biopsy
  - Removal of lid tumours
  - Retropunctal cautery
  - Three-snip operation
  - Tonometry
  - Perimetry
  - Biometry

The optometrist and prosthetist will normally have their clinics in the outpatient department, with the latter working as part of a team, together with the surgeon and the oculoplastic nurse practitioner. The high number of patients attending the outpatient department poses particular problems for the nurse, as she will be unable to learn about each patient's individual needs in detail. She must be aware of those patients who require particular attention in respect of their communication and mobility difficulties, which may result from visual impairment or from other physical impairments – or both. These patients will usually be elderly although not always. The nurse needs to be aware of any special needs or circumstances such as diabetes or registered blind. Clinical governance dictates that confidentiality must be assured, so information should be held discreetly within the notes, not pinned on the top.

It is not possible for the nurse to see every patient as he leaves the department to ensure that he has understood any prescribed treatment or follow-up. However, she must look out for the elderly and hard of hearing in particular, in order to explain any necessary information that the doctor or practitioner may have given. This explanation should be supported by written information.

Some patients will have received bad news from the doctor. Those with dry age-related macular degeneration, for example, will have hoped for treatment to improve their eyesight, only to be told that there is little that can be done apart from providing aids to assist with improving poor vision. Doctors need to communicate with the nurse about such patients so that the nurse is aware of their condition and is available to discuss their concerns and to answer their questions, referring them to a social worker if appropriate.

The ophthalmic trained nurse will be able to give information to the patient due to be booked to come into hospital for an operation. She will be able to inform the patient of the approximate length of the waiting time for the operation, what it entails and the length of the hospital stay. She will be able to answer any queries the patient may have. Patient assessment may be undertaken in the outpatient department at this or a subsequent visit. Pre-assessment should normally be undertaken as near to the operation date as possible to ensure that the information is fully up to date.

It is of benefit to the patient if he can be shown the ward or day case area, as this helps to allay fears of coming into hospital and is especially helpful to children and their parents.

The ophthalmic nurse working in the outpatient department has to deal with many patients in the course of a day, and needs to have sound ophthalmic knowledge to be able to attend to the wide variety of ophthalmic conditions. As the eye condition may be a manifestation of a systemic disorder, she also needs general nursing knowledge in order to give advice and to perform procedures competently. In addition to being competent in carrying out these nursing procedures, she needs to be particularly aware of the special needs of the elderly, the very young, the deaf, the infirm and the anxious.

THE NURSE IN THE ACCIDENT AND EMERGENCY DEPARTMENT

The ophthalmic nurse working in the casualty department is in a similar environment and requires the same sorts of skills as the nurse working in the outpatient department. However, there has recently been a proliferation of nurse-led emergency eye services. The majority of nurses providing these services will have undertaken a recognised ophthalmic nursing qualification and will have undergone a period (usually 1 year) of in-house training under medical and nursing supervision. These ophthalmic nurse practitioners would see any casualty patients presenting with undifferentiated ocular problems. Within the remit of their role, they would diagnose, treat and refer according to protocols. In addition, the ophthalmic nurse must be able to deal with emergencies and to decide on the priority of care. The age of patients attending the casualty department ranges from a few days to more than 100 years old.

As in any emergency setting, the time of one patient's attendance usually coincides with that of many others, and it is essential to have a triage system in place to prioritise the order in which patients will be seen. It should also be borne in mind that patients and health professionals may telephone for advice about attendance. These cases are also triaged and directed to the most appropriate service at the most appropriate time (Marsden 2006).

The following conditions are considered to be ophthalmic emergencies and the patients will require immediate attention:

- Sudden loss of vision due to
  - Central retinal artery occlusion
  - Central retinal vein occlusion
  - Giant cell arteritis
  - Retinal detachment – particularly if the macula is still attached
- Primary acute glaucoma
- Trauma, particularly penetrating or perforating injuries
- Chemical burns
- Orbital cellulitis
- Urgent cases that the nurse may have to deal with, but which are not classed as emergencies, including
  - Corneal ulcer
  - Vitreous haemorrhage
  - Acute dacryocystitis
  - Optic nerve disorders
  - Ocular tumours
  - Acute uveitis

The nurse will need to inform the waiting patients of the approximate waiting time, and she may need to explain that some people require priority care and will be attended to as soon as they arrive in the department. Locally, in response to national targets of any patient waiting longer than 4 hours for treatment (NHS England 2014), many accident and emergency departments have escalation policies that 'kick in' if patient waiting times are getting too long.

It is the nurse's responsibility to take a good history and to decide what priority, if any, the patient should be given. Triage is essential to ensure that real emergencies are given priority. She must take details of the state of the patient's vision on arrival and of the type of injury or eye complaint. The importance of taking an accurate history cannot be overemphasised, as it may give clues to injuries sustained that may not be evident on initial eye examination. The history must include the following details:

- Visual acuity – this may be used for medico-legal purposes, particularly if an accident has occurred at work and damages might be claimed.
- Type of injury must be assessed:
  - If a foreign body entered the eye, determine (1) what the foreign body was; (2) when the accident happened; (3) how it got into the eye – it is particularly important to find out whether the patient was using a hammer and chisel, and if the foreign body hit the eye with force, which might indicate that it had penetrated the eye, in which case an orbital x-ray would need to be ordered; and (4) if protective goggles were being worn at the time of the incident.

- If a fluid or powder substance has entered the eye, determine (1) what the substance is, (2) when the incident occurred, and (3) whether it was washed out immediately.
- If the eye has been scratched, determine (1) what scratched the eye; (2) with what force it did so; and (3) when the incident occurred.

- Type of eye complaint – the nurse must elicit whether the following symptoms are present and their duration:
  - Discharge, especially on waking, noting the colour and consistency. In addition, the age of the patient should be considered as the presence of discharge could be more serious in babies.
  - Watering.
  - Photophobia.
  - Pain or discomfort, its location and nature.
  - Change in vision – (1) blurred vision; (2) floaters; and (3) visual loss (sudden, gradual, total, partial – which visual field is affected and whether it is linked to head injury).
  - Restricted ocular movement.
  - Any degree of exophthalmos/enophthalmos.

The patient should be allocated a triage category and treated accordingly. It should be noted that the ocular trauma could be associated with other injuries and that the latter may need to be treated before the eye injury.

If the patient has had an accident, he may need to be treated for shock. Accompanying relatives or friends may also be shocked and anxious.

Patients suffering from sudden loss of vision will be anxious, as will those who are to be admitted to hospital, especially if this is unexpected. The nurse must help alleviate these fears and anxieties, also offering practical help such as informing relatives or arranging transport.

The nurse will be expected to carry out varied nursing procedures in the accident and emergency department:

- Take and record visual acuity.
- Examine the eye. This may be carried out using a torch or with a slit lamp. Ophthalmic nurse practitioners would be expected to carry out full anterior segment examination of the eye.
- Examine the pupils for relative afferent pupil defect.
- Instill drops and ointment.
- Remove conjunctival and superficial corneal foreign bodies.
- Apply pad and bandage.
- Irrigate the eye.
- Epilate lashes.
- Syringe lacrimal ducts.
- Remove sutures.
- Remove/insert contact lenses.
- Remove/insert prostheses.
- Test urine.
- Record peripheral blood glucose.
- Record blood pressure.
- Take conjunctival swabs.
- Perform tear strip test for dry eyes.
- Provide patient education.
- Provide health and safety advice.

While performing these procedures, the nurse must remember that the patient may feel faint or unwell. Further action is required should the patient's condition worsen.

The nurse in the casualty department must be able to deal with many people and to cope with unexpected situations that might arise. She must have adequate ophthalmic knowledge to be able to recognise urgent cases and to be able to give certain patients priority care. She also needs to be able to perform a variety of ophthalmic procedures competently and knowledgeably.

Time spent in the casualty department is an ideal time to carry out patient education by giving out relevant information leaflets and informing patients on eye protection as appropriate. The nurse in casualty also advises patients over the telephone, so it is vital that her knowledge is accurate and that her communication skills are appropriate.

The management of children with an ocular problem in an eye casualty department requires the ophthalmic nurse to be sensitive to their needs. Very young children can be frightened and anxious in unfamiliar surroundings, and the parents or guardians are often equally anxious. It seems sensible to manage and treat the child quickly to ensure full cooperation during the examination process. Prolonged waiting time before children are seen will increase their fretfulness and anxiety.

THE DAY CASE AND WARD NURSE

While the trend is towards day surgery for the majority of surgical cases, there will be some patients who require inpatient treatment, for example when there are coexisting medical problems, where the treatment centre is some distance from the patient's home and when the patient is admitted for treatment of an ophthalmic condition.

Patients in the ophthalmic day case unit or ward will require pre- and post-operative care, as the majority are admitted for surgery, e.g. cataract extraction, squint surgery, repair of retinal detachment, drainage surgery for chronic glaucoma or following trauma. There may, however, be patients admitted for rest following trauma, for intensive treatment of a severe infection or for treatment of post-operative complications.

Consideration needs to be given to the needs of the ophthalmic patient being nursed in a non-specialist ward (NSW) rather than a dedicated ophthalmic bed. Here the ophthalmic nurse must ensure that the staff on the NSW are given a detailed verbal and written handover to ensure that the patient receives the care and treatment required.

The specific nursing care for each ophthalmic condition is detailed in the relevant chapters. However, a general note on nursing care is given here.

PRE-ASSESSMENT

Patients having day case or inpatient surgery tend to be pre-assessed a few weeks prior to the operation. This assessment is carried out in order to establish the needs of the individual patient so that his short period in hospital can be planned, and also to give the necessary information regarding the surgery and to establish a post-operative care plan with the patient and carers.

Post-operative care will normally involve instillation of drops which, in the majority of cases, will be performed by the patient himself or his carer. Ideally, teaching drop instillation should be instituted at pre-assessment as there is little time for this during admission to hospital. Advising patients to purchase artificial tear drops and to practise at home following instruction is one way of overcoming the lack of time to teach this procedure and to observe the patient's performance.

The nurse has only limited time in which to assess the needs of the patients and must apply all her assessment skills appropriately.

As well as giving the usual pre-operative information to the patient, the nurse may carry out the following procedures and record results and act on findings:

- Testing distance visual acuity
- Tonometry
- Biometry
- ECG
- Focimetry
- Slit lamp examination

Information leaflets regarding the surgery and hospital stay should be given to the patient to support the verbal information and instructions that the nurse will give. These can be translated into languages other than English if necessary. This, together with answering any queries that the patient or carer may have, will help allay fears. Clinical governance requires that patients be actively involved in the production of patient information of any type.

PRE-OPERATIVE CARE

In addition to routine pre-operative care for surgery being performed under either local or general anaesthesia, the nurse may be required to carry out the following procedures, depending on the personal preferences of the ophthalmic surgeon:

- Instilling mydriatic drops prior to cataract extraction or retinal detachment surgery as the pupil needs to be dilated for such surgery to be performed
- Instilling miotic drops prior to trabeculectomy and keratoplasty
- Instilling local anaesthetic drops such as G. oxybuprocaine 0.4%, if the operation is to be performed under a local anaesthetic

These drops are usually administered against a prescription or patient group direction.

POST-OPERATIVE CARE

In addition to the normal post-operative care required by any patient after surgery, the ophthalmic nurse will need to follow a routine such as that described here, although this will vary to some extent according to hospital practice.

EYE CARE

Post-operative eye care involves dressings, cleaning the eye or skin wound, inspection of the eye, instillation of drops and protection of the eye:

- Dressings – eye pads are used but also Cartella shields, with or without a pad, may be in place following surgery. If indicated, as in some types of minor lid surgery, the pad is removed before the patient leaves the unit.
- Cleaning the eye or skin wound – the eye or skin will usually only be cleaned on the day following surgery; subsequent cleaning is usually performed once a day or more frequently if indicated. In the case of some oculoplastic procedures, the pad and bandage will remain untouched for between 5 and 7 days.

- Inspection of the eye and surrounding structures will be undertaken post-operatively.
- Instillation of drops – if prescribed, given accordingly; ointment, if prescribed, may be applied at night. It should be noted that ointment may be prescribed for structures other than the eye, for example, suture lines on the lids.
- Protection of the eye – eye pads or Cartella shields may be worn on the first post-operative day; Cartella shields are usually worn only at night for 1 or 2 weeks following surgery.

DISCHARGE

All patients should be given instructions about care and follow-up:

- Eye drops or ointment – the patient or carer's ability to instil drops or apply ointment should be determined. Ideally, this process will have commenced at pre-assessment. Names of drops or ointment and times of instillation/application must be given verbally as well as written down.
- Cleaning the eye – if the eye is sticky in the mornings, it should be cleaned using cooled, boiled water in a clean receptacle and using cotton wool or gauze. Advise patients to avoid using dry cotton wool near the eye, as fibres can get into the eye.
- General instructions – patients should avoid stooping down too low in case they lose their balance. If appropriate, the patient should be advised to avoid anything causing increased exertion that will raise the intraocular pressure, such as lifting anything heavy. Patients should take care when they wash their hair to avoid getting soap or water into the eye as this would cause irritation that could result in rubbing behaviour. These restrictions should be heeded for 2 weeks initially, but are becoming increasingly less necessary with small incision surgery. Patients must take particular care not to knock or rub the eye, which could cause haemorrhage or cause the iris to prolapse through the wound.
- Outpatient appointment – ensure that the patient has an appointment, usually at 1 or 2 weeks following discharge. Transport may need to be arranged for the day.
- Primary care – the nurse may need to arrange for a community nurse to assist with drop instillation, or may need to organize for the social worker to assess the need for home help or meals on wheels for the patient, prior to discharge.
- Convalescence – not used often, but in some areas recuperation in a convalescent, residential or nursing home can be arranged for patients before they return to their own homes.
- Specialist procedures such as vitrectomy may require a patient to 'posture' in certain positions to ensure a satisfactory surgical outcome. To ensure that the patient complies with the posturing instructions, especially if he lives alone, it may be necessary to involve other agencies such as those provided by social services and primary care.

It is helpful if all the above information and instructions are written down as well as given verbally, as there is often much detail to absorb in the excitement of going home.

NURSING PROCEDURES

The ophthalmic nurse working on the ward and in day case needs to be able to assess the patients and plan their care on an individual basis. She must understand the pre- and post-operative care required for each type of ophthalmic operation. She needs to be able to carry out certain ophthalmic procedures competently and knowledgeably. The nurse must also plan the patient's discharge in advance, ensuring that all relevant agencies are involved. She must be knowledgeable in all ophthalmic aspects in order to discuss relevant points with the patient and relatives so that the hospital stay can be made as easy and as pleasant as possible for all concerned.

THE NURSE IN THE THEATRE

The nurse working in an ophthalmic theatre will need to be familiar with the nursing responsibilities and general duties required of any theatre nurse. In addition, she will need to know the following aspects of ophthalmic theatre nursing, though the details will vary from hospital to hospital. One aspect though that is common to all theatre settings is the implementation of the World Health Organization (WHO) surgical safety checklist (World Alliance for Patient Safety 2008). This helps to ensure that the patient has the correct procedure performed on the correct eye and in an environment where patient safety is ensured.

PREPARATION OF THE PATIENT

Preparation of the patient usually begins in the anaesthetic room where the nurse greets the patient and ensures his comfort on the chair or operating table. She will take a handover report from the day case or ward nurse. The anaesthetic nurse will establish that she has the correct patient by asking name and date of birth and comparing this to the identity bracelet which is, in turn, cross-referenced to the case notes and the surgical procedure for which the patient has given consent. The nurse will ensure that the consent form has been properly completed and will identify the eye to be operated on – which should be marked – and any relevant medical and surgical history, including medications, should be noted.

Once on the operating table, the patient must be positioned safely and correctly, especially if a general anaesthetic is being administered. A Rubens pillow is used to position and support the adult patient's head, with a head ring being used for a child. Local anaesthetic drops, if no general anaesthetic is to be given, may be instilled prior to the operation commencing. If the patient is having a sub-Tenon's anaesthetic, this may be performed by a doctor, anaesthetist or suitably trained nurse.

If the patient is having the operation under a local anaesthetic, it is important that a nurse or a member of the anaesthetic support staff maintains contact with the patient. This can be done by sitting and holding the patient's hand during the procedure. This not only reassures the patient, but can give the nurse an indication of his condition. Intravenous sedatives, e.g. midazolam, may be given to the patient.

During the operation, the patient's face will be covered with a sterile drape. This may make the patient feel claustrophobic and perhaps disoriented. Usually a supply of oxygen at 4 L/min with an air intake or air alone is administered to the patient. If oxygen is being given, the supply must be switched off if cautery is used, as it constitutes a fire hazard.

The nurse holding the patient's hand during local or topical procedures, in order to reassure the patient as well as to establish a communication link to pick up on patient discomfort intra-operatively, is a vital role. She will be able to feel any pressure from the patient's hand indicating that he may be feeling discomfort or pain.

The nurse will also observe the monitoring equipment, noting the pulse rate, blood pressure and oxygen saturation. Any deviation from normal will be reported to the surgeon and recorded in the nursing record.

KNOWLEDGE OF THE INSTRUMENTS

The scrub nurse/operating department practitioner must have a good knowledge of the instruments required for each operation performed. In addition, knowledge of the equipment and how to set this up, use and maintain it, is essential. Many instruments and machine parts are now designed for single-patient use and may not be reused. The suture materials used in ophthalmic surgery tend to be very fine. Owing to microsurgical techniques, some ophthalmic surgery does not require sutures.

TECHNIQUE IN HANDLING THE INSTRUMENTS

Preferably, a non-touch technique is carried out, using forceps to handle the needles and sutures. The tips of the instruments should not be touched with the fingers as this may cause injury and may also damage the instrument.

WEARING SURGICAL GLOVES

Gloves with powder must not be used, as the starch contained in the powder is an irritant to the eye. Surgical gloves containing no powder are available, such as Biogel M worn by surgeons and scrub personnel for microsurgery. Latex-free gloves must be available where there is a known allergy, and the trend is to maximise the amount of latex-free equipment used in the operating theatre.

CARE OF THE INSTRUMENTS

Ophthalmic instruments tend to be small, delicate and expensive, so great care must be taken when handling them. Most instruments and associated equipment are single-patient use only and must be discarded after use. Where non-disposable instruments are used every piece of equipment must have its own identity label, and each set of instruments should be labelled and numbered. Sets of instruments must not be split up. A record of which individual instruments and sets of instruments have been used for a particular procedure must be retained in the case notes. These procedures are vital to enable tracking to take place of equipment for the purposes of audit.

Instruments that are non-disposable should be decontaminated and sterilised in specialist departments and following Department of Health guidelines. This is normally done in a central sterilisation unit. Before instruments are sent for sterilisation, the nurse should wipe micro-instruments with spears dipped in water or balanced salt solution. Enzyme foam spray is used to remove detritus and protein from instruments. This procedure, if followed, will help to prevent the transmission of Creutzfeldt–Jakob disease. Sharps should either be disposable or retractable for safety and to prevent cross-infection. Lumened instruments need to be flushed with sterile water and air according to the manufacturer's instructions. Quick-rinse machines are available commercially for this purpose, delivering 120 mL of water and 120 mL of air.

Instruments are placed in trays lined on the base with lock-down latex-free sheets which serve to hold the instruments securely in place during the wash cycle.

Sterilisation is usually by downward displacement vacuumed autoclave at a temperature of 130°C for 3 minutes, the full cycle lasting 40 minutes in total. Each instrument must be seen to be in good working order, not rusted or damaged, and should be examined under a magnified light source before being sterilised.

THE OPERATION AND USE OF EQUIPMENT

The nurse must be familiar with the equipment used in the ophthalmic theatre:

- The operating microscope used for most intraocular surgery.
- The operating lights.
- The cryotherapy machine used for retinal detachment surgery.
- Phacoemulsifier machines, which are used for extracapsular cataract extractions and for vitrectomy surgery.
- Magnets used for removing intraocular and intracorneal magnetic foreign bodies. Magnetic instruments are used with the magnet and must be demagnetised following use.
- Cautery machines:
  - Bipolar cautery is used on the eye and no diathermy plate is required.
  - Macropolar cautery is used on lids and does require a diathermy plate.
- Laser machines.
- Emergency equipment such as defibrillators and suction.

The nurse working in the ophthalmic theatre must appreciate the delicate nature of the surgery being undertaken. She needs to understand the importance of quietness, speed, attentiveness, cleanliness and sterility. The nurse must also know the particular procedures for each ophthalmic operation at which she will be assisting and must be prepared to develop her knowledge as new procedures, instruments and equipment are introduced.

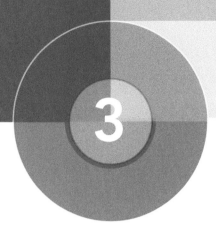

Ophthalmic nursing procedures and investigations

3

This chapter looks at some general principles relating to each procedure and investigation before outlining general and more specific ophthalmic procedures and investigations. Some of the clinical skills have a competency assessment tool provided, to assist you with the assessment of the skill. There is also a generic assessment tool for you to use with the other ophthalmic procedures.

GENERAL PRINCIPLES

Ophthalmic procedures and investigations will vary to some degree between clinical settings. Those listed here can be used as guidelines but local policies must be followed. It is important to remember that all ophthalmic procedures and investigations should take into account the following:

- Patient consent
- Good communication
- Patient education
- Adherence to infection control
- Health and safety
- A holistic approach
- Maintenance of the patient's privacy and dignity

COMMUNICATION

Effective communication is a vital component of patient care, and communication with someone who is visually impaired and who may have other disabilities such as hearing impairment and aphasia can be doubly challenging. Some staff may find it awkward and confusing when trying to communicate with someone with dual or multiple disabilities. The golden rule to remember is to communicate with the person and not the disability. Boxes 3.1 and 3.2 summarise the main points in communication etiquette, and one should take into account the points listed in both boxes when communicating with patients with any kind of disability or specific communication need.

BOX 3.1: Summary of communication etiquette for managing the visually impaired

- Make sure that you are in the patient's field of vision when you approach them to avoid startling them.
- Ensure that when you communicate with the patient that it is done in a well-lit area and preferably in a quiet room.
- Take into account that a patient may have other hidden disabilities of which you may not be aware. For example, following a stroke, head injury or tumour, the patient may experience hemianopia or blindness and a loss of visual awareness as a result of damage to the optic nerve pathway to the brain. The resulting consequence of hemianopia is a loss of one half of the visual field in one or both eyes. There are different types of hemianopia depending on which areas of the brain are affected. Regardless of which type of hemianopia is present, it is important that you approach and communicate from the unaffected side of the patient or from the front.
- Face the patient and speak to them on their level.
- Do not shout or raise your voice. Remember the majority of patients are only visually impaired and have still retained all of their other faculties.
- Remember to speak slowly and clearly and to use non-verbal communication such as body language.
- Ensure that you say who you are when you begin to speak.
- Speak naturally and address the patient and not the carer.
- Where possible, find somewhere quiet as noise can be a distraction for the patient.
- If appropriate, always contact an approved interpreter to interpret for the patient. Where possible, avoid using relatives to interpret to avoid any misunderstanding.
- Before leaving the patient, always inform the patient of your intention. Otherwise the patient will be left talking to himself.

BOX 3.2: Summary of communication etiquette with multiple disabilities such as hearing impairment, aphasia, Alzheimer's and learning disabilities

- If the patient is wearing a hearing aid, ensure that it is turned on and that it is in good working order.
- Stand in front of the patient or where the patient can see you clearly.
- Ask the patient how he would like to communicate. Writing using black bold letters is one option. Some patients who are deaf may prefer to seek the assistance of a signer. Use gestures if it is helpful or use visual objects such as pictures or diagrams to aid communication.
- Be patient and allow the patient plenty of time. Do not rush the patient as it may make him become agitated. Do not second-guess what the patient is trying to say. Allow him plenty of time to express his thoughts and feelings.
- If a patient has difficulty in understanding you, use different words to get your meaning across. Do not attempt to repeat your questions or explanations using the same words. It may also be helpful to use picture cards or drawings.
- Some patients carry communication passports which is a useful way to help you and others understand how someone with learning disability communicates.
- If appropriate, use physical contact, such as a hand on the patient's hand or arm, to convey your care and understanding.

- Only ask one question at a time to avoid confusion. Use key words and repeat them slowly if necessary.
- Avoid invading a patient's personal space. If a patient becomes agitated, a light touch on the arm can be helpful to calm him down although, for some patients, touching can cause offence. Judge each situation and patient individually.
- Do not give lengthy explanations. Always reiterate and check for understanding, especially if a patient is stressed, tired or anxious. Where appropriate, give written information as well. Any written information given should take into account an individual's specific needs.
- If you are having difficulty in communicating with someone with multiple disabilities, be honest and seek help from a more appropriate person.

EDUCATION OF THE OPHTHALMIC PATIENT, INCLUDING CHILDREN

The majority of ophthalmic procedures and investigations carried out can seem extremely daunting to patients, and the patients can be squeamish about any procedures and investigations involving their eyes. It is therefore very important that, prior to any ophthalmic procedures and investigations, the patient is fully informed of the nature and process of the procedure. The explanations given must be clear and concise and must include all possible side effects. Explanations must take into account the patient's learning style and intellectual ability, his physical, mental and emotional state and any sensory deficits. When undertaking an ophthalmic procedure on a child, explanation must be given in a truthful, tactful and sensitive manner and must take into account the child's age, mental capability and other factors such as any pain or discomfort the child might be in. This requires the ophthalmic practitioner to be extra patient and to take into account the whole spectrum of the child's and parents' need, including the psychological and social aspects. A successful outcome of the ophthalmic procedure will be guaranteed if cooperation is obtained from both parties and if any unnecessary trauma to the child and parents can be avoided.

GUIDING A PATIENT WITH VISUAL IMPAIRMENT

PRINCIPLES OF GOOD PRACTICE

Although many visually impaired people can and do find their way around on their own, on occasion, some will require assistance. Follow this advice for approaching and guiding blind or partially sighted people.

Basic principles

Do I need to provide assistance?
Not necessarily…

- Understand that assistance is not always needed.
- Ask what *they* need.
- Do not leave people standing looking lost.
- Ensure the environment is user friendly by avoiding
  - Sharp edges on furnishings
  - Different flooring texture

- Excessive noise levels
- Crowds, if possible
- Let people know when you arrive and alert them to your leaving.
- Extend basic courtesies and sensitivity to the needs of people who are visually impaired.

Hospitals are unfamiliar environments; therefore, attention needs to be given to issues of access for the visually impaired.

- Consider the use of colour and contrast around doors/door frames.
- Use colour contrast for chairs and carpets.
- Design notices on boards with content in 14–16 font and in standard sentence case.
- Use signage that is large enough to see and in a position that is accessible like eye-level height.
- Consider the layout of the room to ensure it is navigable by people with problems with their vision.

1. *Identify yourself and offer help first.* A blind or partially sighted person may well be unaware of you as you approach, so say hello and introduce yourself. Ask politely if the person requires assistance.
2. *Offer your arm.* Offer your arm for the blind or partially sighted person to grip just above the elbow. Keep your guiding arm at your side. Make sure that you are both facing in the same direction and set off. Some visually impaired people prefer to put their hand on the shoulder of the person guiding them.
   a. Communication and trust are key to developing a good rapport.
   b. Be specific with your instructions.
3. *When ascending/descending stairs remember to say step up or step down.* When you reach level ground again take a step forward, then pause to give the person you are guiding time to complete the last step.
   a. If you need to change sides, allow the guided person to trail across your back and find your other arm that you have extended slightly backwards.
   b. When approaching a narrow space, move your guiding arm to the middle of your back, keeping it straight. The guided person automatically will move behind you whilst retaining the grip on your arm.
   c. When guiding a person to a chair, the guide holds the back of the chair and asks the guided person to trail down the grip arm to locate the back of the chair.
4. *Keep your eyes open.* For potential hazards such as parked cars, kerbs, overhanging bushes or rubbish bins.
5. *Do not raise your voice.* Loss of sight does not necessarily mean loss of hearing.
6. *Carefully navigate crowds and traffic.* Take extra care when guiding through crowds or traffic and use pedestrian crossings wherever possible.
7. *Highlight mobility aids.* Let the person you are guiding know of any possible aid to mobility, such as guide rails, especially on buses or trains.
8. *Give attention to parting company.* When the journey is over, make sure the blind or partially sighted person knows where he or she is, the direction in which he or she is facing and where he or she should go next.

Following are some dos and don'ts when encountering guide dogs and other assistance dogs in hospital.

- Guide or assistance dogs are working dogs and should not be patted whilst their harness is in position.
- Always talk to the patient and not the dog.
- Always seek permission from the owner before petting the dog.
- Do not be affronted if you are asked to leave the dog alone.
- Make sure there is a drinking bowl of water available if the dog is with you for some time.
- If a member of staff or patient is frightened of dogs, reassure them and move them away from the dog.

INFECTION CONTROL

Rates of methicillin-resistant *Staphylococcus aureus* (MRSA) in hospitals have fallen significantly in recent years, but over 6% of hospital patients in England still acquire some form of infection during their stay, according to the Health Protection Agency (HPA) in 2012. The report suggests that recent efforts to tackle MRSA transmission in hospitals have been effective at driving down the prevalence of these infections. Many of these are simple yet effective in nature, such as emphasizing regular, thorough handwashing and swabbing patients to test for MRSA as they are being admitted to hospital.

Despite these improvements, the HPA still emphasizes that there needs to be continued focus on these preventative efforts in order to keep the number of these infections low.

Ophthalmic patients not only have to contend with the possibility of succumbing to MRSA and *Clostridium difficile* (*C. difficile*), but also the possibility of other extraocular and intraocular infection. Such infections can have a potentially devastating effect on the patients and their carers. For this reason, the importance of handwashing before and after each patient contact cannot be overemphasized. Infection control also includes other measures such as employing single-use disposable items, correct decontamination and sterilisation of equipment; correct sharps and other waste disposal; and observing standard precautions.

In order to further reduce the spread of infection, some hospitals and clinical practices have adopted the principles of Aseptic Non Touch Technique (ANTT) and incorporated it within ophthalmic procedures. The principle of ANTT aims to prevent microorganisms on hands, equipment and surfaces from being introduced into any susceptible site via intravenous lines, urinary catheter or procedures such as cannulation, venepuncture, wound dressing and administration of intravenous or intracameral drugs.

HEALTH AND SAFETY ISSUES IN OPHTHALMOLOGY

As with any area of medicine, health and safety within ophthalmology is of paramount importance. A system for improving standards of care and maintaining the health and safety of patients is addressed through clinical governance. Clinical governance is a system that ensures that NHS organisations are accountable not only for meeting standards and improving clinical practice, but also have systems in place to safeguard practice. According to RCOph (2014), effective clinical governance within ophthalmology must include the following:

- The continuous improvement of patient services and care should be based on the best available evidence.
- The management of the patient should be patient centred and should take into account the individual needs of a patient.

Table 3.1 The National Patient Safety Agency's (2004–2009) seven steps to patient safety

Stages	Patient safety	Examples of application to practice
Step 1	Build a safety culture	Ensure safety systems are in place in your workplace. For example, risk assessment, incident reporting, induction of workforce, medical alert reporting, root cause analysis of incidents, etc.
Step 2	Lead and support staff in patient safety	Training for new and existing medical devices
Step 3	Integrate risk management	Provide risk-assessment training, including how to assess risk Yearly updates of risk management to all groups of staff
Step 4	Promote reporting of patient safety incidents	Encourage staff to report incidents Online reporting system to simplify reporting mechanisms
Step 5	Involve and communicate with patients and public	Prompt communication in the event of any mishaps and swifter response to complaints, etc.
Step 6	Learn and share safety lessons	Publication and dissemination of lessons-learned bulletins
Step 7	Implement solutions to prevent harm	Appropriate protocols and policies in place and ensuring awareness of staff to the policies and procedures

- Patients should be kept fully informed of their treatment and the management of their ophthalmic condition.
- Patients should be treated with dignity and their privacy must be respected.
- An up-to-date workforce and clinical supervision should be in place.
- There should be a no-blame culture, with the opportunity to learn from errors.

As detailed in Table 3.1, the National Patient Safety Agency (2004–2009) advocates seven steps to patient safety. (See also Department of Health 2008b.)

Other health- and safety-related issues to take into account must also include the following:

- WHO surgical checklist
- Decontamination and sterilisation of equipment
- Medical devices training
- Infection control
- Health and safety in the operating theatre
- Importance of measuring clinical outcomes and effectiveness
- Delivering and monitoring of standards through audits, recording of significant events (critical incident) analysis and complaints monitoring

A HOLISTIC APPROACH

It is sometimes quite easy to regard ophthalmic patients as 'just a pair of eyes' and fail to take into account the patient's physical, mental, social and other health issues and well-being. Visual impairment is a significant cause of physical and psychosocial morbidity, and it is therefore crucial that as healthcare professionals, we take into account the following when dealing with patients with visual impairment:

- Any physical and mental impairment
- Any learning difficulties
- The importance of the psychological and social impact of visual impairment on the patient including the patient's ability to manage any lifestyle changes if the visual impairment is permanent
- Communication with patients and their relatives and involving them fully in the care and management of their eye condition
- Any physical or mental impairment when prescribing treatment which may affect compliance
- The significance of visual impairment for a patient's ability to self-manage any of the patient's other chronic medical conditions such as diabetes

MAINTENANCE OF PATIENT'S PRIVACY AND DIGNITY

Privacy and dignity are two important aspects of care that all patients and carers are entitled to and are now seen as a high priority on the quality-improvement agenda. A patient's privacy and dignity can be compromised through, for example, unnecessary interruptions such as telephone calls, entering consulting rooms without knocking, having gaping curtains and unfastened or poorly fitting theatre gowns and simply not closing the doors of consultation rooms. Asking a patient's personal details or taking telephone messages in a crowded waiting room can also be problematic. It may not always be feasible to take patients away to a quieter and more private area, but privacy and dignity must be maintained in all consultations and treatments, and should be built into the care delivered to patients as well as in the environment in which care is being delivered.

RECORDING VISUAL ACUITY

Visual acuity is the measurement of acuteness of central vision only. An accurate assessment of visual acuity is one of the most important parts of any ophthalmic examination. Visual acuity is a test of the visual system from the occipital cortex to the cornea. Accurate visual acuity testing requires the following:

- Patient cooperation and comprehension of the test
- Ability to recognise the forms displayed
- Clear ocular media and correct focussing
- Ability of the eyes to converge simultaneously
- Good retinal function
- Intact visual pathways and occipital cortex

When all these criteria are present, it is a good test of macula function (North 2001).

GENERAL CONSIDERATIONS WHEN PERFORMING VISUAL ACUITY

When performing visual acuity, a number of general considerations need to be taken into account, including adequate illumination, recording of contact lens wear and the use of methods to avoid patient 'cheating'. Good communication skills (including accurate instructions) and patience are particularly important with patients with any learning disabilities and language difficulties, and also with children.

In order to assess accurately a patient's visual acuity (both distance and near), it is extremely important that the test type or reading material is correctly illuminated, i.e. if using a Snellen box or LogMAR, that all the bulbs are in working order. When testing a patient's near vision, ensure that there is an adequate light source.

It is also important to record if a patient uses contact lenses and if these were worn at the time of testing.

Since each eye is tested separately, it is a good idea to occlude the other eye with his out-patient card or occluder to avoid patient 'cheating' by looking through the gaps between his fingers. Similarly, it is a good idea to rotate the chart round for frequent attendees to the eye outpatient unit to minimise patients memorising the letters on the chart. (As LogMAR has a different chart for testing each eye, this reduces opportunity for remembering all of the letters.)

It is important that the appropriate testing chart, such as the Sheridan Gardner test chart, Kay picture chart or the tumbling 'E' chart (see next section explanations), is used on patients with any learning disabilities and language difficulties. Good communication skills and patience are needed in these circumstances.

The measurement of visual acuity in children also requires special skill and patience, and it is important that an appropriate chart is used on those who are unable to recognise the alphabet.

COMMON CHARTS USED IN THE MEASUREMENT OF DISTANCE VISUAL ACUITY

The most common chart for measuring distance visual acuity in a literate adult is the Snellen chart (Figure 3.1).

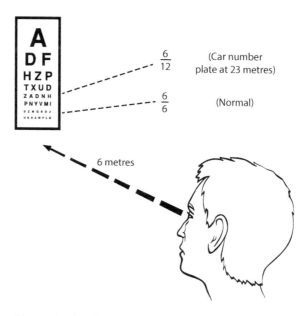

Figure 3.1 Testing distance visual acuity.

Distance vision is tested at 6 m, as rays of light from this distance are nearly parallel. If the patient wears glasses constantly, vision may be recorded with and without glasses, but this must be noted on the record. Each eye is tested and recorded separately, the other being covered with a card held by the examiner.

SNELLEN'S TEST TYPE

Heavy block letters, numbers or symbols printed in black on a white background, are arranged on a chart in nine rows of graded size, diminishing from the top downward. The top letter can be read by the normal eye at a distance of 60 m, and the following rows should be read at 36, 24, 18, 12, 9, 6, 5 and 4 m, respectively.

The patient is seated 6 m from the chart, which must be adequately lit, and is asked to read down to the smallest letter he can distinguish, using one eye at a time.

Visual acuity is expressed as a fraction and abbreviated as VA. The numerator is the distance in metres at which a person can read a given line of letters. The denominator is the distance at which a person with normal average vision can read the same line, e.g. if the seventh line is read at a distance of 6 m, this is VA 6/6. If some letters in the line are read but not all, it is expressed as, for example, VA 6/6 −2, or VA 6/9 + 2.

For vision less than 6/60, the distance between the patient and the chart is reduced by a metre at a time and the vision is recorded accordingly as, for example, 5/60, 4/60, 3/60, 2/60, 1/60.

If the patient cannot read the top letter at a distance of 1 m, the examiner's hand is held at 0.9 m, 0.6 m or 0.3 m away against a dark background and the patient is asked to count the number of fingers held up. If he answers correctly, record VA = CF (count fingers). For less vision, the hand is moved in front of the eye at 0.3 m, record VA = HM (hand movement).

In the case of less vision, test for projection of light by shining a torch into the eye from different directions to see if the patient can tell from which direction it comes. If he sees the light but not the direction, it is noted as VA = PL (perception of light). This test is performed in a dark room. If no light is seen, record no PL, which is total blindness.

USING THE PINHOLE IN THE MEASUREMENT OF VISUAL ACUITY

Occasionally, a patient's visual acuity may be below average, which could be a result of a refractive error not corrected by glasses, or due to the patient wearing an old pair of prescription glasses. One effective, but simple, way to see if distance visual acuity can be improved through spectacles or a change of prescription is a pinhole. A pinhole disc only allows central rays of light to fall onto the macula and does not need to be refracted by the cornea or lens. A 'pinhole disc' is used if the VA is less than 6/6 or 6/9, which may improve VA. If considerable increase in vision is obtained, it may usually be assumed that there is no gross abnormality, but rather a refractive error.

SHERIDAN GARDNER TEST CHART

The Sheridan Gardner test chart can be used for children, patients who are illiterate and patients with learning difficulties. This test type has a single reversible letter on each line, for example, A, V, N. The child holds the card with these letters printed on and is asked to point to the letter on his card which corresponds to the letter on the test type. This test can also be used for very young children as they do not have to name a letter.

KAY PICTURE CHART

The Kay picture chart is again used with patients who are illiterate or with children. Instead of letters, the book contains pictures, which are also of varying sizes. The patient is asked what the picture represents. In order to avoid any misunderstanding amongst patients with language difficulties, it is good practice to ask the hospital's official interpreter to translate for patients.

TUMBLING E CHART

The tumbling E chart again is mainly used for patients who are illiterate. In the chart, the Es face in different directions. The patient is asked to hold a wooden E in his hand and to turn it the same way as the one the examiner is pointing to on the test chart.

It is important to remember to identify in the patient's notes which chart system has been used to test the patient's visual acuity; for example, if the Kay picture chart is used, this must be indicated in the notes.

LOGMAR CHART

The LogMAR chart was designed by Bailie and Lovie and was originally used in the Early Treatment Diabetic Retinopathy Study. The LogMAR chart (Figure 3.2) is expressed as the logarithm of the minimum angle of resolution. LogMAR scale converts the geometric sequence of a traditional chart to a linear scale. It measures visual acuity loss so that positive values indicate vision loss, while negative values denote better or normal vision. It is therefore more accurate than the Snellen's chart and it is gaining more popularity clinically. The chart is designed to be used at various distances such as 4, 3 or 2 m. Unlike the Snellen chart which has 11 lines of block

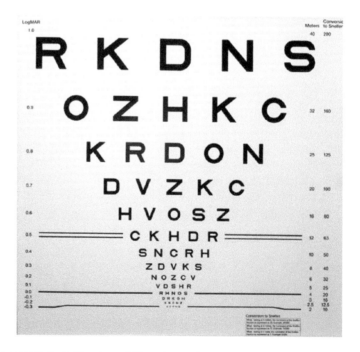

Figure 3.2 LogMAR chart. (Courtesy of Alison Ansons.)

letters and subsequent rows of increasing numbers of letters in decreasing size, the LogMAR uses a special font in which all the lines are of equal thickness and the letter size increases in equal steps of 0.1 LogMAR per line. Bailey and Lovie also advocated that the visual acuity test chart should essentially be the same at each size level on the chart, so that there are the same number of letters on each line and the task of testing for visual acuity is equivalent for each line. The LogMAR chart has five letters of 'almost equal legibility' on each of the rows. Spacing between letters on each row is equal to one letter width, and spacing between rows is equal to the height of the letters on the smaller row. The LogMAR chart thus uses letters of equal legibility, the same number of letters in each row and uniform between-letter and between-row spacing to overcome some of the limitations of the Snellen's chart in which the letters are fairly large and in which there are uneven jumps in the acuity level between the rows. In addition, the crowding of letters on the Snellen's chart also inherently makes it more difficult to read.

LogMAR charts come in 2-, 3- and 4-m types. It should be ensured that the correct chart is selected relative to patient distance from the chart. Different charts should be used for each eye – usually chart 1 for the right eye and chart 2 for the left. LogMAR is also available as a computerised system.

Procedure guideline: Testing distance visual acuity using the LogMAR

1. Seat patient 4, 3 or 2 m away from the test chart, depending upon the chart used.
2. Ensure patient is wearing corrective distance glasses, if worn.
3. Cover the untested eye with an occluder such as tissues or the patient's outpatient card.
4. Instruct the patient, as with the Snellen's chart, to start from the top line and to read the lowest line possible.
5. Ask the patient to read the letters clearly and slowly.
6. Encourage the patient to guess the letters if the patient is uncertain.
7. Ensure that the patient does not lean forward.
8. Use a different chart to test the other eye.

RECORDING LoGMAR ACUITY

The top line of the LogMAR at 3 m gives a score of 1.0 which is equivalent to a Snellen's chart at 6 m, which gives a score of 6/60. Each line will give a score of 0.1 less than the line above so as one moves down each line of the chart, the chart will read 1.0 (as the top line of the chart), 0.9, 0.8, 0.7, 0.6 and so forth so that 0 on the LogMAR chart represents 6/6 on the Snellen's chart. When one goes even further down the LogMAR chart, one will see −0.1, −0.2 and −0.3, which is equivalent to 6/4.8, 6/3.8 and 6/3. LogMAR measures visual acuity loss; positive values indicate vision loss while negative values denote normal or better visual acuity.

Each letter on the chart, regardless of the line concerned, has a score of 0.02. So if a patient reads the top line accurately, which is 1.0, and goes on to read all the letters accurately up to the 0.1 line but cannot get any further and makes one mistake on the 0.0 line, then the LogMAR acuity is 0.02. If the patient gets two letters wrong on the 0.0 line, then the LogMAR acuity will be 0.04; three letters wrong would be 0.06 and so on. If a patient gets all the letters wrong on the 0.0 row, one is then going onto the row above, which is the 0.1 row. If a patient gets one letter wrong on the 0.1 row, the patient's LogMAR reading will be 0.12.

Observe the patient during the test, noting characteristics such as eccentric viewing which could be indicative of vision problems such as macular degeneration, for example.

NEAR VISION

Near vision is tested by cards consisting of different sizes of ordinary printer's type, each card being numbered. The eyes are tested and recorded separately and, if the patient uses reading glasses, these should be worn during the test. The card is held at a comfortable distance (approximately 25 cm) and should be well illuminated by a light from behind the patient's shoulder. The near vision is recorded as the card number of the smallest type size can be most easily read.

UTILISING INFORMATION GAINED FROM VISUAL ACUITY TESTING

The measurement of accurate visual acuity is an important and vital part of any ophthalmological examination. It not only provides the healthcare professional with information on a patient's visual system, but also allows us to gain a realistic insight into a patient's ability to function as a whole. The information gained from measuring a patient's visual acuity allows us to

- Provide a baseline for monitoring of treatment including medical, laser and surgical.
- Monitor the progression or otherwise of the disease.
- Assess a patient's ability to cope and also enable us to provide the most appropriate form of support.
- Provide a measurement tool to assess a patient's vulnerability to trips and falls and to take appropriate measure for their prevention.
- Plan an appropriate form of communication with the patient.
- Prioritise a patient's needs and provide appropriate intervention where necessary, depending on the wishes of a patient – such as social services or district nurses.

The measurement of a patient's visual acuity must never be regarded as a mundane task, and time should be allocated to this important skill. This is an ideal opportunity for the healthcare worker to explore any issues of concern for the patient such as worsening of the ophthalmic condition, inability to cope, issues of compliance with medication and the impact of the eye disease on the patient and his carers. It is also important to document any findings and action taken in the patient's notes.

SPECIAL CONSIDERATION WHEN MEASURING VISUAL ACUITY IN CHILDREN

Assessing and measuring visual acuity accurately in children requires a special skill and takes time, patience and understanding. Young children, especially the very young, often find it difficult to articulate their eye symptoms or their visual disturbance. Depending on the age of the child, various methods of measuring visual acuity should be adapted to suit the child's age, abilities, knowledge, understanding and experience. For example, the measurement of visual acuity in infants, preschool children and children with special needs is not possible with a letter chart. Rather, the Kay picture test chart should be utilised.

Before the commencement of visual acuity testing, it is worthwhile for the ophthalmic nurse to spend a few moments of her time making the child and parents comfortable and for them to become familiar with the visual acuity testing environment. The nurse should create a rapport with the child and parents, talking to the child and finding out his age and interests in order to gain his trust and cooperation. It goes without saying that if a child is crying from fear, discomfort or hunger, the test should be postponed. If required, a demonstration of what the test involves can be helpful so that the parents and child are aware of what is expected in the test.

Depending on the age of the child, the child may feel happier sitting on the parent's lap. Children who normally wear glasses should have their vision tested with their appropriate distance glasses on. If the child does not wear glasses, consideration must be given to ensure that child does not 'peek' out of the eye that is not being tested. Consider purchasing occluder glasses, which are available in bright colours and are available for both left and right eyes. It is often difficult to achieve a complete occlusion with a hand or piece of cardboard.

The child should be asked to keep both eyes open during the test. In order to get the child familiar with the test, one should start off with a 6/60 picture and gradually work down the line. During visual acuity testing using the picture chart, it is important to ensure that the child is familiar with the pictures and is able to articulate. If a child gets a picture wrong, that line should be retested with a different picture. One should ensure that the parents do not inadvertently try to 'assist' the child. At the end of the session, and again depending on the age of the child, coloured stickers and a bravery certificate can be given to the child as a reward and to encourage further cooperating during other examinations that may be necessary.

OPHTHALMIC PROCEDURES UTILISING ANTT PRINCIPLES

An ANTT procedure is achieved by preventing direct and indirect contamination of what are referred to as key parts (e.g. the tip of a syringe or the tip of a drop bottle) or key sites such as the eye or a wound, using a non-touch approach and taking other appropriate infection-control precautions. The principles of ANTT are as follows:

- *Always* wash hands effectively.
- *Never* contaminate key parts or key sites.
- *Touch* non key parts with confidence.
- *Take* appropriate infection-control precautions. (Copyright © 2008 Aseptic Non Touch Technique.)

Procedure guideline: Performing any ANTT procedure

1. Clean hands thoroughly with soap and water or alcohol-based gel.
2. Clean the surface to be used as an aseptic field, e.g. plastic tray or dressing trolley.
3. Collect the equipment for procedure while the tray or trolley is drying.
4. Wash hands again and put on sterile or non-sterile gloves (depending on whether the procedure is clean or sterile). Ask yourself: can I do this procedure without touching key parts or key sites (the eye for example)?
5. Wear a disposable apron if appropriate to do so.
6. Identify key parts of the equipment being used. A key part is a part that needs to remain sterile, such as a syringe tip or the tip of an eye-drop bottle.
7. Prepare the equipment ensuring all key parts are protected at all times when not in use.

8. Prepare the patient, to gain consent and instruct him to tilt his head, or position him as appropriate.
9. Remove gloves, clean hands and reapply new gloves if the patient has been touched.
10. Carry out the procedure ensuring all key parts are protected throughout.
11. Remove gloves and clean hands.
12. Dispose of clinical waste appropriately and decontaminate the tray or trolley before storing.
13. Wash hands and document the procedure.

PRINCIPLES AND PROTOCOL FOR OPHTHALMIC MEDICATION INSTILLATION/APPLICATION

GENERAL PRINCIPLES: INSTILLING DROPS

The aim of all eye medications is to achieve the maximum therapeutic effect from the ophthalmic medications and to minimise the risks, side effects and complications associated with their use. When teaching patients and carers the correct technique for cleaning and instilling drops/ointment to the eye, there are some general principles to follow:

- The medication is delivered in a manner that avoids risk of trauma and/or cross-infection. The latter includes care of drop dispenser and any drop aid used, and instillation technique.
- The drops and ointment should be administered in the correct strength, to the correct patient, into the correct eye, at the correct time and at the appropriate interval.
- All patients must have their drop technique assessed even if they are currently instilling drops for other ophthalmic conditions, e.g. chronic glaucoma.
- The opportunity for self-medication by the patient should be maximised, taking into account his state of well-being. Style and technique will vary between individuals; if the patient is observed to have a drop technique that is adequate, it should not be changed. Where necessary, arrangements for district nurse support should be made.
- In a hospital setting, a record must be kept of all drops instilled and ointment applied.
- Medication that has passed its expiry date must not be used. Any opened drops and ointment must not be used after 7 days in a hospital setting or 28 days in the home care setting. In some settings, single-dose units are used and discarded immediately (British National Formulary 2015).
- Patients need to know the action and the possible side effects of their medication.
- Unless directed otherwise by medical staff, ask the patient to remove his contact lenses prior to instilling drops and ointment. Depending on the patient's ocular problem, it may be necessary to advise the patient to stop wearing contact lenses until the condition has resolved and treatment is completed.
- Patients need to know that drops may sting and some may leave an unpleasant taste in the mouth.
- If patients are on more than one type of drop and/or ointment to the same eye, the order of delivery should be as per pharmacy criteria.
- Normally, one drop is sufficient. Additional drops may reduce the effectiveness as they increase tear-duct stimulation and outflow. It may also increase the amount of systematic

absorption. In addition, any excess drops may overflow onto the cheek and, over a period of time, may cause skin irritation.

- The capacity of the fornix is approximately 30 µL and the average drop size is between 25 and 50 µL. Generic drop bottles may deliver a larger drop than proprietary drop bottles.
- With certain medications, there will be a specific request from the ophthalmologist to occlude the punctum to reduce still further any risk of systemic absorption via mucous membranes of the canaliculi, nose and mouth. However, some medications may be prescribed specifically for their action on the lacrimal apparatus and so punctal occlusion is not desirable. In addition, it is not desirable to occlude the punctum digitally following some types of surgery.
- As the period for effective therapeutic absorption of medication is from 1 to 1.5 minutes, patients should be taught to close their eyes slowly and to keep them closed for a slow count to 60. Keeping the lids gently closed without squeezing reduces lacrimal duct outflow and maximises medication contact with ocular structures.
- An appropriate time interval of approximately 3 minutes is necessary between each drop in order to prevent dilution and overflow.
- All medication should be delivered to the correct location. This is generally the lower fornix but can include the cornea, lids, periocular wounds and the socket.
- Drops must be stored according to the manufacturer's instructions. This includes some drops to be stored in a refrigerator at all times, even before opening, and others that must be stored in the refrigerator only after opening.
- Before using eye drops, patients – or whoever is instilling the drops – should be instructed to shake the bottle to ensure even distribution.
- Pharmacy will label all drop boxes with patient, dose, order and storage instructions. They will also have available upon request large-print labels.
- Certain medications may have an effect on vision. This effect may be transient or may last for the duration of the treatment.

GENERAL PRINCIPLES: APPLICATION OF EYE OINTMENT

- Ointment may be prescribed in addition to drops.
- Ointment should be applied after any prescribed drops have been instilled, leaving approximately a 3-minute interval between medications.
- Ointment may be prescribed for structures other than the eye.
- Ointment may be prescribed for use after first dressing, and this may not happen for up to 1 week in the case of some oculoplastic surgery.
- If requested, visual acuity should be recorded before ointment is applied as ointment clouds vision. Any existing ointment excess is normally removed prior to taking visual acuity measurement.
- A 5-mm strip of ointment should be applied to the inner edge of the lower fornix of the appropriate eye.
- The patient should close his eye and remove excess ointment with a swab.
- The patient should be advised that the ointment is likely to cause blurring of vision because of its viscous nature.
- In the case of wounds on the lids, face or eye socket, ointment should be squeezed directly onto the wound. It may be dispersed using a moistened swab. If requested to do so by the ophthalmic surgeon, the wound or scar should be massaged using the ointment.

GENERAL STAFF PRINCIPLES ON EYE MEDICATION

COMPLIANCE, CONCORDANCE OR ADHERENCE WITH EYE MEDICATION TREATMENT REGIMENS

Compliance relates to how a patient is expected to conform with advice and treatment given by the health professional (i.e. do what the patient is told). This puts a greater responsibility for recovery onto the patient.

Concordance incorporates a partnership between the patient and health professional. An agreement is reached regarding treatment taking into consideration the patient's personal circumstances and allowing for a holistic assessment of the patient's needs. The success of treatment is therefore shared between the patient and health professional. Concordance allows a greater respect for patient autonomy and enables the patient to make informed decisions about their care and treatment. It values the patient's perspective and acknowledges the impact of treatment on quality of life. Patients will be more likely to be concordant if they are involved in shared decision making. This is particularly true for patients suffering from chronic glaucoma.

Adherence is an alternative to compliance that aims to empower the patient to be active in the management of their condition.

- Drops and ointment are drugs, and some eye medications will have a systemic affect other than on the eye.
- All Trust/employer policies for drug administration should be followed in conjunction with these principles. This includes hand hygiene.
- The nurse should explain to the patient what she is going to do and should obtain his consent and cooperation.
- Where appropriate, the patient/partner/carer should be involved. The district nurse should be involved where it is felt necessary to ensure that the eye treatment is delivered.
- Staff should be honest about the effects and side effects of drops, including stinging and discomfort.
- For inpatients – including any day cases – a patient already on glaucoma medication prior to surgery should have it confirmed whether any new medication prescribed is in addition to, or instead of, the glaucoma medication.
- Before the patient is discharged, it should always be ensured that all relevant eye medications, including any that the patient may have been on prior to any ocular surgery, have been prescribed.

GENERAL PATIENT PRINCIPLES ON EYE MEDICATION

- The medical and nursing staff will tell the patient about the drops or ointment used.
- The nursing staff will instruct the patient on when and how to instil his drops and/or apply ointment safely.
- Staff should instruct the patient about the importance of handwashing before and after instilling drops or applying ointment to help prevent infection.
- Staff must ask the patient about any current medication as this could affect the choice of treatment.
- Pharmacy and nursing staff should determine the best way to help the patient distinguish between the different types of drop bottles that have been prescribed.

- Nursing and medical staff should talk with the patient at each visit about how the patient is managing the drops or ointment regimen.
- Staff should advise the patient that devices are available for purchase to help with eye-drop administration. These include bottle attachments to help squeeze the bottle; those to help open the cap; and those to help the patient remember to take the next drop. Information on these devices is available in the hospital pharmacy or community pharmacy. The district nurse or practice nurse may also have the relevant information.
- The patient should be reminded that drops and ointments are prescribed for his use only. Drops and ointments should be stored according to the manufacturer's instructions, which in some cases will be in the refrigerator.
- As with all drugs, advise the patient that medications should be stored in a place out of reach of children and animals.

SPECIAL CONSIDERATIONS FOR INSTILLING EYE MEDICATION IN CHILDREN

Instilling any drops in children can be traumatic for the healthcare professional, the child and parents. Be truthful if a child asks if the drops will sting. Show the drops to the child and, if appropriate, allow the child to handle the drops. If instilling fluoresce in drops, it is helpful to place a drop on the child's hand to demonstrate the colour. Involve the child in the instillation of the drops by giving them some tissues to hold and instruct them to dab the eye after the instillation. If a child refuses to open his or her eyes, instil the drops in the inner canthus of the closed lid and when the child opens his or her eyes, usually some of the drops will flow onto the globe. This latter technique is also helpful when dealing with young babies.

POST-OPERATIVE EYE CARE

The majority of post-operative ophthalmic patients attend for surgery as a day case and, as a result, may be taught to perform their own first dressing at home since some of these patients may not necessarily be reviewed the next day.

GENERAL PRINCIPLES

- The eye should be cleaned only if necessary, e.g. when discharge is present.
- Staff should instruct the patient about the importance of handwashing before and after carrying out any procedure to the eye.
- Cartella shields, if used, should be washed with soap and water if necessary. The shield should be stored dry.

CLINICAL PRACTICE GUIDELINES

Procedure guideline: Procedure for eye-drop instillation or application of ointment

Do not use this procedure for first-day post-operative patients. First-day post-operative patients should follow the procedure listed under 'Procedure guideline: Post-operative eye-drop and eye-ointment instillation'.

EQUIPMENT

- Relevant eye drops/ointment
- Prescription chart/procedure guideline (PGD)
- Access to sink and soap dispenser to wash hands or to apply alcogel
- Tissues

NURSING ACTION

PRE-PROCEDURE

1. Wash hands with soap and water.
2. Gather the eye drops/ointment, boxed tissues and alcohol gel.
3. Check patient identification against request card/patient's notes using patient name band/verbal confirmation from patient.
4. Confirm for which eye the eye drops or ointment has been prescribed.
   Note: Ointment may be prescribed for periocular structures/wounds.
5. Check eye drops/ointment against the prescription/PGD.
6. Check the correct strength (%) of the eye drops/ointment against prescription.
7. Check drops/ointment has not expired. Check the clarity of the drops, i.e. the fluid in the bottle/minim must be clear and not discoloured.
8. Check packaging/bottle/tube seal is intact when first used.
9. Explain the procedure, including any effects and side effects.
10. Identify any allergy to the topical medications.
11. Assess the patient's medical and physical needs and level of understanding, and take into account any cultural needs.
12. Obtain the patient's verbal consent and cooperation.
13. Examine the eye to be treated for the following:
    a. Redness not attributed to surgery or other known causes
    b. No stickiness or pain
    c. No deterioration of vision
14. Check no contact lens *in situ* unless advised to the contrary by doctor such as a bandage contact lens.
15. The patient should be sitting comfortably, ideally in a private area.

PROCEDURE

1. Wash hands.
2. Prepare the eye drops/ointment. *Note*: Before using any bottle of eye drops, shake the bottle first.
3. Gently hold down lower lid with clean tissues, using one hand.
4. Position hand holding the bottle/minims either gently on patient's forehead or just at the lower fornix of the eye. The tip of the bottle/minim/tube must not be in contact with the patient's eyes or anywhere else as this is the key part.
5. Instil only one drop into the lower fornix towards outer cantus or squeeze 5 mm of ointment along lower fornix towards outer cantus.
   Note: Ointment must only be applied after prescribed eye drops.
6. Ask patient to gently close his eyes, counting slowly to 60. This helps to minimise systemic absorption. Punctal occlusion, digital pressure applied to the inner canthus, is an alternative.
7. Wipe away any excess drops/ointment, taking care not to wick away drops from the eye.

8. If further drops are prescribed, wait an interval of 3 minutes before carrying out the procedure. Apply alcogel to hands before instilling the next eye drop.
9. Make the patient comfortable; patients usually appreciate being given a tissue to dab their cheeks.
10. Dispose of clinical waste, cleanse hands and then clean the tray.
11. Document the procedure in the case notes and/or drop chart.

Procedure guideline: Post-operative eye-drop and eye-ointment instillation

This post-procedural pathway is applicable to inpatient day cases, certain outpatient departments and acute ophthalmic patients.

EQUIPMENT

- Plastic tray
- Sterile eye pack
- Alcowipes
- Relevant eye drops/ointment
- Prescription chart/PGD
- Access to sink and soap dispenser to wash hands
- Access to alcohol gel
- Tissues
- Sterile cotton wool (It is appropriate to clean the eye with this as, with most ocular surgery, the wound is on the globe and so linting should not interfere with wound healing; if there is a lid wound, use non-woven swabs.)
- Two sets of non-sterile gloves
- Apron

NURSING ACTION

1. Wash hands and prepare trolley and equipment in accordance with ANTT principles.
2. Check patient identification band against medication chart.
3. Prepare patient for the procedure and obtain consent, giving an explanation of procedure including any side effects of the medication.
4. Assess the patient as before, including ensuring that the drops are not contraindicated.
5. The patient should be seated.
6. Wash hands or use alcogel.
7. Prepare equipment and place in tray, identifying key parts to be protected during the procedure; in this case, the tips of bottles/tubes.
8. Check eye drops/ointment against the prescription.
9. Check the correct strength (%) of the eye drops/ointment against prescription.
10. Check eye drops/ointment have not expired. Check clarity of eye drops, i.e. the fluid in the bottle/minim must be clear and not discoloured.
11. Check packaging/bottle/tube seal is intact when first used.
12. Identify any current allergy to the topical medications.
13. Ensure that the eye drops/ointment are instilled or applied into the correct eye.
    Note: Ointment may be prescribed for periocular structures/wounds.

14. Examine the eye to be treated for the following:
    a. Redness not attributed to surgery or other known causes
    b. No stickiness or pain
    c. No deterioration of vision
    d. Allergies to the prescribed eye drops
15. Check no contact lens *in situ* unless advised to the contrary by the doctor.
16. Remove gloves, clean hands with alcohol gel and reapply non-sterile gloves.
17. Open packaging, ensuring key parts remain protected. *Note*: You may need to open additional packaging if the eye needs cleaning prior to drop instillation, in which case you should proceed to eye cleaning first.
18. Instruct patient to slightly tilt the head back and ask the patient to look up.
    Note: Before using any bottle of eye drops, shake the bottle first.
19. Instil only one drop into the lower fornix towards the outer cantus or squeeze 5 mm of ointment along the lower fornix towards the outer cantus. *Note*: Ointment must only be applied after prescribed eye drops.
20. Ask the patient to gently close his eyes, counting slowly to 60. This helps to minimise systemic absorption. Punctal occlusion, digital pressure applied to the inner canthus, is an alternative.
21. Wipe away any excess eye drops/ointment, taking care not to wick away drops from the eye.
22. If further drops are prescribed, wait an interval of 3 minutes before carrying out the procedure. Apply alcogel to hands before instilling the next eye drop.
23. Make the patient comfortable; patients usually appreciate being given a tissue to dab their cheeks.
24. Dispose of clinical waste, cleanse hands and then clean the tray.
25. Cleanse hands and document the procedure in the case notes and/or drop chart.

Procedure guideline: Taking a conjunctival swab

EQUIPMENT

- Plastic tray or trolley
- Appropriate sterile culture medium and swab stick (different ones are required for bacteria, viruses and Chlamydia)
- Completed request form (paper or electronic)
- Non-sterile gloves

NURSING ACTION

1. Identify patient, utilising local procedure for correct identification of patient.
2. Check request for the type of swab that is required, e.g. bacterial or viral.
3. Wash hands.
4. Clean aseptic surface for carrying out the procedure, i.e. tray or dressing trolley.
5. While tray or trolley is drying, gather equipment for procedure.
6. Wash or apply alcogel to hands, assemble equipment and put it in the tray.
7. If both eyes are to be swabbed, label the swabs 'right' and 'left'.
8. Take assembled tray to patient.

9. Explain to the patient the procedure and obtain verbal consent.
10. Wash or apply alcogel to hands and wait for hands to dry before putting on gloves.
11. Remove the sterile swab from the container and ask patient to look up.
12. Swab firmly along lower fornix from nasal side outwards.
13. Place the stick in culture medium, remove gloves and wash your hands.
14. Ensure the swab is accurately and clearly labelled with patient's name, hospital number, the correct eye, date of birth and date of request of specimen.
15. Dispose of all waste appropriately.
16. Wash or apply alcogel to hands.
17. Clean tray and store dry.
18. Wash hands then document the procedure in the patient's notes.

Procedure guideline: Epilation of lashes

In-growing eyelashes (trichiasis) may be removed by epilation to give temporary relief from symptoms caused by their constant irritation of the cornea and conjunctiva.

EQUIPMENT

- Plastic tray or trolley
- Sterile epilation forceps
- Tissues
- Fluorescein minims
- Slit lamp or good light magnification unit

NURSING ACTION

1. Wash hands and prepare trolley and gather equipment in accordance with ANTT principles.
2. Prepare equipment and place in tray, identifying key parts to be protected during procedure.
3. Check patient identification against request card/notes with patient.
4. Obtain patient's consent and cooperation including explanation of procedure including any side effects.
5. Identify any current allergy to the topical medications.
6. Ensure the patient's head is supported during the procedure.
7. Evert lid slightly – for lower lid ask the patient to look up; for upper lid ask the patient to look down.
8. Remove each of the offending lashes by gripping the lash at the lid margin with epilation forceps and pulling firmly in the direction of the hair growth.
9. Make the patient comfortable; patients usually appreciate being given a tissue to dab their cheeks.
10. Dispose of clinical waste, cleanse hands and then clean the tray.
11. Document the procedure in the case notes and/or drop chart.

The treatment must be repeated as often as required by the patient, e.g. weekly, monthly or as necessary. Patients or carers with good vision may be able to perform epilation themselves at home.

ELECTROLYSIS

Electrolysis is used to remove in-growing lashes by means of a needle electrode applied to the lash follicle. It is a painful procedure, and the lid is first anaesthetised with a local anaesthetic injection.

Procedure guideline: Cryotherapy

Cryotherapy can be used to remove lashes by applying liquid nitrogen to the offending lash follicle. This is usually performed by the doctor or specialist nurse, but the nurse needs to prepare the patient.

EQUIPMENT

- Plastic tray or trolley
- Local anaesthetic drops, e.g. proxymetacaine hydrochloride 0.5% (Ophthaine)
- Local anaesthetic injection, e.g. lignocaine hydrochloride 2%
- 2-mL syringe
- Green and orange needles
- Paraffin gauze
- 'Shoe horn'
- Lubricant (such as K-Y) jelly
- Sterile cotton wool buds
- Dressing towel
- Tissues
- Epilation forceps
- Sterile gloves
- Liquid nitrogen (cryo) container

NURSING ACTION

1. Wash hands and prepare trolley and equipment in accordance with ANTT principles.
2. Check patient identification against request card/notes with patient.
3. Prepare patient for the procedure.
4. Assess the patient as before.
5. The patient should be lying in a recumbent position.
6. Prepare equipment and place in tray, identifying key parts to be protected during procedure.
7. Obtain patient's consent and cooperation giving explanation of procedure including any side effects.
8. Check patient name band against the case notes.
9. Identify any current allergy to the topical medications.
10. Instil prescribed local anaesthetic drops.
11. Prepare and administer local anaesthetic injection.
12. Insert 'shoe horn', well lubricated with jelly, into appropriate fornix.
13. Cover the patient's head with sterile drape leaving appropriate eye exposed.
14. Fill cryo container with liquid nitrogen.
15. Put cotton wool buds into liquid nitrogen and pass to doctor or specialist nurse when ready to assist with procedure.

16. The patient may open or close his eyes during the procedure.
17. Make the patient comfortable.
18. Dispose of clinical waste and clean hands then the trolley.
19. Wash hands and then complete documentation.

The patient should be warned that the lid(s) may become inflamed. Cryotherapy is not used on patients with symblepharon.

TAPING THE LOWER LID TO RELIEVE ENTROPION

As a temporary measure, the lower lid can be taped to relieve an entropion. A piece of hypoallergenic tape about 1.3–2.5 cm (0.25–1 inch) in length is applied just below the lower lid margin and secured on the cheek in such a way as to bring the lower lid into its normal position. Prior to using hypoallergenic tape for this procedure, it is important to ascertain from patients that they are not allergic to hypoallergenics. When the tape is in position on the lower cheek, ask the patient to close his eyes to ensure that the lower conjunctiva is not inadvertently exposed. If the lower conjunctiva is exposed, reposition the tape.

Procedure guideline: Testing for dry eyes using tear strips

The tear strip test is performed to discern if the eyes are dry. It is a test of the quantity not quality of the tear film.

EQUIPMENT

- Tear test strips
- Timer or watch
- Local anaesthetic
- Patient case notes with request

NURSING ACTION

1. Wash hands and prepare trolley and equipment.
2. Confirm patient identification against request card/notes with the patient.
3. Prepare patient for the procedure obtaining consent.
4. The patient should be seated with the head well supported.
5. Prepare equipment and place in tray, identifying key parts and sites to be protected during the procedure.
6. Instil local anaesthetic drops if prescribed or as per PGD.
7. When performed without anaesthesia, this test measures the function of the main lacrimal gland. The irritation from the Schirmer strips stimulates the secretory activity of the main lacrimal gland. When this test is used in conjunction with a topical anaesthetic, it measures the function of the accessory lacrimal glands. Less than 5 mm in 5 minutes is considered abnormal.
8. Prepare strips in accordance with instructions on the packet.
9. Ask the patient to look up and insert the strip in accordance with the manufacturer's instructions. It is helpful to mark the strip R and L as appropriate. The patient may open or close his eyes during the procedure.
10. Make the patient comfortable.
11. Dispose of clinical waste and clean hands then the trolley.
12. Wash hands and then complete documentation.

Procedure guideline: Syringing the nasolacrimal ducts

This is performed to determine whether the lacrimal drainage apparatus is blocked or patent.

EQUIPMENT

- Plastic tray or trolley
- Dressing pack (if used)
- Tray or trolley with
    - One sterile 2-mL syringe
    - One disposable sterile lacrimal cannula
    - One sterile Nettleship dilator
    - One ampule of normal saline
- Local anaesthetic drops, e.g. proxymetacaine hydrochloride 0.5%
- Box of tissues
- Bag for soiled tissues
- Good light magnification unit
- Patient's case notes

NURSING ACTION

1. Wash hands and prepare trolley and equipment.
2. Check patient identification against request card/notes with patient.
3. Prepare the patient for the procedure, obtaining consent.
4. The patient should be seated with the head well supported.
5. Prepare equipment and place in tray, identifying key parts to be protected during procedure. Fill syringe with saline, attach cannula securely and ensure patency.
6. Stand behind or beside the patient, for ease of performance of this procedure.
7. Ask the patient to look upwards/outwards.
8. With the right hand, insert the Nettleship dilator into the punctum vertically 1–2 mm. Then gently turn it horizontally towards the nose and carefully rotate it a few times between the finger and thumb to dilate the first part of the lower canaliculus.
9. Remove the dilator and carefully insert the cannula following the direction of the canaliculus to a maximum of 4–5 mm (when fine disposable cannulas are used, it is not always necessary to dilate the punctum).
10. Inject the fluid slowly. Undue pressure must not be used.
11. Note whether the patient can taste the saline in the back of the throat or if there is any resistance and or regurgitation through the upper or lower punctum.
12. Make the patient comfortable.
13. Dispose of clinical waste and clean hands then the trolley.
14. Wash hands and then complete documentation.

RESULT OF THE PROCEDURE

The result will be one of several outcomes and should be recorded in the patient's case notes:

- The saline may pass easily into the sac, through the nasolacrimal duct and trickle into the nasopharynx. The patient will taste the saline on the back of his tongue and can be told to swallow it. The result is reported as freely patent.

- There may be partial patency with some regurgitation around the cannula.
- The saline may return through the lower punctum around the cannula. This shows an obstruction near the nasal end of the lower canaliculus.
- The saline may return through the upper punctum showing an obstruction in the sac or nasolacrimal duct.
- Mucopurulent discharge may return with the saline if the sac is infected. This should be reported.

Occluding the upper punctum with a second Nettleship dilator is sometimes performed if the saline has returned via the upper punctum. Syringing is repeated to try to remove the obstruction. In this case, an assistant is needed to hold the dilator in place. Syringing must not be performed by a nurse if there is an obvious swelling over the nasolacrimal sac, as infection renders the structures more prone to damage. The medical staff may use a set of lacrimal probes. These are used on infants in theatre, when the saline may be coloured with fluorescein to aid the detection of patency.

Procedure guideline: Subconjunctival injections

Small amounts of fluid (1.5–2 mL) can be injected under the bulbar conjunctiva. This form of treatment is not used as frequently as it used to be for eye infections. Here are some examples of drugs given by this method:

- Mydricaine no. 2 (Moorfields). This contains a cocktail of drugs, all having a mydriatic effect, in a 0.5-mL dose. It is used in uveitis to dilate the pupil when other methods have failed:
    - Atropine sulphate   1.00 mg
    - Procaine hydrochloride   6.00 mg
    - Adrenaline   216 g
- Antibiotics. These are given subconjunctivally to treat or prevent intraocular infection:
    - Cefuroxime   100 mg in 0.5 mL water
    - Gentamicin   10–20 mg
- Steroids. Given to suppress the inflammatory process in cases of uveitis. Steroids used include
    - Betamethasone   4 mg (quick-acting)
    - Methylprednisolone   40 mg (long-acting)
- Local anaesthetics may be given in this manner.

EQUIPMENT

- Tray or trolley
- Dressing pack
- Receiver with
    - 1-mL and/or 2-mL syringe(s)
    - Dark green needle
    - Subconjunctival needle
    - Drugs for injection
- Topical anaesthetic drops
- Gauze squares
- Pad

- Bandage
- Tape
- Sachet of normal saline and alcohol wipe to clean the surface before opening
- A good light source
- Prescribed drops or ointment (if applicable)
- Prescription/case notes
- Tissues

NURSING ACTION

1. Wash hands and prepare trolley and equipment.
2. Check patient identification against request card/notes with patient.
3. Prepare patient for the procedure and obtain consent.
4. Assess the patient as before.
5. Position the patient lying down or sitting in a chair with the head well supported.
6. Cleanse hands and prepare equipment and place in tray, identifying key parts to be protected during procedure.
7. Give prescribed analgesia (if required).
8. Commence instilling local anaesthetic drops as per prescription or PGD, e.g. G. amethocaine hydrochloride 2% or G. cocaine hydrochloride 5%, one drop every 5 minutes over 25 minutes.
9. Apply alcogel to hands and put on non-sterile gloves.
10. Prepare drugs to be injected, identifying key parts to be protected during procedure. Check drugs with second nurse to ensure correct drug(s) are administered. Put subconjunctival needle on syringe firmly and check patency.
11. Once the eye is anaesthetised, commence the procedure.
12. Open dressing pack in usual way.
13. Clean eye if necessary.
14. Hold lower lid down and ask patient to look up (an assistant may be required for this).
15. Hold the syringe horizontally, with the needle bevel uppermost and the fingers in the correct position to inject the drug, to ensure procedure is carried out correctly.
16. Insert the needle under the conjunctiva in the folds of the lower fornix.
17. Inject the drug slowly. The conjunctiva will balloon forwards as it is injected.
18. On completion of the injection, withdraw needle.
19. Apply antibiotic ointment or drops if prescribed, to prevent infection.
20. Apply pad and bandage for 4 hours, for patient comfort.
21. Dispose of clinical waste and clean hands then the trolley/tray.
22. Wash hands and then complete documentation.

NOTES

- Methylprednisolone must not be mixed with any other drug.
- If no assistance is available, it may be necessary to use the following:
  - A speculum to hold the lids open
  - Moorfields forceps to hold up the conjunctiva to ease the insertion of the needle
- Analgesics may be given before the procedure and again once the local anaesthetic has worn off.

Procedure guideline: Removing a dacryocystorhinostomy tube

EQUIPMENT

- Plastic tray or trolley
- Nasal speculum
- Stitch scissors
- Long Spencer Wells forceps
- A good torch/light source

NURSING ACTION

1. Wash hands and prepare trolley and equipment.
2. Check patient identification against request card/notes with patient then prepare the patient for procedure.
3. Assess the patient's needs as before and obtain consent.
4. Position the patient semi-recumbent or sitting in a chair with the head well supported.
5. Cleanse hands and prepare equipment, protecting the key parts.
6. Ask the patient to blow his nose, especially down the nostril on the affected side.
7. Clasp the tube in the nostril with forceps.
8. Cut the tube in the inner canthus and remove from the nostril by pulling with the forceps.
9. Make the patient comfortable.
10. Dispose of clinical waste and clean hands then the trolley/tray.
11. Wash hands and then complete documentation.

NOTE

The snip and blow method used by the ophthalmologist for removal of a dacryocystorhinostomy tube involves instilling topical anaesthetic in the operated eye. Lignocaine spray is sprayed into the nostril and the patient is asked to blow his nose. An endoscope is inserted into the nostril and the tube is snipped from the upper and lower punctum. The tube is gently pulled from the nostril using curved forceps. Occasionally, if there is a lot of mucus which is adherent to the tube, gentle suction can be applied up the nostril prior to removal of the tube.

Procedure guideline: Preparing a patient for fundal fluorescein angiography

NURSING ACTION

1. Ensure that all relevant documentation, i.e. request form for fluorescein angiogram, has been signed.
2. Check patient's details, e.g. date of birth and address, correspond to the fluorescein request form.
3. Explain the procedure to the patient:
   a. Dilating drops will be instilled in the eye/eyes to be photographed. Initially, colour photographs will be taken followed by black and white photographs.
   b. A fluorescein dye will be injected into the antecubital fossa or dorsal aspect of the hand via a butterfly or Venflon.
   c. The dye normally takes about 6–10 seconds before appearing at the fundus.
   d. The patient will be asked to look at a fixation point during the procedure.

e. The patient must be warned about subsequent skin discolouration and the urine being discoloured for 4–6 hours.

f. The patient must be informed about the side effects of fluorescein – ranging from mild nausea, vomiting, urticaria and rash to bronchospasm and anaphylactic shock.

4. Obtain the patient's medical history, with details of medications and allergies, especially shellfish.

5. Obtain written consent from the patient.

NOTES

- Proceed with caution in patients with severe allergies to other dyes or medicines, severe asthmatics or patients with very recent cardiac problems.
- Pregnant women should never be given IV (intravenous) fluorescein.
- Breastfeeding women should be warned that the fluorescein dye will be exhibited in their breast milk, and therefore they should not breastfeed their baby for 24 hours.
- All relevant emergency drugs and equipment must be at hand for any potential complication.
- Extravasation must be avoided as it is extremely painful for the patient.
- Patients who frequently experience nausea or vomiting can be prescribed oral Buccastem, an anti-emetic, half an hour before the procedure. One to two tablets are placed high between upper lip and gum and left to dissolve. All reactions to IV fluorescein should be recorded in the patient's notes.
- Before dilating any ophthalmic patients, check the type of intraocular lens *in situ* (iris clips cannot be dilated). Contact lenses should normally be removed unless specifically instructed not to by the doctor.

PREPARING A PATIENT FOR INTRAVENOUS INJECTION OF INDOCYANINE GREEN DYE

Indocyanine green (ICG) has been used for more than 30 years in tests of cardiac and hepatic functions (Lund-Johansen 1990). The use of ICG in ophthalmology to study the circulation of the retina – and especially of the choroid – is of particular value. ICG angiography, like fluorescein, is generally considered to be a safe procedure but, being invasive, adverse reactions similar to those with fluorescein are known to occur. Reactions range from mild nausea and vomiting, sneezing, urticaria and syncope to severe reactions affecting the cardiac and respiratory systems.

Any patient requiring an ICG angiography should be screened for allergic reactions, especially to iodine, shellfish or previous reaction to ICG. ICG has a 'thinner' feel than fluorescein and enters the body much more quickly than fluorescein.

The recommended dose for ICG is 25 mg in 5 mL of aqueous solvent. A 5-mL bolus of normal saline should immediately follow the injection.

Radioactive iodine uptake studies should not be carried out for 1 week following ICG angiography.

Since ICG is removed from the bloodstream exclusively by the liver, the dye will ultimately be excreted with intestinal contents, so no skin discolouration will occur.

NOTES

- Resuscitation equipment must be at hand as fluorescein and ICG can cause anaphylactic shock.
- The patient must stay for half an hour following the angiogram to enable observation for any reaction to the dye.

Procedure guideline: Preparing a patient for laser treatment

NURSING ACTION

1. Take and record patient's visual acuity.
2. Wash hands at the beginning and end of the procedure, and at any point when they become contaminated.
3. Explain the procedure to the patient:
   a. Mydriatics will be instilled if the retina is to be treated and possibly for a capsulotomy.
   b. Local anaesthetic drops will be instilled.
   c. The patient will have to keep his eyes very still while flashing green lights are emitted from the argon laser; usually nothing is noted by the patient receiving laser treatment from the YAG laser.
   d. Following capsulotomy and trabeculoplasty, the intraocular pressure will be measured 1 hour after the procedure.
4. Wipe eyes following the procedure as lubricating jelly will have been used for the contact lens.

NOTES

- Staff in the laser room should wear protective goggles and adhere to laser safety policies.
- In order to prevent a hypoglycaemic/hyperglycaemic attack during laser treatment, ensure that the patient has had his required intake of food and relevant anti-hypoglycaemic agents.
- Inform the patient of alternative analgesia such as Entonox or peribulbar injection.
- Whilst it is important for the patient to keep still during laser treatment, inform the patient of alternative means of communicating with the doctor during treatment, such as tapping on the laser table to gain the doctor's attention.
- For indirect argon laser, the patient will have to be in the recumbent position on a clinical couch.

Procedure guideline: Preparing a patient for photodynamic therapy

NURSING ACTION

1. Full explanation must be given to the patient.
2. The patient's visual acuity is measured using the LogMAR or Snellen.
3. Wash hands at the beginning and end of the procedure, and at any point when they become contaminated.
4. The patient's blood pressure, pulse rate, height and weight are all accurately measured and recorded. The patient's height and weight is necessary to calculate the dosage of the Visudyne (Verteporfin).
5. An identification bracelet is attached to the patient's wrist, and it is essential that correct details are recorded and the patient wears the band for at least 48 hours following treatment to remind the patient, as well as other health professionals, that he has received Visudyne therapy.
6. The patient's pupil is dilated.

7. The Visudyne infusion equipment is prepared and set up.
8. The Visudyne is given via a cannula.
9. Post-treatment information includes avoiding sunlight for 48 hours, wearing sunglasses and wearing clothing that will fully cover arms and legs. Patients should be warned that their vision might be blurred. Other adverse reactions to the Visudyne therapy include back pain during infusion, severe decreasing vision and reactions around the cannula site, such as pain, swelling, hypersensitivity and leaking of Visudyne.

INTRAVITREAL (IVT) INJECTION

Overview

Intravitreal injection has become an increasingly employed tool in the management of posterior segment diseases. Clinical experience with IVT injections has provided substantial data concerning the safety of this procedure. In a comprehensive review of published clinical studies comprising nearly 15,000 IVT injections, the overall rate of endophthalmitis was 0.3% per injection.

Objectives

Advantages of this mode of administration include targeted delivery of drug to the site of pathology, the ability to bypass the blood/ocular barrier for many drugs, the provision of immediate and therapeutic intraocular concentrations of medications, and the ability to minimize or avoid systemic toxicity of medications. However, IVT injection is an invasive technique. Minimising the risk of infection and avoiding damage to ocular structures play a critical role in optimizing the safety profile.

Procedure guideline: Preparing a patient for intravitreal injection

The intravitreal injection is carried out as per treatment plan. Prior to the injection, assessment of vision is carried out by an optometrist on the patient's first and fourth visit. Optical coherence tomography is also carried out on the first and fourth visit. All IVT injections must be carried out in a clean room specifically set aside for IVT injection. In some hospitals, this is performed in a theatre setting.

EQUIPMENT

- Trolley with sharps bin
- Prescription chart
- Gloves (sterile if high-risk procedure)
- Malosa procedure pack (with drape speculum, gauge and disposable forceps)
- Double-ended scleral marker
- Apron
- 1-mL syringes
- Needles
- Videne 10%
- Sterile water
- Gallipot
- Oxybuprocaine 0.4% minims

- Chloramphenicol minims
- Lucentis/Avastin
- Surgical masks
- Surgical hat
- Medication as prescribed
- Sanicloth 70 wipes
- Access to sink and soap dispenser to wash hands
- Access to sharps container
- Access to alcohol gel
- Injection book

NOTES

- Do not resheath needles.
- Do not replace syringes in paper packets, use needle or bung to protect key parts.

NURSING ACTION

1. Put on apron and wash hands with soap and water as per Trust guidelines.
2. Damp dust room, chair, surfaces, trolley and any equipment in the room working from high surfaces to low surfaces, before the start of clinic using a disposable cloth and general purpose detergent as per Decontamination policy.
3. Dispose of gloves and apron in clinical waste bin.
4. Close the door to the injection room for 5 minutes before using it for the treatment of patients.
5. Put on apron and wash hands as per Trust guidelines with soap and water.
6. Clean metal trolley with a sanicloth 70 wipe and allow to air dry for 30 seconds.
    Note: If tray/trolley is visibly dirty, soap and water must be used for cleaning. The cleaning of plastic trays/trolleys with soap and water must be part of the daily environmental/equipment clean for the clinical area.
7. Decontaminate hands with alcogel as per Trust hand hygiene policy.
8. Whilst the trolley is drying, gather all equipment required to undertake the procedure and place items on the bottom shelf of trolley. Open external packing *only* on age related macular degeneration (AMD) treatment pack.
9. Put on theatre mask, hat and apron and clean hands with alcogel as per Trust policy and put on sterile gloves.
10. Open the blue AMD treatment pack onto the top of the trolley maintaining the sterility of its contents using ANTT.
11. Open a gallipot and syringe on to the non-sterile area of the trolley for the surgeon to mix 5% Videne solution. Ensure that the key parts of the syringe remain sterile.
12. Open all other sterile products onto aseptic field, protecting key parts using ANTT.
13. In a sterile gallipot mix 10% Videne with an equal amount of sterile water to make a 5% Videne solution for the surgeon to instil into the eye.
    Note: 10-mL plastic ampoules of water should be used, clean the neck of the ampoule with an Alcowipe, allow to air dry and empty contents into gallipot. Dispose of the Videne bottle at the end of each session.
14. Assist the patient to put on a theatre hat and bring him or her into the injection room. Make the patient comfortable.

15. Check the consent and identity of the patient and confirm that the eye has been marked in accordance with Trust policy.
16. Instil G. benoxinate × 3 drops over 10 minutes in accordance with Trust ANTT procedure for eye-drop administration.
17. Stay with and make the patient comfortable in a seated position ready for injection.
18. Wash hands with alcogel as per Trust procedure and put on theatre hat, mask and apron.
19. Assist medical or specialist nursing staff with the procedure opening sterile packs as required and pour 10% Videne into the second gallipot to be used for cleansing of the lid and orbit. The gallipot should be placed on the sterile white tray.
20. Open the packaging of Lucentis drug and remove the cap ensuring that the key parts remain sterile. Place the vial on the treatment trolley but *not* on the sterile field.
    Note: The drug must be drawn up immediately once the cap has been removed.
    For Avastin, the syringe is prefilled and sterile. Open the pack and place the syringe onto the surgeon's sterile field.
21. Wash hands with alcogel and apply sterile gloves as per Trust policy to continue to assist with the procedure.
22. Whilst wearing sterile gloves instil antibiotic drops as prescribed by the doctor.
23. Following the procedure, clean the trolley with a Sanicloth 70 wipe and alcogel hands according to Trust policy.
24. Dispose of sharps in the sharps bin as per Trust policy.
25. Dispose of waste as per Trust policies and procedures.
26. Remove gloves, apron and face mask and wash hands as per Trust guidelines with soap and water.
27. Prior to leaving the injection room, remove theatre hat, mask, apron and gloves.

Intravitreal nurse: Expanded role

NURSING ACTION

1. Introduce yourself to the patient, check consent form, ID of patient and that the eye has been marked in accordance with Trust policy. Prior to the procedure check the eyelids for any signs of blepharitis and the eye for any signs of inflammation. (This may have occurred during the initial slit lamp examination.)
2. Put on apron, theatre hat and mask and wash hands as per Trust guidelines with soap and water.
3. Instil G. benoxinate × 3 drops over 10 minutes in accordance with Trust ANTT procedure for eye-drop administration.
4. Instil 5% Videne on to the ocular surface using a sterile syringe and leave for 3 minutes before continuing with the procedure.
5. Surgical scrub hands as per Trust policy and apply sterile gloves.
6. Clean periocular skin and eyelid margins and eye lashes with 10% Videne using sterile gauze and forceps.
7. Check correct drug, dose and expiry date.
8. Apply a sterile drape ensuring that the eyelashes are out of the operative field. If the eyelashes remain in the operative field a new sterile drape must be applied.

Note: Ensure that the surgeon's hands always rest on a sterile surface, that is, not on an undraped forehead. If gloves are contaminated they must be removed and hands should be decontaminated with alcogel as per Trust guidelines and a new pair of sterile gloves applied prior to continuing with the procedure.

9. Insert eyelid speculum or sterile.
10. *Lucentis* – Protecting the key parts, draw up the Lucentis from the vial. The vial must not come into contact with the sterile field. *Avastin* is already prepacked in a sterile syringe. This will be placed on the sterile field by the assisting nurse. Ensure that this syringe remains sterile.
11. Steady the eye with a safe technique/instrument.
12. Insert the needle and inject the drug slowly and carefully at a suggested 3.5 mm from limbus for pseudophakic, 4 mm for phakic eyes.
13. Remove the needle slowly, with suggested application of a sterile cotton bud and applied pressure for 10 seconds.
14. After injection, ensure that the following are done: needle carefully discarded into sharps bin, vision checked and antibiotic drops stat dose instilled.
15. Remove speculum and drapes.
16. Dispose of waste as per Trust policies and procedures.
17. Wash hands with soap and water as per Trust guidelines at the end of the procedure.
18. Remove gloves, apron and mask.
19. Document procedure and drug administration in medical notes.

Procedure guideline: Preparing a patient for ultrasound

NURSING ACTION

1. Take and record visual acuity.
2. Explain the procedure to the patient:
   a. Local anaesthetic drops will be instilled.
   b. Keratometry will be performed prior to an A-scan.
   c. The patient will need to look ahead and keep his eyes still while the scan is being performed.

APPLYING HEAT TO THE EYE

Heat can be applied to the eye in several ways to reduce swelling, encourage the discharge of infected cysts, ease pain and enhance the action of drugs – especially mydriatics. Patients must be assessed as to their ability to safely comply with the procedure.

APPLICATION OF HEAT USING A CLEAN FLANNEL

A clean flannel is put under a hot tap (as hot as the patient's hand can stand). It is wrung out and applied to the closed eyelid. As the flannel cools down, this procedure is repeated a few more times.

Procedure guideline: Removal of sutures

EQUIPMENT

- Sterile receiver with fine scissors, stitch cutter or blade
- One pair of fine forceps
- Sachet of sterile normal saline
- Gallipot
- Dental rolls, cotton wool balls or gauze squares
- The patient's case notes

NURSING ACTION

1. Wash hands and prepare trolley and equipment.
2. Check patient identification against request card/notes with patient then prepare the patient for procedure and obtain consent.
3. Assess the patient's needs as before.
4. Check patient identification against request card/notes with patient.
5. Position the patient in the recumbent, semi-recumbent position or sitting in a chair, with the head well supported.
6. Prepare equipment ready for use following ANTT guidelines, including donning non-sterile gloves.
7. Clean the suture line if necessary.
8. Check the suture line to ensure it is clean and intact/healed, and also to establish the type of suture: individual or continuous.
9. Remove the sutures.
10. Make the patient comfortable.
11. Dispose of clinical waste and clean hands then the trolley/tray.
12. Wash hands and then complete documentation. Record in the case notes the fact that the sutures have been removed, as a permanent record of procedure having taken place.

Procedure guideline: Preparing the patient and equipment for minor surgery

EQUIPMENT

- Trolley
- Relevant sterile instrument set
- Extra instruments
- One sheet of sterile wax paper
- Two sterile linen towels or paper towels
- Eye pad
- Several dental rolls
- Several gauze swabs
- Local anaesthetic drops
- Local anaesthetic injection
- Syringes and needles
- Mediprep or similar skin preparation
- Sutures

- If necessary, a specimen pot with formaldehyde and a pathology form
- Sterile surgical gloves
- Tape

NURSING ACTION

1. Wash hands and prepare trolley and equipment.
2. Check patient identification against request card/notes with patient then prepare the patient for procedure and that written consent has been obtained.
3. Assess the patient's needs as before.
4. Position the patient in the recumbent, semi-recumbent position or sitting in a chair, with the head well supported.
5. Prepare equipment ready for use, including donning sterile gloves.
6. Instil local anaesthetic drops prescribed as per PGD.
7. Prepare local anaesthetic injection.
8. Clean around the eye with Mediprep or similar preparation.
9. Assist the doctor or specialist nurse during the procedure.
10. Support the patient during the procedure.
11. Apply ointment/pad/bandage at the end of the procedure if necessary, which may need to be renewed before the patient goes home.
12. Dispose of clinical waste and clean hands then the trolley and send instruments for sterilisation unless for single patient use, in which case they must be disposed of appropriately.
13. Wash hands and then complete documentation.
14. Make the patient comfortable and offer tea and biscuit before they leave.
15. Give the patient written and verbal post-operative advice about medication; analgesia and post-operative complications, as well as an emergency contact number.
16. Ensure the patient has a follow-up appointment, if appropriate.

NOTE

In some ophthalmic hospitals and units, ophthalmic nurses are performing minor operations such as incision and curettage of chalazion.

Procedure guideline: Insertion of bandage contact lens

EQUIPMENT

- Tray
- Sterile bandage contact lens
- Local anaesthetic drops

NURSING ACTION

1. Wash hands and prepare tray.
2. Check expiry date and open sterile bandage contact lens.
3. Check patient identification against request card/notes with patient then prepare the patient for procedure and obtain verbal consent.
4. Assess the patient for any physical or mental needs that would be needed to be taken into consideration before procedure.

5. Position the patient in the recumbent, semi-recumbent position or sitting in a chair, with the head well supported.
6. Prepare equipment ready for use.
7. Instil local anesthetic eye drops prescribed as per PGD.
8. Wash hands and place sterile bandage contact lens onto your fingertip.
9. Gently hold upper and lower lid open and insert bandage contact lens.
10. Dispose of clinical waste and clean hands then the tray.
11. Wash hands and then complete documentation.

TESTING PUPIL REACTION

Testing the pupils is an important part of the examination especially in a patient complaining of flashing lights and floaters, sudden loss of vision or field loss, orbital cellulitis, widespread retinal disease and optic nerve disease.

The pupil is a space that lies behind the iris and its function is to control the amount of light entering the eye, and it does this by either contraction (miosis) or dilation (mydriasis) under the influence of the autonomic nervous system.

Components of the pupillary reflex pathways

- *Afferent pathway* – Optic disc/nerve, optic chiasm, optic tract and the pretectal nucleus (lying in the dorsal midbrain).
- *Efferent pathway* – This passes through the Edinger–Westphal nucleus before travelling along with the third cranial nerve out to the iris (with a synapse at the ciliary ganglion which sits in the orbit).

It is important to remember that there are several reflexes served by this pathway and each should be examined in turn. Damage at any level of the pathway or abnormalities of the iris itself can cause abnormalities of pupil shape or function.

General observation of the pupil and light reflex test

- Explain to the patient what you are going to do and reasons why.
- Start by general observation of the pupil by noting the shape and size of the pupil in bright light. Size is measured in millimetres and the normal pupil ranges from 1 to 8 mm.
- *Light reflex test (testing for direct and consensual response)* – This assesses the integrity of the papillary light reflex pathway.
- *How to perform the test* – It is important not to stand in front of the patient as the pupil will accommodate to focus on you. Instead, ask the patient to stare at a distant target. Using a bright source of light (an indirect ophthalmoscope is ideal), shine the light in one eye and note the constriction of the pupil. This is known as direct response. Now shine the light in the same eye and watch the other pupil constrict, this is known as consensual response. There should be a brisk, simultaneous, equal response of both pupils in response to light shone in one or the other eye in a patient with no pupillary abnormality.

Swinging flash light test – testing for relative afferent pupillary defect (RAPD)

- *Testing for relative afferent papillary defect* – This test compares the direct and consensual responses in each eye.
- *How to perform the test* – Dim the light in the room. Again use a bright source of light such as an indirect ophthalmoscope and do not stand in front of the patient. Using

the beam from the ophthalmoscope, swing the light rhythmically from just below one eye to the other, making sure that you allow the same amount of light exposure on each eye (about 2 seconds for each eye) and that each is illuminated from the same angle. You should note the pupillary constriction of both eyes when the beam is maintained. If a patient has an RAPD, the affected eye will dilate instead of constricting. If a patient has no RAPD, both pupils will constrict when you shine the light in each eye.

AMSLER GRID

The Amsler grid consists of vertical and horizontal lines used to monitor a patient's central vision. It is a diagnostic tool that aids in the detection of visual disturbances caused by changes in the retina, particularly the macula (e.g. epiretinal membrane), as well as the optic nerve and the visual pathway to the brain. However, the Amsler grid should not be used as a substitute for regular eyesight examination.

Instructions on how to use the Amsler grid

- Explain to the patient the purpose of the test.
- Check if the patient wears any reading glasses and if they do, they will need to wear them.
- Hold the Amsler grid at about the same distance from the patient's eyes that any other reading material would be.
- Check one eye at a time by covering the other eye with the patient's hand. Focus on the dot in the centre and the patient needs to check for the following:
  - Do any of the lines look wavy, blurred or distorted? (All lines should be straight, all intersections should form right angles and all the squares should be the same size.)
  - Are there any missing areas or dark areas in the grid?
  - Can they see all corners and sides of the grid?
- Do not forget to test both eyes.

It is very important to report any irregularity to your eye doctor immediately.

TESTING COLOUR VISION

Ishihara is a colour perception test for red-green colour deficiency. The test consists of a number of coloured plates, called **Ishihara plates**, each of which contains a circle of dots appearing randomized in colour and size. Within the pattern are dots which form a number or shape clearly visible to those with normal colour vision, and invisible, or difficult to see, to those with a red-green colour vision defect, or the other way around. The full test consists of 38 plates, but the existence of a deficiency is usually clear after a few plates. There is also the smaller test consisting only of 24 plates. The plates make up several different test designs. Patients with suspected optic nerve disease will show a defect in their colour vision as this often decreases earlier.

How to check a patient's colour vision

- Explain to the patient the purpose of the test.
- Check if the patient wears any reading glasses and if the patient does, he will need to wear them.
- Hold the Ishihara test type at about the same distance from the patient's eyes that any other reading material would be.

- It is a good idea to test the affected eye first to prevent the patient from memorising the number on the test plate.
- Ask the patient to tell you what the number is on each page. It is also a good idea to document if the patient reads the numbers with ease or if he or she struggles to read.
- Record the number of correct answers out of the total number of pages, for example Right eye 4/17, which is 4 numbers correctly identified out of 17 numbers shown.

TONO-PEN

Tono-Pen is a portable handheld device that measures intraocular pressure (IOP) and is a useful device in measuring IOP in patients who are unsuitable for Goldmann's tonometry. The results correlate well with the Goldmann tonometer, although it slightly overestimates low IOPs and underestimates high IOPs.

Calibration of the Tono-Pen

The Tono-Pen must be calibrated daily to ensure the accurate measurement of IOP.
Calibration must be performed

- Before the first use
- Whenever it is indicated by the LCD display
- When batteries are replaced
- After an unsuccessful calibration

It is not necessary to check calibration prior to each use.
It should be noted that if during operation the Operator's Button is pushed only once and the Tono-Pen displays CAL, the Tono-Pen needs to be calibrated.

The calibration procedure

1. Point the transducer end of the Tono-Pen straight down towards the floor.
2. Depress the Operator's Button twice (rapidly, within 1.5 seconds). The Tono-Pen will 'beep' and display CAL.
3. Wait approximately 15 seconds for the Tono-Pen to 'beep' and display 'UP'.
4. Immediately (within 1 second) invert the Tono-Pen smoothly, pointing the transducer end straight up.
5. A properly functioning Tono-Pen will display 'Good' followed by a 'beep'. Repeat this calibration procedure if 'Bad' is displayed.

Preparing a patient for IOP measurement using the Tono-Pen

Before use, the tip of the Tono-Pen must be covered by a sterile disposable Ocu-Film tip cover. The cover is made out of latex which may cause an allergic reaction in patients. The patients must always be questioned on latex allergy before performing the test. Tono-Pen must not be used on any patients with suspected latex allergy.

1. Explain to the patient what the test entails.
2. Ensure that the patient is in a comfortable sitting position.
3. Instill a drop of topical anesthetic in the eye to be tested.
4. Ask the patient to look straight ahead at a distance object.
5. Hold the Tono-Pen as you would a pencil.
6. Position yourself to facilitate viewing of the probe tip and patient's cornea where contact will be made. For normal corneas, central corneal contact is recommended.

7. Brace the heel of your hand on the patient's cheek for stability while holding the Tono-Pen perpendicular to and within 1.3 cm of the patient's cornea.
8. To initiate an IOP measurement, depress the Operator's Button once, and only once.
9. Once activated, and a 'beep' tone is heard, touch the Tono-Pen XL unit to the cornea lightly and briefly, then withdraw. Repeat several times. The corneal surface needs only to be momentarily contacted: indentation is not required and may lead to inaccurate readings.
10. A chirp will sound and a digital IOP measurement will be displayed each time a valid reading is obtained. The single horizontal bar at the bottom of the LCD, indicating statistical reliability, will not be displayed with each single IOP measurement.
11. After four valid readings are obtained, a final beep will sound and the averaged measurement will appear on the LCD along with the single bar denoting statistical reliability.
12. Document your reading.

OPTICAL COHERENCE TOMOGRAPHY (OCT)

Optical coherence tomography (OCT) is a non-invasive imaging test that uses light waves to take cross-sectional pictures of the retina.

AUTOREFRACTION

An autorefractor is a machine used to measure a person's refractive error and prescription for eyeglasses or contact lenses. This is achieved by measuring how light is changed as it enters a person's eye. The automated refraction technique is quick, simple and painless. The patient takes a seat and places his chin on a rest. One eye at a time, the patient looks into the machine at a picture inside. The picture moves in and out of focus as the machine takes readings to determine when the image is on the retina. Several readings are taken which the machine averages to form a prescription. No feedback is required from the patient during this process.

SPECULAR MICROSCOPY

This is a non-invasive procedure used to observe, monitor and document the number, density and quality of endothelial cells that line the back of the cornea. The endothelium of a young, 10-year-old, healthy cornea has approximately 3500 cells per square millimeter. Normal ageing causes the cells to gradually decrease over time. By age 60, most people have approximately 2500 cells per square millimeter.

Reasons for performing specular microscopy

- To screen for corneal diseases such as Fuchs' dystrophy, keratoconus, trauma and other types of corneal dystrophies.
- To evaluate localized oedema, haze, trauma and diseases caused by contact lenses/ phakic intraocular contact lenses (IOLs).
- To observe and document the backside of human cornea of the eye, corneal endothelial cell layer, *in vivo* at high magnification.
- To provide a simple and quick way of acquiring repeatable, accurate information unobtainable with standard biomicroscopy or corneal topography.

CORNEAL TOPOGRAPHY

Also known as videokeratography, corneal topography is a process for mapping the surface curvature of the cornea, similar to making a contour map of land. The cornea is a clear membrane that covers the front of the eye and is responsible for about 70% of the eye's focussing power. To a large extent, the shape of the cornea determines the visual ability of an otherwise healthy eye. A perfect eye has an evenly rounded cornea, but if the cornea is too flat, too steep or unevenly curved, less than perfect vision results.

The purpose of corneal topography is to produce a detailed description of the shape and power of the cornea. Using computerized imaging technology, the three-dimensional map produced by the corneal topographer aids an ophthalmologist in the diagnosis, monitoring and treatment of various visual conditions.

How corneal topography works

The corneal topograph is made up of a computer linked to a lighted bowl that contains a pattern of concentric rings. The patient is seated in front of the bowl with his head pressed against a bar while a series of data points are generated on a placido disk, which has been projected on the cornea. Computer software digitizes these data points to produce a printout of the corneal shape, using different colors to identify different elevations.

The procedure itself is painless and brief. It is a noncontact examination that photographs the surface of the eye using ordinary light. The greatest advantage of corneal topography is its ability to detect conditions invisible to most conventional testing.

The uses of corneal topography

Corneal topography is not a routine test. Rather, it is used in diagnosing certain types of problems, in evaluating a disease's progression, in fitting some types of contact lenses and in planning surgery. It is commonly used in preparing for refractive eye surgery. The corneal topography map is used in conjunction with other tests to determine exactly how much corneal tissue will be removed to correct the visual defect.

Corneal topography is used in the diagnosis and management of various corneal curvature abnormalities and diseases such as

- Keratoconus, a degenerative condition that causes a thinning of the cornea
- Corneal transplants
- Corneal scars or opacities
- Corneal deformities
- Contact lenses fitting
- Irregular astigmatism following corneal transplantation
- Planning for refractive surgery
- Post-operative cataract extraction with acquired astigmatism

Steps in the acquisition and analysis of videokeratoscopy information require that the

- Patient is positioned correctly.
- Patient fixates on target.
- Placido disc is illuminated.
- Mires are reflected from the corneal surface.
- Clinician focusses and aligns the mires.
- Clinician triggers image acquisition.
- CCD video camera records the image.

- Frame grabber captures the image. Image is digitised.
- Position of mires is identified.
- Reference point is established.
- Data points are located.
- Algorithm is applied.

PACHYMETRY

Pachymetry is the measurement of corneal thickness. The accurate measurement of IOP is a cornerstone of the diagnosis and management of glaucoma. The influence of corneal thickness in IOP measurements using Goldmann Applanation Tonometry measurement is well recognised.

Research has shown that a thick cornea can cause an elevated IOP reading while a thin cornea can give a false low reading. A cross-sectional observational study by Felipe et al. (2002) concluded that patients classified as having ocular hypertension but with visual field loss detected by short-wavelength automated perimetry had significantly lower central corneal thickness measurements than the ocular hypertension patients with normal visual fields results. These results suggest that central corneal thickness should be taken into account when assessing risk for the development of glaucomatous damage among ocular hypertension patients.

When performing pachymetry, take into account the following:

- As there are a number of different pachymeters available, each student needs to ensure that he or she is familiar with his or her own machine.
- Ensure that the person teaching you is fully trained in the use of the machine.
- Choose a cooperative patient to practice on.
- Follow your own local hospital policy on cleaning and disinfecting the pachymeter probe.

HEIDELBERG RETINAL TOMOGRAPHY

Heidelberg retinal tomography (HRT) is a procedure used for precise measurement, documentation and diagnosis of the optic nerve head. The HRT uses a confocal scanning laser microscope to build up a three-dimensional scan of the optic nerve head and its surrounding structures.

While glaucoma is managed primarily through managing the pressure of the eye, it is important to remember that it is in fact a complex disease of the optic nerve, whereby progressive damage to the nerve fibre layer results in gradual loss of visual information leaving the brain. As such the tomogram produced by the procedure and its ability to detect small changes in the structure of the nerve provide a valuable tool in monitoring and detecting the early changes of glaucoma before visual loss takes place by objectively assessing loss of the neuroretinal layer and progression of cupping.

The test is noninvasive and does not usually require dilation of the eye. It is carried out by placing the patient comfortably on the head and chin rests and then asking the patient to look towards the fixation target (a small green light) that will be seen to the opposite side of the eye that is being tested, i.e. when testing the patient's right eye, they will need to look approximately 10° to the left of primary position. Align the light from the laser with the patient's pupil, aiming to be a few millimetres away from the lids, lashes or cornea. When the patient is properly aligned you should be able to see an image of the optic nerve head on the screen. Adjust the focus dial on the front to obtain the clearest, brightest possible image, using cylindrical lenses if needed. Fine-tune the alignment of the laser, and then press the trigger button.

During the procedure it is important that the patient remains steadily fixated on the target light and blinks as little as possible; it is wise to keep minims of saline handy for those with dry eyes. The actual scanning of the laser usually takes around 6 seconds and during this time you should watch the live feed to ensure the image remains clear and steady.

Once the procedure is completed and the computer has processed the image, you will be able to view the results of the scan. In new patients you will be asked to plot the rim of the optic nerve head. This is done simply by placing points around the rim itself and can be confirmed by switching to the three-dimensional model.

The accuracy of the test is displayed as the test standard deviation (SD), with lower values indicating a more accurate scan. If the standard deviation is over 30 it is advised that the test be repeated to try and improve the results. There will also be a false coloured overlay on a picture of the nerve head which shows the cupped area in red. Also available on the report is the global classification of the disc which compares segments of the nerve head as normal, borderline or outside normal limits based on Moorfield regression analysis.

DIPLOPIA – ASSESSING IF IT IS BINOCULAR OR MONOCULAR

Double vision or diplopia is a symptom with many potential causes that can involve many different structures. An anatomic and systematic approach to the clinical evaluation of diplopia can lead you to refer the patient for an orthoptic assessment and to an accurate diagnosis.

There are generally two types of diplopia – binocular and monocular. Binocular diplopia is defined as the disappearance of diplopia with either eye occluded, and monocular diplopia is defined as double vision still present in the affected eye while the other eye is occluded.

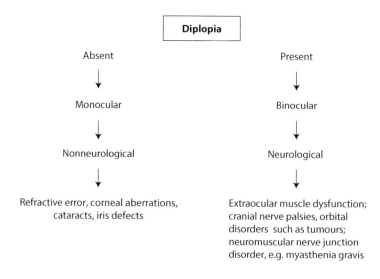

KERATOMETRY

Keratometry is used to measure the greater and lesser curvatures of the cornea, usually in conjunction with biometry, to discover the strength of the intraocular lens required by a patient following cataract extraction. As biometry involves contact with the eye, which may distort it slightly, keratometry should be performed before biometry. Each eye is tested separately. A number of machines are used, but the principles of each are similar. The patient should be sat comfortably with his chin and forehead on the rests and asked to look down the barrel of the keratometer. The patient must keep as still as possible. The nurse looks through the eyepieces and may need to adjust the machine until she sees the cornea clearly, as well as certain points that must be aligned before a reading can be taken.

BIOMETRY

Biometry uses an A-scan to measure the axial length of the eye. As a probe touches the eye, a local anaesthetic must be instilled in the patient's eye. The patient is positioned comfortably with his chin supported on a rest such as a slit lamp and is asked to fix his gaze. The nurse must also ensure that she is comfortable and within easy reach of the footplate. Once the patient's eye is aligned, the nurse gently places the probe on the cornea. A steady hand is required, as the probe must make contact in order to measure correctly. Excess pressure, however, will indent the cornea and give a false reading, which the nurse must be able to identify.

By measuring both eyes, a comparison can be made to further prove accuracy, as it is unusual to find a marked difference between the axial lengths of the two eyes. It may be easier to obtain a reading after the pupil has been dilated. The information gained from the keratometry and biometry is fed into a computer, which produces the desired intraocular lens power for the individual patient.

CONFRONTATIONAL TEST FOR VISUAL FIELDS

This is a quick and basic check of a patient's visual field to give you some indication if further tests are required such as Goldman or Humphrey perimetry:

1. Sit opposite the patient.
2. Ask the patient to cover his right eye with his right hand and vice versa with the other.
3. Cover your own left eye in order to compare your own peripheral vision to that of the patient.
4. Ask the patient to stare at your right eye.
5. Hold up two fingers midway between yourself and patient. Wriggle your finger and ask if the patient is able to see it.
6. Do this for all four quadrants of the visual field – upper left, upper right, lower right and lower left.
7. Repeat this to the other eye.
8. Document your findings and refer for other investigations if appropriate.

PERIMETRY (VISUAL FIELD TESTING)

The purpose of visual field testing, or perimetry, is to provide information critical to

- Diagnosing ocular diseases, especially glaucoma
- Evaluating neurological diseases
- Monitoring the progress of ocular diseases

Visual field testing can lead to early detection and treatment of disease. In the case of glaucoma, visual fields play a major role in identifying visual field defects and evaluating the efficacy of the therapy used to control the disease process. The machine of choice at many centres is the Humphrey field analyser.

Humphrey field analyser

The Humphrey field analyser gives a wide choice of testing options, from very basic screening tests like the C-40 screening test to complex strategies such as the C24-2 SITA standard.

The choice of test strategy is always an important starting point. There would be little point in choosing a central 40-point screening test to check for glaucoma because the points tested would be too far apart and would only test at one intensity of light. Normally the central 24-2 SITA test would be selected to test fully the appropriate areas of the visual field.

Patient data need to be entered into the perimeter analyser, and the most important piece of information entered is the patient's age. Every point tested during the procedure is age related, which enables the perimeter analyser to calculate the results, giving an overall view of how the vision of that patient compares to the vision of other people of the same age. The patient's name and hospital number are also entered, along with the prescription details of any refractive error.

Before the patient can begin the test, an explanation of what is required of the patient is needed. The simpler this explanation is kept, the easier it is for the patient.

The patient needs to fixate on a yellow light at the back of the testing bowl (having the patient look at only one spot throughout the test ensures that we are testing accurately his peripheral vision; if the patient moves his eye, he moves his field of vision). The ophthalmic nurse should try to avoid calling the light a 'bright' yellow light; it may be a bright light to her, but if the patient is suffering from cataracts say, then the light will not be bright to him.

While the patient is looking at the yellow light, the perimeter analyser will present white stimuli onto the testing bowl or, if preferred, will flash 'white lights'. Whenever the patient sees a 'white light', he should respond by pressing a button. (Whenever the patient responds, the stimuli will return to the same point of the eye tested and will be fainter, so the more the patient responds to light, the fainter that light gets until the patient no longer sees it. At this point the perimeter analyser records the intensity of the last stimuli seen.)

The patient should always be advised (if not encouraged) to blink, as the more the patient blinks, the more focussed his vision is and the lower the chance of tear build-up affecting the result.

Unless a binocular test is to be performed, the patient will need to have one eye occluded.

The correction lens should be in place and the patient brought up to the perimeter. The patient needs to place his chin on the chin rest and his forehead forward against the headrest. Once the patient is in position, it is worth standing back to carry out an overall assessment of the patient prior to the test to ensure the patient's comfort, safety and cooperation. Consider the following:

- Is the patient's back straight? A patient not sitting straight will very soon get lower back pain.
- Is the patient crouching into the perimeter? Again, this will cause back pain, and eventually the patient will try to sit up straighter thereby taking his eyes off the centre of the perimeter bowl.
- Is the patient straining to rest his head against the headrest? If this is the case, the patient will be falling away from the perimeter bowl throughout the test, causing discrepancies in the printed result and thus rendering the test result invalid.

The patient should be sat comfortably at the perimeter analyser, with the response button in his hand on his lap and the corrective lens brought up as close to the eye as possible without it touching the eyelashes.

The patient should be given a brief refresher of what is required of him during the procedure, remembering to ask if he is comfortable and ready to begin the test.

During the test, the perimeter analyser will be constantly monitoring the patient's fixation. It does this by plotting the patient's natural blind spot; this is the point where the optic nerve connects to the back of the eye, and the perimeter analyser flashes a light into this spot. If this point has not been plotted correctly, then the perimeter analyser will record the patient's responses as fixation errors, making the test results unreliable and wasting the time of the ophthalmic nurse, the patient and the doctor. The blind spot can be re-plotted at any time during the test by pressing the 'fixation' button. Care must be taken by the tester to ensure that the patient is indeed looking straight ahead at the yellow fixation light and is not in fact looking at the white stimuli being presented in the bowl. A gentle reminder to the patient that he should always keep looking straight ahead is always useful.

As the test progresses, the patient should be checked for signs of fatigue such as starting to 'sag' in the chair, head leaning to one side, etc. Encouragement should be given throughout the test, including giving praise to the patient. In order to further improve compliance with the test, it is also a good idea to inform patients of the estimated completion time of the test.

When the first eye has been tested, the result should be printed out before commencing on the second eye. This extra time also gives patients a breathing space to compose themselves before commencing on the second eye. Patients should always be given another brief reminder to keep looking straight ahead and to blink before starting with the second eye.

After the visual field test, patients may be reviewed in the clinic or may be given another appointment to be reviewed in clinic with the test results.

The test results contain a variety of other information apart from the obvious greyscale picture.

The print-out contains the following information:

- All the patient information entered before the test began.
- Fixation losses, i.e. how many times out of a given number of presentations the patient saw a light presented in the blind-spot area. A high number of losses are due to either an incorrectly plotted blind spot or to poor fixation from the patient which has not been dealt with. Patients who have let their heads tilt or who have moved away from the head rest will also build up fixation losses.
- False-positive errors are recorded when the patient responds but no stimuli have been presented. Some patients will get concerned that they have not seen any stimuli; these patients should be assured that they will not always see stimuli during the test and that they should only respond when they have seen stimuli.
- False-negative errors. Occasionally during the test, a stimulus is repeated at a level much brighter than has already been seen. If the patient does not respond to these stimuli, it is recorded as a false-negative error.
- On the left along the lower half of the print-out are the total deviation plots; the numerical values on top represent the difference in decibels (dB) between the patient's results and the age-corrected normal values below. The lower plot (probability plot) translates the values into shaded symbols. The darker the symbol, the less likely is the field normal in that point.
- On the right along the lower half of the print-out are two further plots. Pattern deviation plots aim to separate out localised field defect and to take into account

the patient's age and overall reductions in sensitivity due to factors such as cataracts or small pupils. Again, the darker the symbol, the greater is the deviation from the age norm.

GOLDMANN BOWL PERIMETRY

Goldmann bowl perimetry is the kinetic measurement of the visual field as opposed to the static measurement performed with the Humphrey visual field analyser. Goldmann bowl perimetry is the ideal choice for patients with neurological defects, gross defects or for patients who simply find automated perimetry too difficult.

Procedure guideline: Goldmann bowl perimetry: Testing the patient

NURSING ACTION

PRE-PROCEDURE

1. Welcome the patient to the room and show him to the testing seat.
2. Explain to the patient the test you are about to perform. The patient, as with automated perimetry, should always fixate on the spot at the back of the bowl. Fixation is monitored from this point on the tester's side of the perimeter.
3. Explain that the patient will see moving white lights and that, as these lights appear in the patient's vision, they should respond by either pressing the response button provided, or using a pen to tap the table with. (The use of the pen provides a much more sensitive response from the patient. If the patient sees the stimuli clearly, you will recognise that the patient responds with the same tap. If the patient is unsure of what he has just seen, he invariably responds with a softer tap, giving the tester an indication that this area may need more investigation.)
4. The patients should be reminded that they must blink to prevent the build-up of tears in their eyes, which could inadvertently affect the test. Again, the patients must be reminded to look ahead at the fixation point and not look for the stimuli. If the patient has previously had automated perimetry, then a brief explanation of why the test has been changed to a different perimeter analyser may be advantageous.

POINTS TO REMEMBER

If a neurological defect is suspected, then this could fall outside of the tested area of the automated perimetry and so testing on the Goldmann will encompass the whole island of vision.

If the patient is suffering from a gross defect, for instance end-stage glaucoma, then testing on the Goldmann is easier as the stimuli are directed at the area of vision in a much slower presentation than automated perimetry, and a much bigger stimuli may be used. The Goldmann would also be able to plot any useful vision that falls outside the limits of automated perimetry.

If the patient has performed poorly with automated perimetry, then he will find the Goldmann a much easier test to perform. There is much more interaction with the patient, the test is performed at a slower speed and losses in fixation are dealt with much more easily.

Last, a patient suspected of hysterical field loss should be tested on the Goldmann to provide a 'spiral' result if this is the case. The eye not being tested should be occluded with a patch.

NURSING ACTION

PROCEDURE

1. Turn on the perimeter analyser. The switch is on the tester's right.
2. Begin the test by slowly moving the arm from the edge of the testing area towards the centre of the chart. This should be done at an advised speed of 10° every 3 seconds. As soon as the patient responds, then the chart should be marked with a pencil, then, again, the arm should be moved to the edge of the testing area and brought in again until the patient responds. This is repeated until the peripheral vision has been plotted.
3. The optic nerve needs to be plotted as an aid to fixation. This can be found at around 15° on the same side of the chart as the patient's eye being tested, i.e. right eye, right-hand side of the chart.
4. Once the whole peripheral vision and optic nerve have been plotted, a spot check of the vision should be conducted with each stimuli used. All four central quadrants should be checked, and random points on either side of the vertical line should also be checked. Any resulting scotomas should also be plotted.
5. Once it is certain that everything has been plotted with the chosen stimuli, then it should be 'joined up' with the corresponding coloured pencil:
   a. V/4e brown
   b. IV/4e green
   c. I/4e red
   d. I/3e black
   e. I/2e blue
   f. Any other stimuli – purple
6. This process continues, making the stimuli smaller and fainter each time. If the patient requires a reading addition lens, then everything that is tested with this lens in place should be recorded as tested with lens.

See Appendix 3 for assessment of skills audit tools for many of the procedures in this chapter.

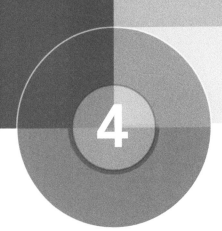

Ocular history taking and slit-lamp examination

4

This chapter looks at ocular history taking and procedures used in emergency-care settings, including examination of the eye.

OCULAR HISTORY TAKING

Taking an accurate ocular history is a crucial part of the examination of a patient with an ocular problem and helps the clinician to perform the appropriate investigation, rule out differential diagnoses and arrive at an accurate ophthalmic diagnosis. Good history taking also eliminates the need to perform unnecessary investigations and allows the clinician to focus on relevant and pertinent clinical examination. Before taking a history, it is important for you to commence the observation of your patient when you initially call your patient into the consultation, such as any physical, apparent mental or learning difficulties, general demeanor such as holding their eye so as to suggest pain or photophobia, any sign of agitation or fear.

TAKING A HISTORY

Introduction – Identify yourself by name and professional job title. Confirm the patient's details such as date of birth and address to ensure that you have the correct patient. Identify anyone accompanying the patient and determine that their presence is acceptable to the patient. Similarly, if you have a student with you, introduce the student and establish whether the patient is happy for the student to be there at the consultation. Explain to the patient and carer the purpose of history taking.

Confidentiality – Ensure patient's confidentiality by closing the consulting room door to maintain privacy. Be sensitive to patient's needs especially when questioning about ocular problems associated with sexually transmitted diseases.

Documentation – Be concise and document only relevant information. Be systematic and methodical in your questioning to avoid any omission in your history taking (James et al., 2007). Write legibly and note down any concerns the patient may have expressed. Document facts and remember that patients have a legal right to have access to their medical records.

Communication – It is important to put the patient at ease so smile and make eye contact. Make small talk if it helps to 'settle' the patient down before the consultation. Ensure that you have the patient's consent before you begin. Observe for non-verbal communication and 'listen' to what the patient is not telling you.

Questioning – Start with some open questions such as, 'What problems are you having with your eyes?' This will paint a bigger picture for you and your patient. Directed question such as 'how long have you had the problem' will enable you to 'home in' on the problem. Closed (forced choice) questions such as 'if you closed one eye, has the double vision disappeared' will provide you with more clues. Avoid confusing the patient by asking multiple questions such as 'has your eye been red and watering?' (see Figure 4.1).

Communicating with children – Communicating with children requires a very different communication style. Children are often frightened of hospital and this is made worse if they are in pain. It is also a good idea not to keep a child waiting for too long before he is seen as a fractious child is an uncooperative child. Put the child at ease by making small talk such as asking the child's name, the child's age and the child's favourite toy. During questioning, observe the behaviour of the child. Observe if the child is in pain, rubbing his eyes or if the child is agitated. If it is a small child, ask the carer to sit the child on the carer's knee. Introduce yourself to the child and explain to the child what you are going to do. Depending on the age of the child, it may be appropriate to either talk to the child or accompanying adult. Whether you examine the child on the slit lamp or examine the child using a direct or indirect ophthalmoscope will be dependent on the presenting complaint and the cooperation of the child. Always praise the child for being good

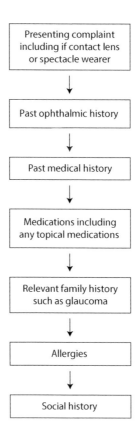

Figure 4.1 Stages of questioning.

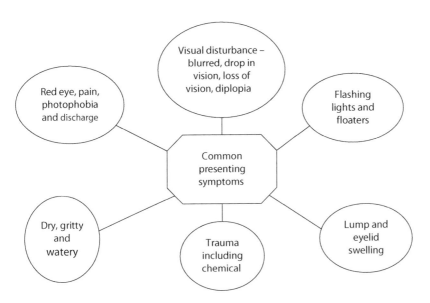

Figure 4.2 Common presentation of symptoms to eye casualty.

(even though he might not be) and promise to give the child a treat such as an 'I am good' sticker at the end of the examination.

Taking an ophthalmic history – Ocular history taking is similar to taking a medical history. If a patient has been referred by another healthcare professional such as optometrist, GP or from another hospital, establish the reason for referral and clarify with the patient that this is his understanding, too.

Start off with asking open-ended questions to set the scene. As stated previously, discourage the patient from giving you a diagnosis such as 'I have an eye infection' and instead ask them to describe their symptoms. Once again, if the patient presents with unilateral eye problems, remember to ask about the other eye (see Figure 4.2).

PRESENTING COMPLAINT

Duration – When did it start getting worse, better, the same; is it sudden or gradual onset?

Location – Which eye and if it is unilateral, is one eye worse than the other? Which part of the eye is affected – for example, the eyelids, orbit, sclera, retina or other?

Redness and distribution of redness – Has the eye been red? Is the redness localized/sectorial or generalized redness? Does light bother you?

Pain – What type of pain is it – is it aching or is it a sharp pain? Is it intermittent or continuous? Is it relieved by analgesia? Is it worse on movement?

Any disturbance in vision – Is it blurred, double vision, flashing lights or floaters?

Discharge – Is there a discharge and type and colour of discharge – watery, mucopurulent?

Other associated symptoms – Such as itching, burning, stinging, watering, soreness, grittiness.

Timing – Are the symptoms identified such as redness, pain or discharge, there all the time or only on waking up?

Context and potential cause – What were you doing at the time – were you at work – grinding, hammering, or chemical, playing sports, no reason?

Onset – Was it sudden, gradual, started in one eye and spread to other?

Modifying factors – What makes it better or worse?

Associated factors – Generally unwell, nausea, recent cold or cough, recent viral infections, headache – location of headache such as temporal, history of migraine?

PAST OPHTHALMIC HISTORY

This includes any previous ophthalmic history such as cataract operation, retinal diseases or operation, laser surgery for retinal and macular conditions, laser surgery to correct short-sightedness, previous yttrium aluminium garnet (YAG) laser, previous injury, previous iritis, corneal ulcers, posterior vitreous detachment, chronic glaucoma and other relevant ophthalmic conditions.

PAST MEDICAL HISTORY

This includes any medical problem such as diabetes, cerebrovascular accident, hypertension, respiratory disorders, cardiovascular disorders, arthritis, previous infections, autoimmune disorders, serious operations and any systemic conditions which may contribute to the ocular disorders.

MEDICATIONS

Enquire about medications intake including any current topical medications.

RELEVANT FAMILY HISTORY

Check for any family history of glaucoma or other inherited ocular diseases such as retinitis pigmentosa and any family history of strabismus, refractive error or amblyopia that may aid diagnosis when presented with a squint in a child.

ALLERGIES

Record all adverse drug reactions and how they affected the patient. Remember that some systemic drugs can cause ocular side effects. Topical drugs may also stimulate an allergic reaction which may be the cause of a patient presenting with a red eye.

SOCIAL HISTORY

The depth of social history questioning will be dependent on whether the patient is seen for a routine appointment such as for pre-operative assessment or if a patient has presented as an emergency referral. Patients attending for pre-operative assessment will need a more in-depth social history assessment in order to plan for a safe and uneventful recovery and discharge of patient home (suitability of a patient for day case surgery). It is important to include questions such as driving, reading, day-to-day activities which may have functional and social repercussion for the patients. It is important to remember that any degree of visual impairment whether permanent or temporary (as a result of dilating drops), patients must be given the appropriate advice. As part of your assessment, patients with a visual disability and who live alone must be assessed for falls risk.

EXAMPLES OF AREAS OF SPECIFIC QUESTIONING

The Red Eye

Duration of symptoms

Unilateral or bilateral

Is there any preorbital swelling

Context – at work, sports, gardening

Any visual disturbance – blurred vision

Ascertain if contact lens wearer

Any pain and type of pain – aching, sharp pain

Is the pain intermittent or continuous?

Any discharge and types of discharge

Any photophobia

Check intraocular pressure

General well-being such as any nausea, vomiting

Loss of Vision

Duration of symptoms

Unilateral or bilateral

White or red eye

Sudden or gradual

Transient or permanent

Painful or painless

Any associated symptoms – curtains, flashing light, floaters

General well-being – jaw claudication, scalp tenderness, night sweats, shoulder ache

Check pupillary reaction

Check colour vision

SUMMARY

Accurate history taking is essential for correct diagnosis and treatment planning. Staff must be knowledgeable and skilled in these procedures. Obtaining maximum data from GPs and optometrists and cross-checking with patient data improves quality and decreases risk. Documentation must be accurate, legible and thorough to ensure a robust assessment process.

SLIT-LAMP EXAMINATION

An introduction to the slit lamp and basic examination techniques is presented here.

USING THE SLIT LAMP

It is important to practise and familiarise yourself with the controls of the slit lamp. It is like driving a car and getting used to the clutch and the gear stick, etc. and gradually gaining in confidence. Find a willing volunteer to sit on the other side and go through the practical skills.

THE PRINCIPLE

A narrow 'slit' beam of very bright light is produced by a lamp. This beam is focussed onto the eye, which is then viewed under magnification with a microscope.

BASIC KEY POINTS IN SLIT-LAMP EXAMINATION

- The patient's and your own comfort at the slit lamp are of utmost importance.
- Good explanation and reassurance of this procedure will ensure the patient's cooperation.
- Be systematic and methodical in your slit-lamp examination to ensure that nothing gets omitted.
- Ensure that your eyepieces are properly adjusted prior to commencing, e.g. your refractive errors (if any) are accounted for and that you have adjusted the pupillary apertures accordingly.
- All findings should be accurately and legibly documented.

USES OF SLIT LAMP

- Observation of ocular adnexa and structures, including cornea, anterior chamber, iris, lens and anterior vitreous face
- Monitoring of signs and symptoms of anterior segment disease or injury
- Examination of posterior segment of the eye by the use of auxiliary lenses
- Further 'special' investigations
  - Goldmann tonometry
  - Van Herrick's estimation of anterior chamber depth
  - Gonioscopic examination of the angle

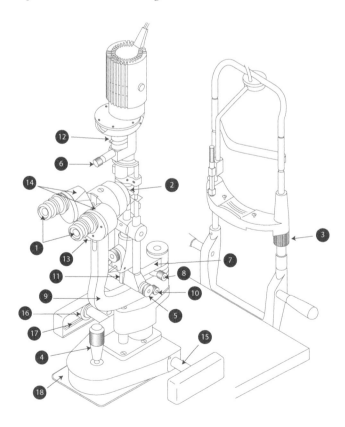

Components of the Slit Lamp (Cordero 2010)

1. Viewing eyepiece
2. Emission of light
3. Chin rest adjustment
4. Joystick
5. Slit controls – slit width
6. Slit control – slit length
7. Illumination rotation arm
8. Locking screw
9. Microscope rotation arm
10. Locking screw for microscope arm
11. Illumination tilting latch
12. Filter changing knob
13. Magnification lever
14. Pupillary distance adjuster
15. Rod connecting two geared wheels
16. Geared wheels
17. Rails supporting wheels
18. Base of slit lamp

THE MICROSCOPE AND ADJUSTMENT OF OCULAR EYEPIECES

The slit lamp has binocular microscopes, which means that it gives the examiner a three-dimensional view of the eye and surrounding structures. The advantage of a three-dimensional view is that ocular abnormalities can be detected with greater precision.

The viewing system of the microscope can be adjusted to account for any refractive error. If you normally wear glasses, you need to make a decision as to whether to keep them on or take them off for examining the patients. If you wish to remove your glasses to examine the patient, the viewing system should be set up to accommodate your refractive correction. If you are unsure what your refractive correction is, a focussing rod (supplied with the slit lamp) can be used to measure your refractive error. Slide off the footplate and insert the focussing rod with the flat side facing you. Turn on the slit lamp and, using a slit beam of light (about 1–2 mm in width), focus the light onto the rod. Close one eye and, with the other eye, look through the slit lamp and start turning the wheel of the ocular eyepiece from the plus side of the scale and stopping immediately as soon as the image of the light through the eyepiece is clear and in focus. Where possible (if you know your own refraction readings), check whether the scale readings in dioptres actually correspond to your own spectacle correction.

You will also need to adjust the inter-pupillary distance for your own eyes as some people's eyes are more widely spaced apart or closer set than others. In order to adjust the eyepieces to suit your inter-pupillary distance, first take a look down the binocular eyepieces of the slit lamp. You must not be aware of seeing any black shading in your field of vision. If black shading is noted, you will need to adjust the interpupillary aperture, either by squeezing the eyepieces together or by pulling them farther apart. When the pupillary apertures are correctly set, you should have an unobstructed view with both eyes when looking down the slit lamp.

Attached to the binoculars of the microscope are settings for magnification. Depending on your slit-lamp model, the magnification changer can be altered either by flipping a lever just at the bottom of the ocular eyepieces or by turning a knob which is attached a little distance from the eyepieces. If your magnification changer is a lever switch, you will have two different settings – 10× and 16×. If your magnification changer is a knob, you will have five different magnification settings – 6×, 10×, 16×, 25× and 40×. Magnifications of 10× and 16× are adequate for most examination purposes.

SLIT-LAMP POSITION CONTROLS

The movement of the slit lamp is by using the joystick. The joystick is situated on the base of the slit lamp and, by moving the joystick left to right and back to front, movement of the slit lamp is achieved. In addition, twirling the joystick clockwise will elevate the slit lamp, and turning the joystick anticlockwise will lower the slit lamp.

Further adjustment to the slit lamp can be achieved by a lever located at the base of the slit-lamp table. By releasing the lever, the height of the whole table (including the slit lamp) can be adjusted to accommodate the height of the individual patient.

The patient's comfort at the slit lamp can be further achieved by moving the chin rest up and down by means of a lever adjustment knob located on the side frame of the slit lamp. When the patient is in the correct position, the patient's outer canthus is aligned with a black mark or notch on the headrest bar and the patient's forehead against the forehead rest.

Turn on the slit lamp and, using a slit beam of light (about 1–2 mm in width), focus the light onto the rod. Close one eye and, with the other eye look through the slit lamp and start turning the wheel of the ocular eyepiece from the plus side of the scale and stopping immediately as soon as the image of the light through the eyepiece is clear and in focus.

Familiarise yourself with the controls, switch the machine on. Start off with using the lowest voltage setting on the slit lamp to minimise patient's discomfort at having a very bright light in his eyes.

The joystick moves the whole slit lamp – the illumination system as well as the binocular – up and down and left and right. These various movements allow you to examine the eye at various positions and depth. It also allows both eyes to be examined with ease. When the slit lamp is not in use, secure the slit lamp to the table by turning the screw, which is situated on the right-hand side of the base of the slit lamp. If the slit lamp is not securely fastened, the microscope may roll forward, causing the whole slit lamp to topple forward, jarring not only the delicate optics and illumination system but also potentially crushing the patient.

THE ILLUMINATION ARM

At the top of the arm, the first circle on the left-hand side represents unfiltered bright white light. You should never use this first light as, in theory, you could burn the retina. The second circle with slashes in the centre represents the heat filter, while the third circle is the grey filter. The last circle is for accommodating an additional filter.

Note: You use the green light to make red objects black, thus increasing their definition.

The blue filter is used for examination of corneal integrity and for applanation tonometry. It is necessary to instil topical fluorescein to observe if the cornea is compromised and a combination of topical local anaesthetic and fluorescein for the measurement of intraocular pressure.

Procedure guideline: Step by step to a good basic slit-lamp examination

NURSING ACTION

PRE-PROCEDURE

Good explanation to the patient is vital in order to ensure cooperation.

1. Explain to the patient that, although the machine may look formidable, it is only a glorified microscope used to magnify the different structures of the eye.
2. Inform the patient that he needs to ensure that his forehead must rest against the bar, that his chin must be in the chin rest and that his mouth must be closed.

3. Warn the patient that the light from the slit lamp can be bright.
4. Tell the patient to keep both eyes open.

NURSING ACTION: POSITIONING THE PATIENT

The position of the slit lamp is equally important to ensure cooperation. Be patient with the elderly and the very young. If the patient is in a wheelchair, where possible transfer him to your examination chair. If it is not possible, manoeuvre the slit lamp as close as you can to the patient by removing the arm and footrest of the wheelchair. For shorter patients or children, it is possible to examine them standing right in front of the slit lamp. Women with large breasts can have considerable difficulty in leaning forward, and you may experience difficulty in pushing your slit lamp all the way forward. In this scenario, place the examining chair away from the slit lamp and get the patient to lean forward and into the chin and headrest. Patients with head tremors should have their head supported from behind. Above all, be patient.

1. Align the black marker to the patient's outer cantus.
2. Correct positioning can be achieved by moving the whole slit lamp (including the table) up or down using the lever situated underneath the table and manipulating the knob of the chin rest.
3. Make yourself comfortable.

TIPS FOR USING THE SLIT LAMP

- Fixation – ask the patient to look at your right ear when you examine his right eye and vice versa: some machines have a fixation light; this is useful when you are removing foreign bodies.
- The wheel moves the chin rest up and down.
- The latch tilts the slit lamp, which is useful for posterior examination work or if you want to see the depth of a foreign body penetration.
- Set your slit lamp on the lower magnification and turn on the control box on to the lowest voltage.
- Usually one hand is used to operate the joystick and the other hand to operate the illumination arm. If examining the patient's left eye, have the illumination unit on the left-hand side and vice versa.
- In order to focus the light on to the slit lamp, you can look at the patient's eyes by looking from the side of the slit-lamp machine and grossly aligning the eye. Once the eye is grossly aligned, look through the oculars and fine-tune the focus by using the joystick and by movement of the illumination arm. The second method of alignment is to look through the oculars from the beginning and, by using the joystick, to move the slit lamp and illumination arm until the eye is in focus. For the beginners, this may require some practice before you get the hang of it. Do not despair if you do not get it the first few times. It gets easier with practice.
- Be methodical in your examination. In this way, you are less likely to miss something.

SLIT-LAMP ILLUMINATION TECHNIQUES

The slit lamp offers the option of various illumination to examine the different structures of the eye. The following is a suggestion as to the way a routine technique should be performed – it is by no means the only way to perform a slit-lamp routine and indeed not all practitioners will do so. A good routine is one that you feel comfortable with and that allows you to detect and investigate any irregularities and note the normal condition (baseline data) of the eye.

The examiner uses one hand to operate the joystick and the other to control the magnification, fixation light position and the type and angle of illumination, merging from one method to another until the examination is complete. The setting up and use of each kind of illumination must be practised until the proceedings become automatic. *Note*: Regardless of the type of illumination used, to examine the entire cornea/sclera/lens you must ask the patient to look up, down, right and left (holding the upper or lower lid when necessary).

The various types of illumination are

- Broad/diffuse
- Parallelepiped
- Optic section
- Conical beam
- Retro
- Sclerotic
- Specular reflection

DIFFUSE ILLUMINATION

Set the microscope straight ahead and the illumination arm at 30°. Set the magnification at low setting (10×). Use low voltage setting.

PARALLELEPIPED ILLUMINATION (BROAD BEAM)

This illumination allows the observer to see a three-dimensional block of cornea. In order to do this,

- Decrease the width of the beam to 1–3 mm wide.
- Set the illumination arm approximately 30°–45°.
- Instruct the patient to look straight ahead and scan the cornea. When you reach the apex of the cornea, swing the illumination arm to the other side, set at a proper angle and continue scanning.
- Ascertain the depth of foreign bodies, corneal abrasion.

OPTIC SECTION ILLUMINATION (NARROW BEAM)

This illumination is used for estimation of the depth of the anterior chamber and also location of the depth of an opacity within the lens. In order to do this,

- The biomicroscope should be directly in front of the patient's eye.
- Illumination source is at 45°.
- Slit width is almost closed (0.5–1.0 mm wide by 7–9 mm high).
- Low magnification is used.
- Once cornea is in sharp focus, scan the cornea from temporal limbus to nasal limbus.
- Again, move the illumination source to the opposite side when crossing the midline of the cornea.

ASSESSING THE ANTERIOR CHAMBER DEPTH USING THE OPTIC SECTION ILLUMINATION (VAN HERRICK)

The optic section illumination can be used to grade the anterior chamber depth. This illumination uses an optic section placed near the limbus with the light source at 60°.

- Place the biomicroscope directly before the patient's eye.
- To assess anterior chamber depth, compare the thickness of the cornea with the dark section seen between the front of the iris and the back of the cornea.
- Grade 4 – wide open angle – Angle chamber depth (ACD) (shadow) is equal to or greater than corneal thickness.
- Grade 3 – moderately open angle – ACD is between 1/4 and 1/2 the corneal thickness.
- Grade 2 – moderately narrow angle – closure possible – 1/4 to the corneal thickness.
- Grade 1 – extremely narrow angle – less than 1/4 the corneal thickness.
- 0 – very narrow slit or no anterior chamber angle.

CONICAL BEAM: METHOD OF LOCATING AND GRADING CELLS AND FLARE

- Reduce the beam to a small circular pattern and increase magnification.
- Light source 45°–60° temporally and directed into the pupil.
- Position the slit lamp in front of the patient's eye with bright illumination and high magnification. Allow yourself a period of time to dark adapt.
- The conical beam is focussed between the cornea and the anterior lens surface and observation is concentrated on the dark zone between the out-of-focus cornea and lens. This zone is normally optically empty and appears totally black.
- Flare (protein escaping from dilated vessels) makes the normally optic empty zone appear gray or milky when compared to the uninvolved eye. Cells (white blood cells escaping from dilated vessels) will reflect the light and be seen as white dots.
  - 0: no cells; optically empty
  - 1: 2–5 cells; faint haze
  - 2: 5–10 cells; moderate but iris detail still clear
  - 3: 10–50 cells scattered throughout beam; iris details becoming hazy
  - 4: > 50 more than you can count; dense haze with obvious fibrin collecting on iris

RETRO-ILLUMINATION FOR DETECTING IRIS DEFECT

- This uses a parallelepiped that bounces unfocussed light off one structure while observing the backlighting of another.
- Biomicroscope and light source are placed in direct alignment with each other.
- The slit width is 1–2 mm wide and 4–5 mm high. They are both positioned directly in front of the eye to be examined.
- Focus the slit just off the edge of the iris and on the front of the lens.
- If there are defects or atrophy of the iris they will be seen as a retinal 'orange' glow coming back through each defect or hole.

USING THE BLUE FILTER

- This is used in conjunction with fluorescein drops for the examination of epithelial defects and evaluation of dry eyes. Lignocaine/fluorescein is used for applanation tonometry.

- In eyes with an epithelial defect, a bright green hue occurs in the Bowman's layer and the extent of the abrasion or superficial punctuate erosion can be evaluated.

GOLDMANN APPLANATION TONOMETRY

Goldmann applanation tonometry measures the intraocular pressure indirectly by measuring the force necessary to flatten a 3.06-mm diameter portion of the corneal surface. The higher the intraocular pressure, the greater is the force required.

MEASURING PRINCIPLE (DEVISED BY IMBERT-FICK)

The cornea is flattened with a plastic prism which has a flat anterior surface and a diameter of 7 mm. The prism is brought into contact with the cornea by advancing the slit lamp. The measuring drum, which regulates the force applied to the pressure arm, is turned and the tension on the eyes is increased until a surface of known and constant size of 3.06 mm is flattened. The intraocular pressure (in millimetres of mercury [mmHg]) is found by multiplying the drum reading by 10.

The correct end point is when the inner edges of the two fluorescein semicircle images just touch.

Procedure guideline: Nursing action and rationale

1. Ensure that the slit lamp is switched on and that the eyepieces are correctly focussed. This ensures accurate reading of intraocular pressure.
2. Switch on the blue filter and bring into the beam of the slit lamp.
3. Adjust the angle between the illumination and the microscope to about 60°.
4. Insert the tonometer into the slit-lamp base plate. The instrument can be used in either of two positions; observation is monocular with either the right or left microscope.
5. Bring the pressure arm into the notch position so that the axis of the prism and the microscope coincide.

NURSING ACTION: PREPARING THE PATIENT

1. Identify the patient in order to ensure the correct patient receives the treatment and to obtain the patient's consent and cooperation.
2. Check if the patient is wearing contact lenses and, if so, remove them before commencing the procedure. It is not possible to perform tonometry with contact lenses *in situ*.
3. Wash hands and instil topical anaesthesia into both eyes in order to reduce discomfort.
4. Instil fluorescein stain by means of fluorescein paper strips or fluorescein drops, to ensure accurate reading and to prevent too much fluorescein in the eye.
5. Instruct the patient to look straight ahead with both eyes wide open. If necessary, the patient's eyelids should be held apart by the examiner without pressure being applied to the eyeball.

NURSING ACTION: MEASUREMENT

1. The prism is brought into contact with the centre of the cornea, by advancing the slit lamp. A blue light illuminates the limbus when contact is made. The examiner looks through the microscope at this point.

2. Upon contact, a thin circular outline of fluorescein is produced. The prism splits the circle into two semicircles coloured green. Any necessary adjustment is made by the control lever or height adjustment control on the slit lamp, until the flattened area is seen as two semicircles of equal size in the middle of the field of view.

3. The pressure on the eye is increased by manually adjusting the measuring drum on the tonometer, until the inner borders of the two fluorescein rings just touch each other. The inner border of the ring represents the demarcation between the cornea flattened by applanation and the cornea not flattened.

4. The amount of force required to do this is translated by the scale into a pressure reading of millimetre of mercury (mmHg), which is found by multiplying the drum reading by 10.

  Tonometry can also be performed using the handheld Perkins' tonometer or a Tono-Pen.

Notes

- It is good practice to calibrate the tonometer daily. Any errors in reading should be reported and documented.
- The use of disposable Tonoshield or Tonosafe is encouraged to prevent the spread of infection.

EXAMINING THE EYE

Although the main focus in this section is on examining the eye, it is good nursing practice to take a holistic approach to patient care. Ensure that the patient you are going to examine is made comfortable and pain free. For any patients with a traumatic eye injury, ensure that the patient is not suffering from shock and has not sustained any other injuries. Always consider the patient's age and psychological state.

Patients attending with an acute eye problem should always have their ophthalmic history taken first to ascertain the nature and acuteness of the problem. For example, for patients attending with a chemical injury, treatment should always be instigated prior to examining the eye.

When examining a patient's eye, first look at the patient's face as a whole to determine facial symmetry and note any obvious palsy, ptosis, proptosis, obvious trauma, ocular movement or allergic reactions.

The eye is always examined from the outside inwards. If only one eye is affected, inspect the 'good' eye first for comparison.

Ask the patient to open both eyes as this is easier than opening one. Use a slit lamp or a good pen torch. Ensure that the patient's head is well supported. If the patient is experiencing ocular pain, topical anaesthetic drops may be necessary. However, the patient's pain must be assessed before administering any topical anaesthetic. The patient's pain can be assessed using a pain-rating tool such as the verbal pain scale. Care should be taken not to 'misuse' the topical anaesthetic in controlling a patient's corneal pain since this can actually delay corneal epithelial healing. *On no account* must these drops be given to the patient to take home. If the patient is in a great deal of pain, more effective oral analgesia or a non-steroidal anti-inflammatory such as Voltarol can be prescribed.

If there is a history of glass or fibreglass in the eye or the history indicates possible penetrating injury or perforation, local anaesthetic should not be instilled. The reason for the former is to more easily identify if the glass/fibreglass has been removed, and the latter to avoid the drug entering the eye.

EYELIDS

Look for

- Ptosis
- Swelling
- Discoloration
- Discharge/crusting
- In-growing lashes (see Figure 4.3)
- Entropion
- Ectropion
- Laceration

CONJUNCTIVA

The upper palpebral conjunctiva must also be examined by everting the upper lid. Look for

- Injection (redness)
- Degree of injection
- Position of injection
  - Limbal/ciliary
  - Localised – with or without dilated episcleral vessels
  - Generalised
- Subconjunctival haemorrhage
- Chemosis (swelling)

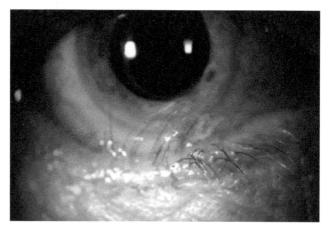

Figure 4.3 Trichiasis with cicatricial pemphigoid.

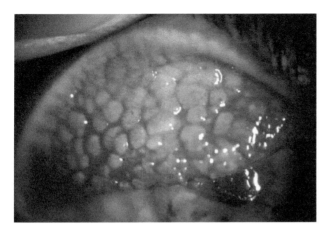

Figure 4.4 Cobblestone papillae.

- Foreign body
- Laceration
- Cysts
- Pinguecula
- Pterygium
- Follicles
- Papillae (see Figure 4.4)

CORNEA

Look for

- Clarity
- Corneal curvature, e.g. keratoconus
- Pannus (superficial vascularisation of the cornea)
- Foreign body/penetrating injury (see Figure 4.5)

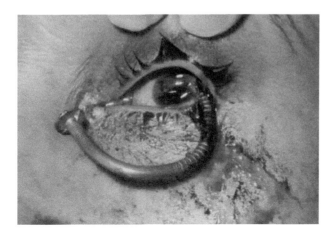

Figure 4.5 Penetrating injury.

- Abrasion
- Laceration
- Ulcers

Using a slit lamp, examine the layers of the cornea and note any abnormalities such as sub-epithelial opacities, corneal oedema, Descemet's folds or breaks, fresh or old keratitic precipitate or pigment on the endothelium.

ANTERIOR CHAMBER

Assess depth (should be deep but compare with other eye). Look for

- Hyphaema (see Figure 4.6)
- Hypopyon
- Flare and cells (using slit lamp)

IRIS

Assess the following:

- Colour – compare with other eye
- Clarity and pattern

Look for

- Iridodialysis
- Iris prolapse

PUPIL

Assess the following:

- Shape (should be round – an irregular pupil could indicate synaechiae; an oval pupil could indicate acute glaucoma).

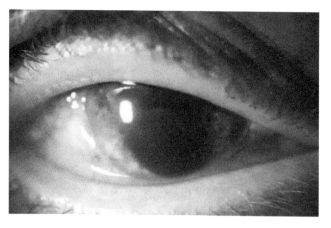

Figure 4.6 Hyphaema.

- Size.
- Reaction.
- RAPD (relative afferent pupil defect).
- Position (should be central).
- Colour – usually black: The red reflex may be noted (a white or grey pupil suggests the presence of a cataract; a white pupil in a baby/child indicates a cataract or retinoblastoma or imperforate pupil membrane).

Procedure guideline: Everting the upper lid

The upper lid is everted to inspect the palpebral conjunctiva over the sub-tarsal area. Foreign bodies, conjunctival follicles, papillae or concretions may be present.

EQUIPMENT

- Cotton bud
- Slit lamp or illuminated magnification unit

NURSING ACTION

1. Wash hands and prepare trolley and gather equipment in accordance with Aseptic Non Touch Technique (ANTT) principles.
2. Prepare equipment, identifying key parts and key sites to be protected during the procedure.
3. Check patient identification against request card/notes with patient.
4. Obtain patient's consent and cooperation. Explain procedure, including any side effects. Warn patient that there will be a peculiar sensation during the examination.
5. Ask the patient to look downward.
6. Take hold of the lashes of the upper lid with one hand and gently pull forward and downward.
7. With the other hand, place cotton bud vertically over tarsal plate (mid-lid area). Do not apply any pressure on the globe.
8. Push gently into the tarsal plate, at the same time the hand holding the lashes everts the lid, discard the cotton bud.
9. Remind the patient to keep looking down.
10. Inspect the sub-tarsal conjunctiva.
11. Repeat for other eye if required.
12. Release the lid and ask the patient to rest back.
13. Dispose of waste appropriately, cleaning hands, tray/trolley as before.
14. Document the procedure in the patient's notes, adding time, date and signature.

REMOVING A CONJUNCTIVAL OR CORNEAL FOREIGN BODY

The majority of foreign bodies (such as metal) found either on the conjunctiva or especially on the cornea are usually well embedded. Removal of such foreign bodies should *never* be attempted by inexperienced staff, nor without the slit lamp. Attempted removal by inexperienced staff or without the slit lamp can cause a great deal of damage to the cornea and may result in the creation of a larger corneal injury, infection and even perforation of the cornea.

Using the slit lamp for removal of a corneal foreign body by experienced staff allows a thorough examination of the eye before and after removal. Prior to removing either the conjunctival or corneal foreign body, the following steps should be taken.

Procedure guideline: Removing a conjunctival or corneal foreign body

1. Take and record the patient's visual acuity in order to assess the extent of visual disturbance and to provide a baseline measurement.
2. Take and document the relevant patient history. The history must include the presenting complaint; the patient's description of his presenting signs and symptoms; the nature of the injury (e.g. while grinding, hammering, chiseling); an assessment of any pain or discomfort; any subjective loss of vision; the use of any appropriate eye protection at the time of injury; any previous ophthalmic problems; allergies; and any systemic and topical medications. Note if the patient wears contact lenses. This is to accurately assess the patient prior to examination and removal of any foreign body.
3. Examination of the anterior segment of the eye must take into account location, type of foreign body and depth of penetration. A careful search including a sub-tarsal search of the eye must be undertaken to locate any other foreign bodies or injuries to other parts of the eye and surrounding structures. Examination techniques such as iris transillumination and Seidel test must be carried out to exclude any intraocular penetration by the foreign body. However, it is unlikely that if a corneal foreign body is located in the anterior segment of the eye, there is any ocular penetration.
4. Sit patient back from slit lamp and explain your findings to him. Explain the procedure for removal of conjunctival/corneal foreign body. This is to reassure the patient and to obtain the patient's consent and cooperation regarding the procedure.

Procedure guideline: Equipment needed

- Plastic tray or trolley
- Slit lamp
- Sterile green needle firmly mounted on a cotton bud
- Sterile wet (minims normal saline) cotton bud
- Local anaesthetic drops
- Minims of fluorescein drops
- Minims of lignocaine/fluorescein drops

NURSING ACTION

1. Wash hands and clean the tray and trolley as before.
2. Gather equipment needed and assemble in the tray. The key parts should be identified.
3. Prepare patient for procedure by assessment of patient, which should include the following: medical and physical issues; level of understanding; cultural and other needs.
4. Instil topical anaesthetic such as G. tetracaine hydrochloride (Amethocaine) or oxybuprocaine hydrochloride (G. benoxinate).

5. Bring patient back into the slit lamp and ensure that he understands the need to keep his eyes completely still during the procedure. To maintain fixation, it is a good idea to ask the patient to fixate his other eye on an object in the room.
6. Hold the patient's upper lid with your hand away from the cornea.
7. Increase the magnification on the slit lamp to get a better view.
8. Using the sterile green needle firmly mounted on a cotton bud, gently dislocate the foreign body. It may be necessary to gently swab the foreign body off the conjunctiva/cornea with a sterile wet cotton bud.
9. Continue to examine the anterior segment of the eye for signs of infiltrate. Take appropriate action if any signs noted. Note extent of injury by using a topical fluorescein. If the foreign body is metal, a rust ring may be noted. If it is difficult to remove the rust ring at that visit, the patient must be given an appointment in 2 days to have the rust ring removed. Meanwhile, a broad-spectrum antibiotic is prescribed to prevent infection. The antibiotic ointment will also soften the rust and make it easier to remove.
10. It is good practice to measure the patient's intraocular pressure as part of the examination, to detect any abnormalities in intraocular measurement.
11. Dispose of waste appropriately, cleaning hands, tray/trolley as before.
12. Document the procedure in the patient's notes, adding time, date and signature.

APPLYING PAD AND BANDAGE

Pads are now seldom applied to patients with corneal abrasions as it is known that the corneal epithelium healing rate was significantly improved without a pad. Patients with large abrasions may find a pad, and perhaps a bandage, afford more comfort if applied firmly as the eyelid is prevented from irritating the abrasion (Marsden 2006).

If a pad is to be applied, it is important that the eye is firmly closed under the pad to avoid corneal abrasion. In some instances, it is useful to apply a piece of paraffin gauze over the eyelids, then a pad or half a pad folded in two, and finally a pad applied flat over the eye. This method is useful in the casualty or outpatient departments but should not be used on post-operative patients as it will put too much pressure on the globe, unless pressure needs to be applied post-operatively, e.g. to seal a leaking wound. Secure the pad with three pieces of tape. For the right eye, the first piece of tape should be placed over the centre of the pad, diagonally from 1 to 7 o'clock. For the left eye, it is placed diagonally from 11 to 5 o'clock. The second and third pieces of tape are placed each side of this central piece, parallel to it. Position the ends of each piece of tape on each other so that removal is easier and kinder to the patient. Pads may be applied to post-operative patients undergoing certain oculoplastic procedures. Cartella shields are now in common use in most ocular surgical cases instead of a pad.

In cases of chemical injury, the eye should *never* be padded.

DISADVANTAGES OF EYE PADS

Eye pads have several disadvantages:

- Corneal abrasion can be caused if the eye is not closed under the pad.
- Pads create a good medium for bacterial growth.
- Pads are flammable.
- Pads are uncomfortable to wear.

- If the lids are swollen, a lid abrasion may occur.
- The corneal healing rate is reduced.

BANDAGING

There are several different methods of applying an eye bandage. One method is described here, which provides a secure, comfortable, effective result. You should hold the bandage barrel uppermost with the tail to the right or left depending on the eye to be covered.

Procedure guideline: Bandaging

NURSING ACTION

1. Take the bandage twice around the forehead.
2. Bring it up under the ear on the affected side and over the centre of the eye pad.
3. Repeat this twice, covering the eye pad above and below the first central turn.
4. Take the bandage once more around the forehead and secure it.
5. Take care when bandaging not to occlude the 'good eye' or the patient's ears.

REMOVING A CORNEAL RUST RING

Use the same technique as removing corneal foreign body. Note that when all the rust has been removed, you will observe some rust staining on the cornea. This can be safely left alone. Ensure that there is no sign of corneal infiltrate.

TESTING FOR TEAR FILM BREAK-UP RIME: ASSESSING THE QUALITY OF TEARS

The quality of tears can be measured by applying a drop of fluorescein to the lower bulbar conjunctiva and asking the patient to gently close his eyes, and position the patient on the slit lamp. The patient is asked to open his eyes and to refrain from blinking. Using the blue filter of the slit lamp, the tear film is scanned and the operator starts counting from one until the appearance of the first dry spot. The time that elapses before the appearance of the first dry spot is the tear film break-up time. The normal break-up time is about 10–15 seconds. The break-up time is shorter in eyes with aqueous and mucin tear deficiency.

IRRIGATING THE EYE

Irrigation of the eye is performed to clean the eye thoroughly of all foreign substances, especially corrosive matter. As an emergency measure, speedy dilution of any substance is very important, and irrigating the eye immediately with the nearest tap water may greatly reduce the amount of damage to the tissues.

Procedure guideline: Irrigating the eye

EQUIPMENT

- pH indicator
- Irrigation set
- A bottle of sterile water or sodium chloride
- Local anaesthetic drops
- Desmarres lid retractor
- Paper tissues
- Protective plastic bibs or cape
- Paper towels
- Receptacle for paper towels
- Receiver

NURSING ACTION

1. Prepare self and equipment as previously indicated.
2. Establish patient identity against request card/notes with patient and obtain verbal consent.
3. Assess the patient as previously identified.
4. Sit the patient in a chair with his head well supported and turned slightly to the affected side.
5. Test pH of conjunctival sac to ascertain length of time for which eye needs to be irrigated. Post-irrigation pH should be between 7.3 and 7.7.
6. Instil anaesthetic drops as per procedure guideline.
7. Place a protective bib and paper towels around the patient's neck.
8. Place the receiver against the patient's face on the affected side. Ask the patient to hold it if no other help is available.
9. Initially, run a stream of fluid up the cheek towards the eye to prepare the patient for fluid entering the eye.
10. Evert the lower lid, asking the patient to look up, and irrigate the lower fornix.
11. Evert the upper lid, asking the patient to look down, and irrigate the upper fornix.
12. Double-evert the upper lid using Desmarres lid retractor if necessary. This is to ensure that no solidified material (e.g. cement) is in the upper fornix.
13. Complete the irrigation by asking the patient to move his eye from side to side and up and down, holding the lids open.
14. These steps ensure all anterior surfaces of the eye, especially the fornices, are irrigated.
15. Retest the pH of the conjunctival sac. Allow approximately 5 minutes between irrigation and pH testing; testing sooner than this would mean that you are testing the irrigation fluid still in the eye and not the tear film.
16. Repeat irrigation as required until the pH is normal.
17. Wipe patient's face dry, for patient comfort.
18. Wash hands.
19. Dispose of clinical waste; clean and store equipment as before.
20. Document results and date and sign the entry in the patient's notes.

Notes

- Do not hold the irrigation nozzle too close or too far away from the eye – about 2.5 cm is best. If too close, it may touch the eye; if too far away, the stream of fluid may not be sufficient to reach the eye.
- It may be necessary to instil local anaesthetic drops over the everted upper lid.

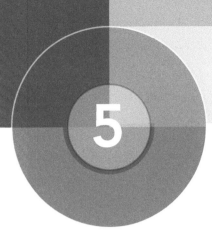

The globe: A brief overview

5

This chapter is deliberately brief to avoid repetition, as more detailed descriptions can be found in the individual chapters on each structure. Its aim is to enable the ophthalmic nurse to see the interrelationships between the various structures.

The globe or eyeball is situated in the bony socket or orbit, which affords it protection. Also in the socket are nerves, muscles, blood vessels and fat.

Anteriorly, the globe is also protected by the upper and lower eyelids, which contain muscles, secretory glands and eyelashes.

The lacrimal gland sits in the upper-outer aspect of the frontal bone of the orbit and produces tears, which drain into the lacrimal drainage system. This is composed of an upper and lower punctum situated on the inner aspects of the upper and lower lid margins, the upper and lower canaliculi and the lacrimal sac, which opens into the nasal duct.

There are six extraocular muscles, which move the eye in the direction of gaze, four recti muscles and two oblique muscles.

The conjunctiva lines the lids (the palpebral conjunctiva) and overlies the sclera (the bulbar conjunctiva), terminating at the cornea.

The globe (Figure 5.1) is approximately 2.5 cm in diameter by the age of 3 years. It has three layers:

1. The outer protective layer comprises the sclera for approximately its posterior five-sixths and the cornea for its anterior one-sixth. The cornea is clear to allow light rays through and is highly sensitive. The sclera is composed of tough white fibrous tissue.
2. The middle layer is the pigmented vascular uveal tract. The choroid forms approximately the posterior four-fifths and the ciliary body and iris the anterior one-fifth. The iris is a diaphragm allowing varying amounts of light to enter the eye through the pupil in its centre. The ciliary processes produce aqueous humour and the ciliary muscles control the shape of the crystalline lens for focussing. The choroidal blood vessels supply the underlying outer layers of the retina.
3. The inner layer is formed by the retina and is the nerve-ending layer containing rods and cones, which receive the light stimulus that is sent via the optic nerve to the occipital cortex for interpretation.

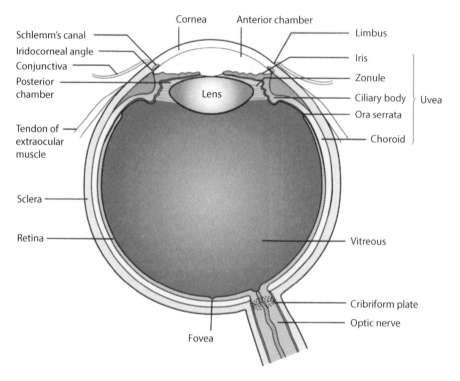

Figure 5.1 Basic anatomy of the eye. (From James, B., Chew, C., Bron, A., *Lecture Notes: Ophthalmology*. 10th edition, Blackwell Publishing, UK, 2007, reproduced with permission.)

Aqueous humour is produced by the ciliary processes, which are part of the ciliary body, and flows into the posterior chamber, through the pupil, into the anterior chamber and drains through the trabecular meshwork and the canal of Schlemm in the angle of the anterior chamber. Some drainage also takes place via the uveo-scleral route. It nourishes the crystalline lens and cornea.

The anterior chamber is the area between the cornea and the iris. The posterior chamber is the area between the posterior surface of the iris and the anterior surface of the crystalline lens.

The crystalline lens is suspended by the suspensory ligaments (zonules) from the ciliary body and lies behind the iris. It is clear to allow light rays to pass through unhindered. It changes shape so light rays can be focussed on the retina for near vision, a process known as accommodation.

Vitreous humour is a clear gelatinous substance, which fills the posterior segment of the eye between the crystalline lens and the retina.

NERVE SUPPLY TO THE EYE

The oculomotor or third cranial nerve supplies the

- Levator palpebral superioris muscle
- Superior rectus muscle
- Inferior rectus muscle

- Medial rectus muscle
- Inferior oblique muscle

Its branch, the short ciliary nerve, supplies the

- Sphincter muscle of the iris
- Ciliary muscle

The trochlea or fourth cranial nerve supplies the

- Superior oblique muscle
- Trigeminal or fifth cranial nerve

The first division of the trigeminal nerve is the ophthalmic division. This division has three branches:

- Lacrimal branch, supplying the lacrimal gland
- Frontal branch, supplying the skin of the forehead
- Nasociliary, with two branches:
  - Infratrochlea supplying the inside of the nose
  - Long ciliary supplying the dilator muscle of the iris, the conjunctiva and the cornea

The abducens or sixth cranial nerve supplies the lateral rectus muscle. The facial or seventh cranial nerve supplies the orbicularis muscle.

BLOOD SUPPLY TO THE EYE

The ophthalmic artery and its branches supply the blood to the eye. Drainage is via the ophthalmic vein and its branches:

- The central retinal artery and vein supply and drain the retina.
- The short posterior ciliary artery and choroidal vein supply and drain the choroid.
- The long posterior ciliary artery supplies the ciliary body.
- The anterior ciliary artery supplies the
  - Ciliary body
  - Conjunctiva
  - Corneal limbus
- The arterial circle of the iris, supplying blood to the iris, is formed from the
  - Long posterior ciliary artery
  - Anterior ciliary artery
- The anterior ciliary vein drains the
  - Ciliary body
  - Iris
  - Conjunctiva
  - Corneal limbus
- The conjunctival artery and vein supply and drain the conjunctiva.
- The superior and inferior medial palpebral artery and vein supply and drain the
  - Conjunctiva
  - Eyelids
  - Lacrimal sac
- The episcleral artery and vein supply and drain the sclera.

- The lacrimal artery and vein supply and drain the
    - Lacrimal gland
    - Eyelids
- The supraorbital artery and vein supply and drain the upper eyelids.
- The muscular artery and vein supply and drain the extraocular muscles.
- The nasal artery and vein supply and drain the lacrimal sac.
- The frontal artery and vein supply and drain the forehead.
- The four vortex veins drain the ciliary body, iris and choroid leaving the globe at its equator to drain into the ophthalmic vein.

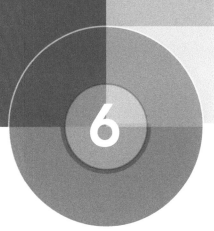

The protective structures, including removal of an eye

6

This chapter explores some of the issues associated with orbital conditions.

THE ORBIT

The eyeball or globe is protected by the bony socket or orbit in which it sits (Figure 6.1). The orbit is composed of seven bones:

- Maxilla
- Frontal
- Lacrimal
- Ethmoid
- Sphenoid
- Zygomatic
- Palatine

Each orbit has four walls: a floor, roof, lateral wall and medial wall. The two medial walls are parallel to each other and the two orbits diverge to allow for a greater field of vision. The orbits are pyramid shaped with the apex posteriorly.

AREAS OF THE ORBIT

- *Roof* – Triangular shaped and made up of the frontal bone anteriorly and part of the sphenoid posteriorly
- *Floor* – Triangular shaped and made up of the maxilla anteriorly, part of the zygomatic laterally and the palatine posteriorly
- *Lateral wall* – Composed of the zygomatic anteriorly and the sphenoid posteriorly
- *Medial wall* – Composed of four bones; from the front backwards: part of the maxilla, the lacrimal, the ethmoid and part of the sphenoid

Three apertures are situated at the apex of each orbit:

1. The optic foramen through which passes
   a. The optic nerve (second cranial nerve) leaving the orbit
   b. The ophthalmic artery entering the orbit, running underneath the optic nerve

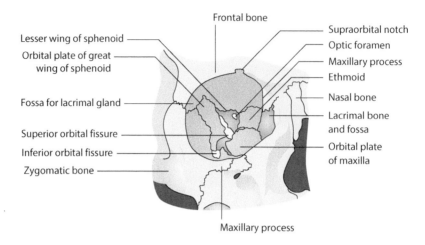

Figure 6.1 The anatomy of the orbit. (From James, B. et al., *Lecture Notes: Ophthalmology*, Blackwell Publishing, 2007, reproduced with permission.)

2. The superior orbital fissure through which pass
   a. Nerves
   b. Oculomotor (third cranial nerve) – superior and inferior branches
   c. Trochlea (fourth cranial nerve); trigeminal (fifth cranial nerve) – three branches of the first division (ophthalmic division): lacrimal, frontal and nasociliary
   d. Abducens (sixth cranial nerve)
   e. Blood vessels
   f. Ophthalmic vein – superior and inferior branches
3. The inferior orbital fissure through which pass
   a. The infraorbital artery
   b. The trigeminal nerve – some branches of the second division (maxillary division)

Surrounding the globe in the socket are muscles, ligaments, blood vessels, nerves and fat. Tenon's capsule is a thin membrane which encircles the globe from the margin of the cornea to the optic nerve, adhering closely to the sclera beneath it.

THE EYELIDS

The functions of the eyelids are to protect the globe and to lubricate its anterior surface (Figure 6.2). The top lid, the larger of the two, closes over the globe to protect it. By blinking, the tear film is spread over the anterior surface thus lubricating it.

AREAS OF THE LID

These are illustrated in Figure 6.3:

• Palpebral conjunctiva lining the under-surface.
• Tarsal plate – a band of connective tissue lying posteriorly forming a stiff plate.
• Skin on the outer surface.
• Grey line – inter-marginal sulcus, where the skin joins the palpebral conjunctiva on the lid margin.

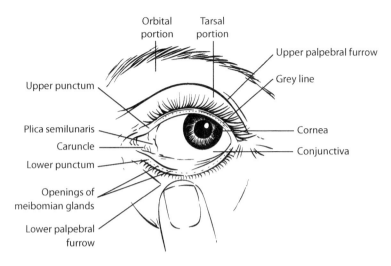

Figure 6.2 The outer appearance of the eye and eyelid.

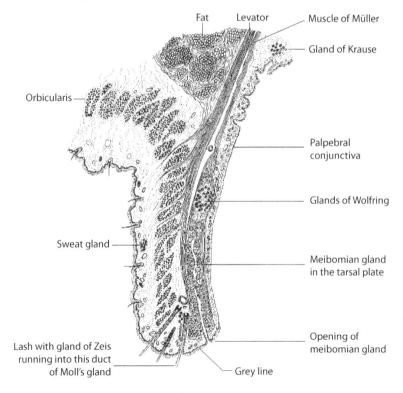

Figure 6.3 Vertical section through the upper lid.

- Hair follicles – lashes, near the grey line.
- Fat – surrounding the structures.
- Glands.
- Meibomian glands. There are 20–30 meibomian glands in each lid, contained within the tarsal plate, their ducts opening through the palpebral conjunctiva just behind

the lashes. They produce a sebaceous substance which creates the oily layer of the tear film.

- Glands of Moll – These are sweat glands producing sebum.
- Glands of Zeis – These are modified sebaceous glands which open into the lash follicles.
- Glands of Krause and Wolfring – These are situated in the fornices and are accessory tear glands.
- Sweat glands – These open directly onto the skin of the outer surface.
- Muscles – there are three muscles supplying the eyelid:
  - Orbicularis:
    - Origin – lacrimal bone
    - Insertion – deep in the fascia around the lacrimal sac
    - Function – to close the lids and to screw up the eyes
    - Nerve supply – facial nerve (seventh cranial nerve)
  - Levator palpebral superioris:
    - Origin – Annulus of Zinn (a ring tendon surrounding the optic nerve at the apex of the orbit)
    - Insertion – into the tarsal plate, palpebral ligaments and skin of the upper lid
    - Function – to lift the upper lid
    - Nerve supply – oculomotor (third cranial nerve)
  - Müller's muscle (this is a smooth muscle):
    - Origin – in the levator palpebral superioris muscle
    - Insertion – tarsal plate
    - Function – to provide extra elevation to the upper lid
    - Nerve supply – sympathetic nervous system

SENSORY NERVE SUPPLY

Sensory nerve supply is as follows:

- Upper lid – Ophthalmic division of the trigeminal nerve (fifth cranial nerve)
- Lower lid – Maxillary division of the trigeminal nerve

BLOOD SUPPLY

The blood supply to and drainage from the eyelids is via:

- Lacrimal artery and vein
- Supraorbital artery and vein (upper lid)
- Superior and inferior medial palpebral artery and vein

CONDITIONS OF THE ORBIT

ORBITAL CELLULITIS

Orbital cellulitis (Figure 6.4) is an acute purulent inflammation of the cellular tissue of the orbit. An ophthalmic emergency because of optic nerve compression, it is more common in children and is usually unilateral. It is usual to involve the ear, nose and throat specialist team in the joint care and management of the patient; indeed the patient may have been seen by them

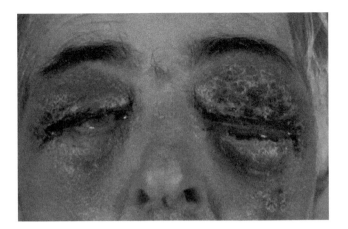

Figure 6.4 Bilateral orbital cellulitis.

first and treatment already commenced. It is classed as an ophthalmic emergency and requires immediate treatment.

Condition guideline: Orbital cellulitis

CAUSES

- Spread of infection from neighbouring structures, e.g. nasal sinus
- Sepsis following penetrating injuries
- Following septic operations, e.g. enucleation
- Facial erysipelas
- Spread of pyaemia – causative organisms: pneumococcus; *Staphylococcus*; *Streptococcus*

SIGNS

- Proptosis of the affected eye, pushed forward by the inflamed tissue within the orbit, behind the eyeball
- Red and inflamed lids
- Chemosis of conjunctiva
- Formation of abscess over the upper eyelid
- Reduction in visual acuity
- Reduction in colour vision
- Malaise and fever
- Relative afferent pupil defect
- Possible double vision
- Limitations and painful ocular movements
- Possible signs of optic nerve dysfunction in advanced cases

PATIENT'S NEEDS

- Admission to hospital if necessary.
- All suspected cases of orbital cellulitis will need to have a computed tomography (CT) scan to look for any sight/life-threatening subperiosteal and orbital collections.

The scan will also show evidence of any adjacent sinus disease. If adjacent sinus disease is not located but intraconal opacity is seen on the CT scan, trauma or foreign body should be suspected.

- Relief of symptoms:
  - Pain – especially on eye movement
  - Nasal congestion; fever – there may be rigors
  - Anorexia
  - General malaise

NURSING ACTION

1. Admit patient to ward if necessary.
2. Arrange urgent CT scan of paranasal sinuses orbits and brain.
3. Arrange urgent referral to ear, nose and throat specialist.
4. Take blood for full blood count, urea, electrolytes and glucose, blood cultures.
5. It is important to liaise with microbiologist, especially if local changes in sensitivity and resistance occur.
6. Give prescribed analgesia for pain. Local heat application may be comforting.
7. Fan and/or tepid sponge patient to bring down temperature.
8. Administer prescribed antibiotics:
   a. Oral, e.g. clindamycin which is effective against Gram-positive cocci such as streptococci, dose for adults 150–300 mg 6 hourly and, where the infection is severe, 450 mg 6 hourly. Child doses are calculated based on 3–6 mg per kg of body weight 6 hourly and Ciprofloxacin 500–750 mg BD for adults (British Medical Association and Royal Pharmaceutical Society of Great Britain 2009). Oral antibiotics may be continued for up to 6 weeks.
   b. Eye drops, e.g. G. chloramphenicol 0.5%, to be given 2–4 hourly.
   c. In severe cases, intravenous antibiotics may be prescribed.
9. Administer nasal decongestant spray as prescribed, e.g. xylometa-zoline hydrochloride 0.1%.
10. Give nourishing fluids and a light diet.
11. Provide general nursing care of an ill patient.
12. Dress abscess if this forms.
13. Prepare for, and give, post-operative care of patient following drainage of abscess in the sinuses or orbit. Send a pus sample from the drainage for analysis.
14. Monitoring of optic nerve function hourly or as directed by the doctor:- testing distance visual acuity, pupillary reactions, assessing colour vision using the Ishihara colour vision chart and light brightness appreciation (Kanski et al. 1996).
15. Prolapsed conjunctiva requires a Frost suture and lubricants.

COMPLICATIONS

- The infection may spread backwards into the brain causing:
  - Cavernous sinus thrombosis
  - Meningitis
  - Brain abscess
- Possible occurrence of panophthalmitis
- Sinus formation, if the cause is a sinusitis

- Optic atrophy due to pressure on the nerve
- Subperiorbital abscess
- Central retinal vein or artery occlusion
- Raised intraocular pressure
- Exposure keratopathy

Where orbital cellulitis occurs in a child, referral to an ear, nose and throat specialist is usual, as the cause is invariably from ethmoidal/maxillary sinus.

PRESEPTAL CELLULITIS

Preseptal cellulitis is infection of the eyelids only, i.e. preseptal, anterior to the orbital septum. Preseptal cellulitis is often preceded by infection of the teeth or sinuses, by trauma or by infected lid chalazion (inflammatory cyst). The infection does not spread beyond the orbital septum of the upper lid into the orbit. The signs and symptoms are similar to orbital cellulitis, but the condition is not so dangerous.

If a child presents with an obvious lid cyst, treat with oral antibiotics and consider drainage. The child must be reviewed daily until improvement is seen. The child is to be admitted if unwell, if in pain, if it is due to trauma, if no clear history, if parental understanding is poor or if significant ptosis is obstructing examination.

CAVERNOUS SINUS THROMBOSIS

The cavernous sinus is situated near the pituitary gland. Through it pass many of the veins draining structures around the face, including the orbit, globe, nose, mouth, sinuses and the meninges. Thus infection can spread from any of these structures into the cavernous sinus. It may also spread from a general infectious disease or septic focus elsewhere in the body. It is a serious condition. Fifty percent of cases are bilateral.

Condition guideline: Cavernous sinus thrombosis

SIGNS

Signs are as for orbital cellulitis, plus some others:

- Paralysis of the extraocular muscles, as their nerves pass through the cavernous sinus and are thus involved
- Dilated pupil(s), usually non-reactive due to the trigeminal nerve being involved as it also passes through the cavernous sinus
- Anaesthetic cornea due to the involvement of the trigeminal nerve
- Reduced visual acuity due to pressure
- Papilloedema due to pressure
- Signs of cerebral irritation

PATIENT'S NEEDS AND NURSING ACTION

1. Patient's needs and nursing action are as for orbital cellulitis.
2. The antibiotics will be administered by the intravenous route in large doses.
3. Anticoagulants may be prescribed.

THYROID EYE DISEASE (GRAVES' OPHTHALMOPATHY)

Graves' disease describes the most common cause of hyperthyroidism and is thought to be due to an autoimmune problem and some associated environmental factors. It usually affects women between the ages of 20 and 45 years who have signs and symptoms of thyrotoxicosis together with ophthalmic signs. Ophthalmic signs can occur in patients who are clinically euthyroid and, in these cases, the disease is referred to as ophthalmic Graves' disease. The signs and symptoms tend to be similar.

Condition guideline: Thyroid eye disease

SIGNS

- Exophthalmos – Unilateral or bilateral. Inflammatory cytokines and plasma cell infiltration of the orbital fat and extraocular muscles lead to engorgement and swelling which within the confines of the bony orbit, push the globe forward.
- Lid lag – When looking downwards, the top lid normally moves with the eye. In this condition, the lid moves very slowly down or not at all. This is possibly due to sympathetic overactivity of Müller's muscle and mechanical restriction due to proptosis.
- Lid retraction – The upper lid retracts, giving the typical 'stare' associated with thyroid eye disease. The sclera above the cornea is visible. This is probably due to involvement of the levator muscle and mechanical restriction due to proptosis.
- Corneal exposure – Corneal exposure occurs because
    - The lids are unable to close over the protruding globe.
    - Defective blinking occurs because of involvement of the lid muscles.
- Exophthalmoplegia – This is the inability to move the eye in the fields of gaze because the extraocular muscles are involved due to infiltration and later fibrosis. Diplopia results.
- In hyperthyroidism, signs of thyrotoxicosis such as tachycardia, proximal myopathy and muscular tremors may be present.

PATIENT'S NEEDS

- Protection of the exposed cornea – which is the most important factor, for example temporary suture tarsorrhaphy.
- Prevention of complications, which can result in loss of vision.
- Investigation and treatment of thyroid state by an endocrinologist.
- Correction of diplopia.
- Treatment of lid lag.
- In severe cases, rapid relief of orbital pressure.
- Psychological care – The patient may be frightened and in need of reassurance.
- Smoking cessation – Smoking exacerbates the disease process as much as sevenfold.
- Encouragement to take selenium.

NURSING ACTION

1. Corneal exposure – The nurse will
    a. Instruct the patient in application of prescribed ointment such as simple eye ointment or Oc. chloramphenicol 1% at night.
    b. Prepare the patient for a tarsorrhaphy, which may be necessary; the edges of the eyelids are sewn together, usually in the lateral aspect, to protect the cornea.

   c. Instruct the patient in the use and care of a bandage contact lens; this is a large contact lens which covers the whole of the cornea, thereby giving protection (see Appendix 2: Contact Lenses).

2. Explain the investigations needed for thyroid function estimations.
3. Explain to the patient that diplopia can be treated by wearing glasses with prisms in the lenses. A squint operation may be carried out when the thyroid state is stable.
4. Treatment for lid lag – the nurse will prepare the patient for lid surgery when Müller's muscle will be divided.
5. In severe cases, where emergency treatment is required to reduce the orbital pressure, the nurse will
   a. Give the prescribed high doses of systemic steroids.
   b. Prepare the patient for orbital decompression – Part of the lateral wall of the orbit is removed so the orbital contents can prolapse and therefore relieve the pressure on the optic nerve.
   c. Prepare the patient for radiotherapy.

COMPLICATIONS

- Corneal ulceration due to exposure keratitis
- Visual loss due to optic nerve compression, central retinal artery and vein occlusion
- Cataract formation due to metabolic disturbance to the lens
- Secondary glaucoma due to compression on the globe by the orbital contents, causing the intraocular pressure to rise

REMOVAL OF AN EYE

An eye is removed if it is blind and painful – usually as a result of chronic or secondary glaucoma, if there is severe infection or malignancy, or following severe trauma. Three operative procedures can be used for removal of an eye. The decision of the surgeon to opt for a particular method is determined by the nature of the pathology.

1. *Enucleation.* Enucleation is the surgical removal of the eyeball itself. The extraocular muscles and remaining orbital contents are conserved. The muscles are utilised to create movement of the prosthetic eye. It is performed when the eye is blind and painful; following trauma to the globe; or for malignancy which is confined to the globe, such as a malignant choroidal melanoma or retinoblastoma. In cases of malignancy, a length of optic nerve must be removed as well to ensure that the disease has not spread along the nerve fibres. If the nerve is found to be involved, radiotherapy will be given to the socket. Cases where the patient has enucleated their own eye, while rare, do happen. Such patients usually have underlying psychological or psychiatric problems. The void left after removal of the eye is usually replaced with an orbital implant: bioceramic, hydroxyapatite or baseball implant.
2. *Evisceration.* Evisceration is the removal of the contents of the globe, leaving the sclera intact. This is performed following trauma and in cases of severe infection, the sclera being left *in situ* to prevent infection spreading into the brain via the optic nerve and ophthalmic blood vessels. The sclera provides scaffolding for any subsequent implant and prosthetic eye.

3. *Exenteration*. Exenteration is the removal of the total contents of the orbit and, if necessary, the eyelids, plus any involved bone. This is performed for malignancy that is outside the eyeball, such as a basal cell carcinoma of the eyelid that has eroded structures behind it.

Removal of the eye should never be performed before a second opinion is obtained as to its necessity.

PATIENT'S NEEDS

Some patients will already be in hospital following trauma or infection when the decision to remove the eye is taken. Others will need to be admitted. If the eye is blind and painful, the patient may be relieved at the thought of its removal. Some people, though, resist having the eye removed despite severe pain, preferring to rely on analgesics or nerve blocks for pain relief. It may be worth pointing out to these patients that a blind eye gradually shrinks (phthisis bulbi) and becomes unsightly.

Removal of an eye is an emotive subject, and most patients will be highly anxious about the social, physical and psychological effects and will need much support. The patient's reaction to having an eye removed will vary according to his individual personality, family support, age and gender as well as the circumstances surrounding the cause of the removal.

A very young child will not understand fully what is happening and may quickly adapt to a prosthesis as he will have known little else. However, the parents will be feeling very differently, requiring a great amount of support. They may be suffering from acute feelings of guilt, especially if the child had an accident for which they blame themselves. Siblings and friends may also be upset, especially if they have been involved in, or caused, the accident.

All patients of any age will go through a period of loss for their eye, including feelings of anger and resentment, while coming to terms with their condition. Teenagers may be particularly concerned about their appearance and body image, which may prevent them from socialising with their peers. All age groups and both sexes will be very aware of their changed appearance. They will be much more critical of their prosthesis, noting minute differences to their other eye. It is worth pointing out to them that no two natural eyes in the same face are the same.

Some families and friends will be able to give the patient the necessary support, but others may not feel able to. Some family members may require help from the nurse to come to terms with the patient's loss.

Procedure guideline: Removal of an eye

NURSING ACTION

1. Admit the patient to hospital.
2. Give psychological and practical help. Explain about prostheses (see below) to the patient, pointing out that these days they are very good matches and need not be removed. It may be helpful to put him in touch with a patient who already has a prosthesis. A visit by the prosthetist before the operation will result in the patient having a better understanding of the processes involved in creating the artificial eye. The patient needs to understand that the prosthesis will not be placed in the socket at the time of surgery but at a later stage. In addition, patients should be advised that post-operatively they will have a dressing of pad and bandage, worn undisturbed

for 1 week. First dressing takes place in the outpatient setting. They should be advised also that it is not unusual to suffer nausea and vomiting immediately post-operatively. They should be reassured that the nurse will give analgesia and anti-emetics as required (Waterman et al. 1998). Pain can be a significant problem in this group of patients; it may be beneficial to involve the pain team if possible to help manage this. If the patient is a child, the parents must be totally involved in his care.

3. Give pre-operative care.
4. Give post-operative care:
   a. Remove pressure dressing at the first dressing, clean socket and instil prescribed antibiotic ointment. It is common practice to place a conformer (temporary shell) in the socket at the time of surgery to protect the underlying tissue and prevent conjunctival prolapse. Subsequently, the socket will be cleaned regularly and the ointment instilled. No further dressing is applied.
   b. The temporary shell may need to be checked and the patient informed of its presence.
   c. Teach the patient or parents to remove, clean and replace the shell, and instil antibiotic ointment.
5. On discharge, ensure that the patient has an appointment with the prosthetist and give him the assurance that he can return at any time to the hospital if there are any problems with the shell.

COMPLICATIONS

- The socket may become infected at any stage following removal of the eye. This requires cleaning of the socket and antibiotic treatment, usually ointment.
- The socket may shrink with time, causing the prosthesis to protrude and making it appear much larger than the other eye. A new prosthesis will need to be made.

PROSTHESES

Once the initial socket dressing has been removed following surgery and the socket is clean, a temporary shell is inserted into the socket to maintain the shape of the eyelids and to prevent them retracting. The patient is taught to remove, clean and replace this temporary shell and to make sure that the socket is clean.

At 4–6 weeks following surgery, a permanent individualised prosthesis will be made from an impression of the socket (Figure 6.5). The colour of the sclera, the pattern of the conjunctival vessels, the colour and pattern of the iris and the position of the pupil will be painted on by hand, carefully matching the other eye. Prosthetists are perfectionists who pay attention to the smallest of details.

Prostheses are nowadays made of an inert plastic material which can remain in the socket for up to 1 year. If there are no problems, the prosthesis is cleaned and polished annually to smooth any rough surfaces.

A prosthesis will need to be removed if it becomes too big for the shrinking socket or if the colour of the other eye changes – as it does with age – the sclera becoming less white and the conjunctival blood vessels more pronounced. The iris may change colour and an arcus senilis may appear.

Prostheses are made to measure and, with careful matching of the other eye, it is often dif-ficult to tell an artificial eye from a real one. Sometimes, the movement of the prosthesis is not as good as in a normal eye. Following an evisceration, movement should be nearly normal as

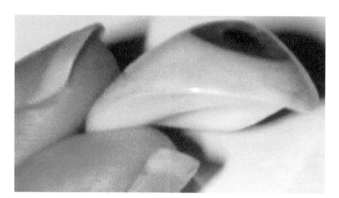

Figure 6.5 Artificial eye. (Courtesy of Louise Edwards.)

the extraocular muscles are still in place and can move the prosthesis. During an enucleation, the extraocular muscles are cut from their insertion in the sclera and sutured to the orbital implant. This affords some movement of the prosthesis. Implants can be rejected, and they tend to extrude after about 20 years, requiring removal. Some surgeons may cover the orbital implant at the time of surgery with an additional layer to prevent rejection, commonly using autologous sclera or temporal facia patch graft. Hydroxyapatite implants, being a naturally derived material from coral, with a similar structure to bone, are not as commonly rejected by the body. The body tissue actually grows into the implant.

Patients who undergo orbital exenteration surgery require considerable psychological support as well as considerable input to the socket's wound care requirements. It is common practice to line the socket with a split thickness skin graft harvested from the thigh. It may take several months for the socket to heal with a number of visits to the out patient department (OPD). The patient will need time to adjust and support from groups such as Changing Faces can provide help. Once the socket has completely healed it may be possible to have an artificial prosthesis fabricated to fill the socket.

Procedure guideline: Inserting/removing a prosthesis/shell

NURSING ACTION: INSERTING A PROSTHESIS/SHELL

1. Explain to the patient what you are going to do to gain informed consent.
2. Wash hands at the beginning and end of the procedure, and at any point when your hands become contaminated.
3. Pull up the upper lid and insert the prosthesis into the upper fornix.
4. Evert the lower lid and slip lower border of the prosthesis into the lower fornix.

NURSING ACTION: REMOVING A PROSTHESIS/SHELL

1. Explain to the patient what you are going to do to gain informed consent.
2. Wash hands at the beginning and end of the procedure, and at any point when your hands become contaminated.
3. Evert the lower lid and ease the prosthesis out. A small plastic spatula may be required to assist in the removal. The prosthesis then slips out.

CONDITIONS OF THE EYELIDS

Condition guideline: Chalazion

A chalazion is a swelling of one of the meibomian glands due to a blockage of its duct (Figure 6.6). It can affect either the upper or lower lid. It may become infected, when it is sometimes called an internal hordeolum. Staphylococci are commonly the cause of the infection. The swelling may fluctuate in size during the course of the condition. Some chalazions point to the skin surface. Some people appear to be prone to this condition and should be examined to ensure that they are not diabetic. Some chalazions are so large as to obstruct vision and, by pressing on the cornea, cause astigmatism.

PATIENT'S NEEDS

- Relief of swollen eyelid, which is causing pain and discomfort
- Relief of sticky discharge, which may be present

NURSING ACTION

1. Instruct the patient to apply steam/hot bathing to the eye.
2. Instruct the patient in the use of the antibiotic ointment which will be prescribed if the chalazion is infected. Chloramphenicol 1% is the usual ointment. This is used three to four times a day after the eye has been steamed. This should be continued for 14 days.
3. Instruct the patient to keep the eyelids clean by, twice a day, using warm water to wash off any crusts and discharge.
4. Instruct the patient to return if the swelling does not subside, as the simple operation of incision and curettage can be performed once the infection has cleared up, to remove any remaining material.
5. Sometimes for persistent or multiple chalazia an oral antibiotic course may be recommended, e.g. doxycycline.

Condition guideline: Oedema of the lids

Oedema of the lids is a common condition and, because of the looseness of the tissue, the swelling can be so great as to close the eye.

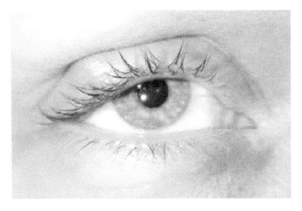

Figure 6.6 Meibomian cyst. (From Marsden, J., *Ophthalmic Care*. Wiley, Chichester, 2006, reproduced with permission.)

CAUSES

- Insect bites/stings
- Dermatitis
- Stye
- Chalazion

Oedema of the lids is associated with

- Orbital cellulitis
- Conjunctivitis
- Dacryocystitis
- Drug allergy

PATIENT'S NEEDS

- Reduction of swelling
- Treatment of cause
- Analgesia as required

NURSING ACTION

Explain to the patient the methods that should be used to reduce the swelling:

1. Cold compress
2. Bathing eyelid with sodium bicarbonate solution

Explain to the patient the treatment of the cause of the condition. Antihistamine ointment and/or tablets may be used to treat insect bites/stings.

Condition guideline: Blepharitis

Blepharitis can be an acute or a chronic inflammatory condition of the lid margins and is usually bilateral (Figure 6.7). It can be classified as anterior blepharitis or posterior blepharitis (that is anterior or posterior to the grey line). Blepharitis, and particularly posterior blepharitis, is often undetected, even when the eyes have been examined for other reasons.

CAUSES

- Staphylococcal – chronic infection
- Seborrhoeic – excessive secretion of lipid from meibomian glands
- Possible association with dandruff, poor hygiene, eczema or allergy to make-up, or drugs
- Acne rosacea

SIGNS

- Red, swollen lid margins
- Scales on lashes
- Eyelid irritation
- Burning sensation
- Itching
- Loss of eyelashes

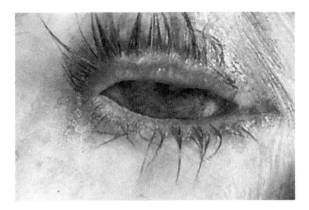

Figure 6.7 Staphylococcal blepharitis. (From Leitman, M., *Manual for Eye Examination and Diagnosis*, 7th edition, Blackwell Publishing, 2007, reproduced with permission.)

PATIENT'S NEEDS

The patient requires relief of the following symptoms:

- Itchiness around eye
- Discharge if an infective cause
- Burning sensation

NURSING ACTION

Instruct the patient on the treatment:

1. Cleaning the eyelids:
   a. Clean lid margin and lashes with diluted baby shampoo (as this does not cause stinging) or diluted sodium bicarbonate (half a teaspoon to half a cup of cooled, boiled water) twice a day. Use good-quality cotton buds or wrap a clean face cloth round your first finger to scrub the lid margins.
   b. There is an abundance of blepharitis treatments now available over the counter to aid with prevention and cleaning.
   c. Some patients prefer to scrub their eyelids while having a shower, in which case they should use the baby shampoo on a clean face cloth.
   d. Apply antibiotic ointment along the lid margin two or three times a day, if severe.
2. Dandruff – treat dandruff with antidandruff shampoo.
3. Make-up – stop using make-up or change the brand used: at the end of the day, remove all traces of make-up. It is advisable to dispose of eye make-up including mascara every 3 months.
4. Eczema – eczema may be treated with steroid ointment.
5. Drugs – stop using the offending drug.
6. Poor hygiene – instruct the patient on improving general hygiene, especially to hair, face and hands.
7. For the relief of soreness and itching, moisten clean face cloth under hot (as hot as you can stand) running water. Wring it out and place over closed eyelids. Repeat as the heat goes out of the face cloth.
8. Patients who are dependent on carers for their other hygiene needs should also be shown the technique of lid hygiene and general facial cleanliness.

Inform the patient that the treatment will need to continue for several weeks, if not for life, as it is a chronic condition, although the frequency of treatment can be reduced. Encourage him not to give up the treatment, even if it does not appear to be working in the initial stages.

COMPLICATIONS

Complications can occur following blepharitis caused by infective organisms that result in ulceration of the lid margin:

- Conjunctivitis
- Trichiasis and its sequelae due to chronic ulceration, which, when healed, contract the skin in that area, causing the lash(es) to turn inwards
- Entropion or ectropion of the lower lid in particularly severe cases
- Corneal ulcer

Condition guideline: Stye or external hordeolum

A stye or external hordeolum is an inflammation of a gland of Zeis that opens into the lash follicle. An abscess forms, which usually points near an eyelash.

SIGNS

Signs of a stye or external hordeolum are swelling, often with pointing on the lid margin situated near a lash.

PATIENT'S NEEDS

The patient requires relief of pain and swelling.

NURSING ACTION

1. Explain the treatment, which is similar to that for a chalazion.
2. Incision and curettage is not necessary for a stye. Removal of the affected lash will cause the abscess to drain, but this action is momentarily very painful.
3. If styes recur, the patient should be investigated for diabetes mellitus.

Condition guideline: Trichiasis

Trichiasis is a condition in which the lashes grow inwards and rub on the cornea. This may follow, for example, blepharitis, trauma or surgery to the lids. Often the cause is unknown.

PATIENT'S NEEDS

The patient requires removal of the offending lash(es) which is(are) causing irritation to the eye.

NURSING ACTION

1. Remove the lash by
   a. Epilating it using epilation forceps: this will need to be repeated regularly.
   b. Assisting the doctor or specialist nurse to use electrolysis, when an electrode is introduced to each offending lash follicle to destroy it.
      i. Prepare local anaesthetic injection and drops.
      ii. Instil antibiotic ointment to the eye following the procedure.

    c.   Assisting the doctor to apply cryotherapy (liquid nitrogen) to the lash follicle to destroy it:
        i.   Prepare local anaesthetic injection and drops.
        ii.   Instil antibiotic ointment following the procedure.
        iii.   Warn the patient that the eye will be uncomfortable for a few days following cryotherapy.
    d.   Assisting the doctor to apply argon laser to the offending lash.

2. Check the cornea for abrasions from the ingrowing lash(es) by staining lashes with G. fluorescein. If abrasions have occurred, instruct the patient to use the prescribed antibiotic ointment three times a day for 3 or 4 days.
3. Instruct the patient to return for further lash epilation as soon as he feels that the eye is becoming irritated, so that complications can be avoided by prompt treatment.

COMPLICATIONS

- Corneal abrasions
- Corneal ulceration
- Superficial corneal opacities
- Vascularisation of the cornea

Unfortunately, treatment is rarely completely successful and usually needs to be repeated at regular intervals.

Condition guideline: Entropion

Entropion is the turning inwards of the eyelid, usually the lower lid (Figure 6.8).

CAUSES

- Spastic entropion occurring in old age when spasm of the orbicularis muscle occurs, causing the lid to turn inwards
- Cicatricial contraction of the palpebral conjunctiva following trauma or disease to the lid or conjunctiva

PATIENT'S NEEDS

The patient requires relief of symptoms of irritation in the eye.

NURSING ACTION

1. As a temporary measure, strap the lower lid to pull it outwards. Care must be taken not to leave the globe exposed as this could cause complications such as exposure keratitis.
2. Prepare the patient and equipment for surgery to evert the lid. Care must be taken when performing entropion surgery to avoid an ectropion resulting.
3. Entropion operations include
    a.   Cautery
    b.   Transverse lid everting suture
    c.   Wies procedure – lid splitting and marginal rotation
    d.   Lower eyelid tightening by a lateral tarsal strip (LTS) procedure (often associated with a lower eyelid retractor reinsertion)
    e.   Shortening of lower lid retractors

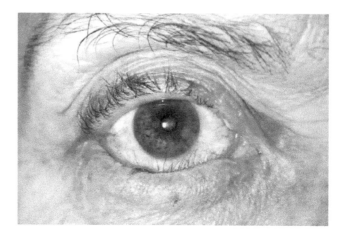

Figure 6.8 Spastic entropion. (From Olver J. and Cassidy, L. *Ophthalmology at a Glance*, Blackwell Publishing, 2005, reproduced with permission.)

COMPLICATIONS

The complications for entropion are the same as those for trichiasis.

Condition guideline: Ectropion

Ectropion is the turning outwards of the eyelid, usually the lower lid (Figure 6.9).

CAUSES

- Senile ectropion due to relaxation of the orbicularis muscle, turning the eyelid outwards
- Cicatricial ectropion due to scarring following trauma or chronic disease of the lid or conjunctiva, pulling lid outwards
- Paralytic ectropion occurring with palsies of the seventh cranial nerve
- Floppy eyelid syndrome

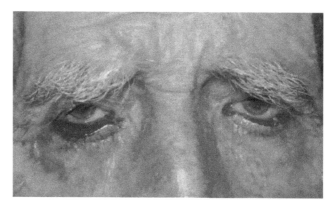

Figure 6.9 Ectropion. (From Marsden, J., *Ophthalmic Care*. Wiley, Chichester, 2006, reproduced with permission.)

Because the punctum is not in apposition to the bulbar conjunctiva when an ectropion is present, the tears cannot flow through the punctum and into the lacrimal drainage system. They therefore spill over the lid margin and down the cheek.

PATIENT'S NEEDS

The patient requires relief of symptoms:

- Watering eye
- Irritable sensation
- Discharge, which may be present
- Sore skin area over maxilla from constantly wiping away tears

NURSING ACTION

Prepare the patient and equipment for surgery to invert the lid:

1. Lower or upper eyelid wedge procedure (removing a section of the eyelid).
2. Retropunctal cautery and/or medial spindle.
3. Canthotomoy and cantholysis.

Care must be taken when performing ectropion surgery to avoid an entropion resulting.

Condition guideline: Ptosis

Ptosis is drooping of the upper lid (Figure 6.10). It may be unilateral, bilateral, constant or intermittent.

CAUSES

Congenital ptosis is caused by failure of development of the levator muscle. It is usually bilateral. The child with bilateral congenital ptosis has to tilt his head backwards to be able to see properly. This will prevent amblyopia developing. There is a danger that amblyopia will occur with unilateral ptosis.

Acquired ptosis is caused by

- Mechanical failure – Abnormal weight on lid due to oedema, tumour, scarring.
- Muscle involvement – Trauma to muscle. Disease involving muscles, e.g. muscular dystrophy, myasthenia gravis. If, following an injection of neostigmine, an anticholinesterase drug, the ptosis is temporarily relieved, myasthenia can be diagnosed.
- Paralysis of nerves supplying the upper lid (third nerve palsy).

PATIENT'S NEEDS

- Correction of lid, if it obscures sight
- Treatment of underlying disease

NURSING ACTION

Explain and prepare the patient for any of the following treatments:

1. Lid surgery, levator aponeurosis advancement, the most common procedure but also to resect the levator muscle or remove growths if present

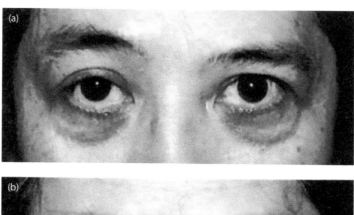

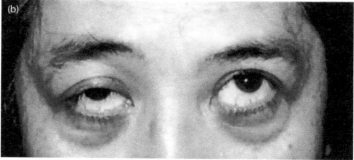

Figure 6.10 Left ptosis. (a) Primary position of gaze. (b) Upward position of gaze. (From Leitman, M., *Manual for Eye Examination and Diagnosis*, 7th edition, Blackwell Publishing, 2007, reproduced with permission.)

2. Wearing of special glasses or contact lenses with 'ptosis edge' to hold the lid up (rarely used)
3. Treatment of causative or underlying disease, e.g. myasthenia gravis

BELL'S PALSY

Bell's palsy is due to paralysis of the seventh nerve with resulting incomplete lid closure and corneal exposure. As a result of ineffective lid closure and corneal exposure, patients may present with a painful, red watery eye. The early management of Bell's palsy is aimed at the painful red eye. Initially copious topical lubricant and taping of the eyelid at night is all that is required. The patient will need constant reassurance and support at every stage. If corneal exposure is severe, a temporary lateral tarsorrhaphy may be needed. Lateral tarsorrhaphy joins the upper and lower lids laterally in order to reduce the palpebral aperture and protect the cornea. The long-term management of poor lid closure may include the implantation of gold weights into the upper lid. This procedure allows a better lid closure and a more natural blink. Possible complications may include extrusion or migration (Collin and Rose 2001).

BLEPHAROSPASM

Blepharospasm is a condition that causes forceful, painful spasm eyelid closure resulting in difficulty in opening the eye. Photophobia is present and the condition is exacerbated by bright lights, stress and excessive movement around the person. It can cause the individual concerned to become socially isolated and unable to work. There may be some accompanying contraction of the lower facial muscles. Treatment is by injections of botulinum (Bowling 2015) into the orbicularis muscle. This is repeated every 2–3 months.

Condition guideline: Tumours

Growths on the eyelids can be either benign or malignant.

BENIGN

- Papilloma
- Warts
- Granulomas
- Xanthelasma

MALIGNANT

- Basal cell carcinoma (see Figures 6.11 and 6.12)
- Squamous cell carcinoma
- Melanoma

PATIENT'S NEEDS

- Removal of tumour is required urgently, especially if it is thought to be malignant.
- Mohs' micrographic surgery (where available) is used in the management of periocular basal cell carcinoma. Mohs' micrographic surgery allows each cancerous layer to be visualised through the microscope. Excision of the cancerous layer continues until cancer-free layers are obtained.

NURSING ACTION

1. Prepare the patient and equipment for removal of the tumour. Skin grafting or flaps may be necessary depending on the size and position of the tumour.
2. Send specimen to the laboratory for histology.

Surgery to the lids must be performed with great care to avoid an ectropion, entropion or trichiasis resulting.

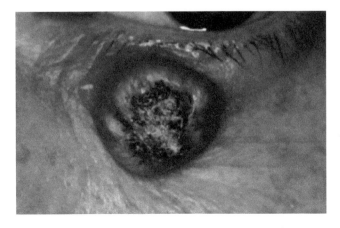

Figure 6.11 Rodent ulcer.

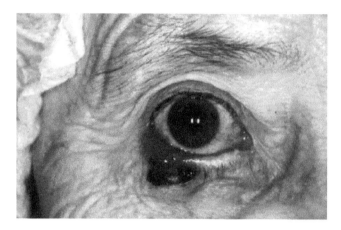

Figure 6.12 Basal cell carcinoma.

Reflective activity

Consider a patient whom you have seen recently with a problem associated with the protective structures:

- What were the presenting signs and symptoms?
- Was there any associated systemic disease or diseases?
- What tests and investigations were carried out and why?
- How did you arrive at a diagnosis?
- What was the treatment plan?
- Outline the care and management of the patient.
- If there were any challenges in caring for the patient, what were they?
- Was any other member of the multidisciplinary team involved in the care and what was their input?
- Utilising a recognised health-promotion framework, how would you explain the condition and treatment to the patient in order to ensure that he adheres to the treatment?
- What was the clinical outcome?
- What local or national policies, guidelines or protocols influenced the care and management of this patient?
- On reflection, would you have done anything differently and, if so, what?

Your completed case study can be used to contribute to your continuing professional development portfolio for Registration and your Knowledge and Skills Framework or appraisal review.

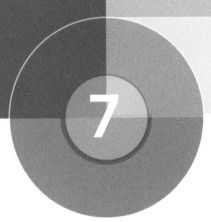

The lacrimal system and tear film

7

This chapter provides an overview of the gross anatomy and physiology and associated conditions and treatment.

INTRODUCTION

The lacrimal system (Figure 7.1) consists of

- The lacrimal gland
- The lacrimal drainage system comprising
  - Puncta
  - Canaliculi
  - Lacrimal sac
  - Nasolacrimal duct

LACRIMAL GLAND

The lacrimal gland is situated in the upper, outer quadrant of the orbit, in the lacrimal fossa of the frontal bone. It is almond shaped and is divided into two lobes by the levator palpebral muscle:

- Superior or orbital lobe
- Inferior or palpebral lobe

There are 10–12 drainage channels leaving the lacrimal gland to convey tears to openings in the upper fornix.

BLOOD SUPPLY

The lacrimal artery and vein supply and drain blood to and from the lacrimal gland.

NERVE SUPPLY

The nerve supply to the lacrimal gland is via the lacrimal nerve, the first branch of the ophthalmic division of the trigeminal nerve.

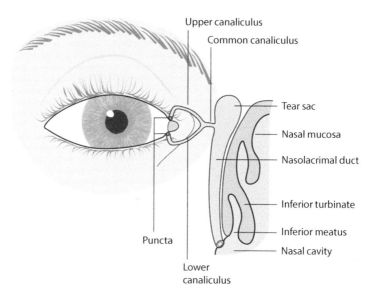

Upper canaliculus
Common canaliculus
Tear sac
Nasal mucosa
Nasolacrimal duct
Inferior turbinate
Inferior meatus
Nasal cavity
Puncta
Lower canaliculus

Figure 7.1 The major components of the lacrimal drainage system. (From Marsden, J., *Ophthalmic Care*. Wiley, Chichester, 2006, reproduced with permission.)

FUNCTION OF THE LACRIMAL GLAND

The function of the lacrimal gland is to produce tears in response to stimulation of the trigeminal nerve through, for example, emotion; foreign body on the cornea or conjunctiva; or noxious fumes, such as smoke or peeled onions.

LACRIMAL DRAINAGE SYSTEM

PUNCTA

The upper and lower puncta are small round or slightly oval apertures situated on the lid margin on a slight elevation called the lacrimal papilla. This is a pale area, due to the presence of few blood vessels, about 6 mm from the inner canthus. Both puncta are normally turned inwards towards the bulbar conjunctiva so tears can drain into them. Fibres of the orbicularis muscle surround them.

CANALICULI

The upper and lower canaliculi are narrow ducts passing from each puncta vertically for 1.5–2.0 mm, which then turn medially and travel horizontally for 10 mm. They usually unite to form a common canaliculus for about 1 mm before opening out into the lacrimal sac.

LACRIMAL SAC

The lacrimal sac is situated in the lacrimal fossa of the lacrimal bone. It is blind-ended superiorly, 5 mm wide and 12–14 mm in length. Fibres of the orbicularis and Horner's muscles surround the sac.

NASOLACRIMAL DUCT

The nasolacrimal duct is a downward continuation of the sac for 12–24 mm before opening into the inferior meatus of the nose beneath the inferior turbinate bone. The valve of Hasner, a mucosal fold, covers part of the opening. All the passages of the lacrimal drainage system are lined with epithelium.

BLOOD SUPPLY

Blood is supplied to the nasolacrimal duct via the nasal artery and the superior and inferior medial palpebral artery. Drainage is via the nasal vein and the superior and inferior medial palpebral veins.

NERVE SUPPLY

The infratrochlear nerve, a branch of the nasociliary nerve, which is the third branch of the ophthalmic division of the trigeminal nerve, provides the nerve supply for the nasolacrimal duct.

LYMPHATIC DRAINAGE

Lymph is drained from the nasolacrimal duct via the submaxillary nodes.

TEAR FILM

The tear film is a mixture of secretions from the accessory tear glands of Krause and Wolfring, the goblets cells of the conjunctiva and the meibomian glands of the eyelids. The tear film is a constant film of fluid bathing the conjunctiva and cornea. The lacrimal gland produces excess tears.

THREE LAYERS OF THE TEAR FILM

These layers are illustrated in Figure 7.2:

1. *Oil* – The outer layer, produced by the meibomian glands of the tarsal plates and also the glands of Moll and Zeis. The oily layer prevents evaporation and spillage of tears over the lid margin.
2. *Aqueous* – The middle layer, the 'tears proper', produced by the lacrimal gland and the glands of Krause and Wolfring.
3. *Mucin* – The inner layer, produced by the goblet cells of the conjunctiva, is a wetting substance for easy spread over the cornea.

COMPOSITION OF TEARS

Tears are composed of

- Water (98%)
- Protein (2%–5%)
- Glucose
- Urea

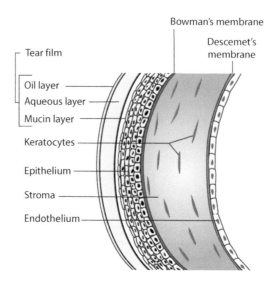

Figure 7.2 The structure of the cornea and precorneal tear film (schematic, not to scale – the stroma accounts for 95% of the corneal thickness). (From James, B., Chew, C., Bron, A., *Lecture Notes: Ophthalmology.* 10th edition., Blackwell Publishing, UK, 2007, reproduced with permission.)

- Sodium
- Potassium
- Retinol
- Chloride
- Lysozyme – an antimicrobial enzyme
- Immunoproteins and antimicrobial agents
- Normal pH is between 6.5 and 7.6 (Forrester et al. 2002)

FUNCTION OF TEARS

Tears have the following functions:

- Refraction – to provide an optically smooth surface to the cornea
- Lubrication of the front of the eyeball
- Cleansing action by washing away dust particles from the eye
- Protection from infection by secreting the enzyme lysozyme, immunoproteins and antimicrobial agents

FLOW OF TEARS

Tears flow across the front of the eyeball into the lacrimal drainage channels as a result of the following factors:

- Gravity itself assists tear flow.
- Blinking – Lid movements assist the flow of tears across the front of the cornea and conjunctiva.
- Capillary attraction into the puncta and canaliculi.
- The lacrimal pump – The contraction of orbicularis and Horner's muscles around the puncta and lacrimal sac dilate these structures and draw in the tears.
- Some tears are lost as a result of evaporation into the atmosphere.

CONDITIONS OF THE LACRIMAL SYSTEM

Condition guideline: Dacryoadenitis

Dacryoadenitis is a rare acute or chronic inflammation of the lacrimal gland. Causes include

- Acute:
  - Complication of systemic infections such as: mumps, measles, infectious mononucleosis or influenza
  - Trachoma
  - Herpes zoster
  - Staphylococcal infection
  - Following injury to the lacrimal gland
- Chronic:
  - Sarcoidosis
  - Tuberculosis
  - Syphilis
  - Lymphatic leukaemia
  - Lymphosarcoma

SIGNS AND SYMPTOMS

Acute:

- Pain – Swelling and redness of the upper lid, especially in the upper temporal aspect
- S-shaped curve to the upper lid

PATIENT'S NEEDS

- Relief of pain must be a priority. Measure pain and the effect of analgesia using an appropriate pain-assessment tool.
- Admission to hospital may be necessary if condition is severe.
- Incision of abscess should be performed where necessary.
- Application of warm compresses (as hot as the patient can tolerate without causing heat trauma) can provide some relief.
- Active infection should be treated with appropriate antibiotic.
- The underlying cause should be treated, if possible.

NURSING ACTION

1. Admit patient to hospital if condition is severe.
2. Give/advise the patient:
   a. To instil antibiotic drops and ointment, usually for 7–10 days
   b. To take any prescribed oral antibiotics for the duration of the course
   c. To take analgesics or apply local heat for pain relief
3. Prepare patient and equipment for incision of abscess.
4. Chronic – Normally painless and develops slowly. Treatment is usually with warm compresses and antibiotic therapy.

Condition guidelines: Dacryocystitis

Dacryocystitis is an acute or chronic inflammation of the lacrimal sac (Figure 7.3). It is a rare condition but is more common than dacryoadenitis. It is usually unilateral and is associated with obstruction to the lacrimal drainage system.

CAUSES

ACUTE

- Most causes of acute dacryocystitis are unknown
- Following chronic dacryocystitis
- Causative organisms include – staphylococci, streptococci and pneumococci

CHRONIC

- Following trauma to the lacrimal system
- Following chronic conjunctivitis, e.g. trachoma

INFANT

This may occur due to failure of canalisation of lacrimal ducts following birth.

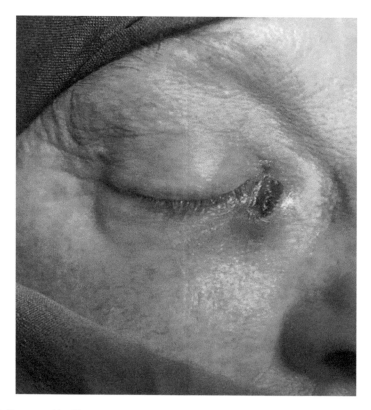

Figure 7.3 Dacrocystitis. (Courtesy of Keith Barton.)

SIGNS

ADULT ACUTE AND INFANT

- Pain
- Red, tender swelling over the lacrimal sac
- Pus regurgitating through the punctum
- Conjunctivitis
- Watering eye (epiphora), which may cause visual disturbance

CHRONIC

- There may be swelling over the lacrimal sac, which can be recurrent.
- Pus may emerge from the punctum when pressure is applied to the sac.
- Epiphora may be present, which may cause visual disturbance.

PATIENT'S NEEDS

ACUTE

- Relief of pain, which can be severe, with appropriate analgesia; warm compresses can effect some relief of pain. Measure pain and the effect of analgesia using an appropriate pain-assessment tool.
- Lid hygiene can be used to address the problem of discharge and watering eye.

CHRONIC

- Relief of watering eye due to blockage of drainage channels
- Diagnosis and treatment of obstruction

INFANT

- Relief of pain
- Lid hygiene to address the problem of discharge and watering eye
- Admission to hospital for probing of ducts if initial treatment fails

NURSING ACTION

ACUTE ADULT

1. Apply/instruct the patient how to apply warm compress to the inflamed area (clean face cloths rinsed under a warm tap can provide some relief).
2. Give/instruct him to take the prescribed analgesia, e.g. paracetamol 500 g and antibiotics, e.g. amoxicillin 250 mg three times a day for 7–10 days.
3. Clean/instruct him how to clean the eye if sticky and instil prescribed antibiotic drops or apply ointment, usually chloramphenicol or Fucithalmic.

CHRONIC ADULT

1. Perform lacrimal sac washout to detect area of blockage. *Note*: This is never carried out on a patient with an acute infection of the sac as the inflamed walls are easy to perforate.
2. Prepare patient for dacryocystogram. This is an x-ray using radio-opaque dye, which is introduced into the lacrimal drainage system to show up any blockage. Warn the patient that it is an uncomfortable procedure and that he should be accompanied home following this test as he may feel unwell.

3. Admit and prepare the patient for surgery to correct the blockage. Dacryocystorhinostomy (DCR) is performed to open up a new drainage channel into the nasal cavity. This may be performed using an endoscope or a more traditional external approach through the skin. Sometimes a tube is left *in situ* (DCR and tubes) for 3–6 months to maintain the patency of the new drainage channels. These tubes should not interfere with the cornea unless they extrude.

POST-OPERATIVE CARE

- Pain should be managed effectively, ideally using a pain-assessment tool to plot the severity of the pain and the degree of relief obtained following the administration of analgesia.
- In the immediate post-operative period, the patient must be monitored carefully for any epistaxis (nosebleed). Blood loss from this can be catastrophic. The haemorrhage may be overt or could be via the back of the throat. For this reason, pulse, blood pressure and respiratory rate should be monitored and, where used, an early warning score recorded. Where appropriate, urgent medical assistance must be obtained.
- A pressure dressing will remain in place until the dressing the morning after surgery. This should be observed for signs of haemorrhage.
- In the case of endoscopic DCR, a nasal pack will be *in situ*. This too must be observed for haemorrhage. It usually is removed the next day.
- Standard DCR:
    - Clean the eye and suture line.
    - Instil antibiotic drops; occasionally antibiotic cream is prescribed to be applied to the suture line. The surgeon may recommend that this is gently massaged in to reduce scarring.
    - Remove sutures 5–7 days post-operatively (usually in outpatient department).
    - Instruct the patient not to blow his nose vigorously as this could cause bleeding and will dislodge the tubing.
    - If a tube is present, it will be removed in the outpatient department. The procedure is relatively painless and does not warrant surgery.

INFANT

- Instruct the parent/guardian to instil topical antibiotic drops, e.g. G. chloramphenicol.
- Instruct the parent/guardian to massage over the lacrimal sac area to remove the accumulated mucus, which may lead to a patent duct.
- Admitting the child to hospital should be considered if these methods fail to open the canaliculus.
- A thorough pre-operative assessment as well as review by the anaesthetist should be completed. Parental or legal guardian's consent must be obtained.
- Probing of the tear ducts will be done under general anaesthetic.
- Give standard pre-operative care prior to probing of the ducts.
- Give post-operative care, including analgesia: instil antibiotic drops.

COMPLICATIONS

Following acute dacryocystitis, fistula formation may develop. DCR is not always successful in curing the watering eye.

Condition guideline: Epiphora

Epiphora is watering of the eye (increased lacrimation).

CAUSES

Causes of epiphora include

- Acute or chronic dacryocystitis
- Ectropion
- A small, tight or absent punctum
- Increased secretion of tears due to reflex stimulation of the lacrimal gland, e.g. by wind, smoke, onions, or a foreign body in the eye
- Allergy, e.g. hay fever

PATIENT'S NEEDS

- Explanation of the condition, its cause and prognosis
- Dilation of a small or tight punctum
- Removal of causative agent of increased stimulation
- Treatment of hay fever

NURSING ACTION

1. A careful history should be carried out of the presenting complaint, systematic examination of the eyelids, conjunctiva and the cornea.
2. If a foreign body is present, remove this appropriately.
3. If the cause is a small or tight punctum, this needs to be dilated regularly over a period of several months. This is usually performed every week or so using for example, a Nettleship dilator, holding it in place in the punctum for 5 minutes.
4. Prepare patient and equipment for a one, two or three-snip operation, which will be carried out if the dilation fails. During this procedure, performed under local anaesthetic, snips are made behind the punctum to release the muscle around the punctum.
5. Prescribe topical antihistamine drops such as lodoxamide 0.1%.

Condition guideline: Dry eye syndrome (keratoconjunctivitis sicca)

Dryness of the eye results from any disease associated with deficiency of any of the layers of the tear film as well as lid or corneal surface abnormalities. Its name (dry eyes) appears to imply a non-significant condition. This is not the case. In addition to being very uncomfortable, it has the potential to be sight threatening.

CAUSES

- Lacrimal gland failure
- Oil deficiency
- Exposure – proptosis, facial palsy
- Hot, dry climate/environment
- Lid damage
- Blepharitis

- Meibomianitis
- Aqueous deficiency
- Sjögren's syndrome (arthritis, dry eye, achlorhydria)
- Removal/absence of glands
- Trachoma
- Chronic dacryoadenitis
- Drugs – beta-blockers, diuretics
- Old age
- Menopause
- Mucin deficiency
- Chemical burns
- Chronic conjunctivitis
- Antihistamines
- Stevens–Johnson syndrome
- Xerophthalmia
- Other causes – deficient blinking; corneal scarring

SIGNS

- Usually a normal-looking eye.
- Damaged epithelial, corneal and conjunctival cells stain with fluorescein drops.
- Breaks in the tear film are seen when stained with G. fluorescein. The normal tear break-up time is usually over 10 seconds.

PATIENT'S NEEDS

- An adequate explanation of the condition
- Recognition that it causes ocular disturbance
- Advice that this is a chronic condition and treatment is about relieving symptoms or preventing symptoms from occurring
- Relief of symptoms that include
  - Gritty feeling
  - Itching
  - Burning sensation
  - Inability to produce tears
  - Pain around and in the eye
  - Sometimes a red eye
  - Difficulty in opening eyes on waking and moving lids
  - Excessive watering eye (if the outer oil layer of the tear film is deficient, tears will spill over the lower lid margin)
- Investigation and treatment of underlying cause, if possible
- Treatment with replacement tears

NURSING ACTION

1. Perform tear production test. In some centres, tear osmolality is also tested.
2. Instruct the patient to use the prescribed artificial tears, e.g. G hypromellose. These drops can usually be used as often as the patient requires, keeping the eye feeling comfortable, and will probably need long-term use.
3. Cautery to the punctum or insertion of punctal plugs may be employed to prevent what little tears are produced from draining into the punctum.

COMPLICATIONS

- Chronic conjunctivitis due to loss of the protective function of the tear film and lysozyme
- Corneal scarring and vascularisation
- Corneal ulceration, thinning and perforation
- Eventual loss of the eye through recurrent infections

Reflective activity

Consider a patient that you have seen recently with a condition affecting the lacrimal system or tear film:

- What were the presenting signs and symptoms?
- Was there any associated systemic disease or diseases?
- What tests and investigations were carried out and why?
- How did you arrive at a diagnosis?
- What was the treatment plan?
- Outline the care and management of the patient.
- If there were any challenges in caring for the patient, what were they?
- Was any other member of the multidisciplinary team involved in the care and what was his or her input?
- Utilising a recognised health-promotion framework, how would you explain the condition and treatment to the patient in order to ensure that he or she adheres to the treatment?
- What was the clinical outcome?
- What local or national policies, guidelines or protocols influenced the care and management of this patient?
- On reflection, would you have done anything differently and, if so, what?

Your completed case study can be used to contribute to your continuing professional development portfolio for Registration and your Knowledge and Skills Framework or appraisal review.

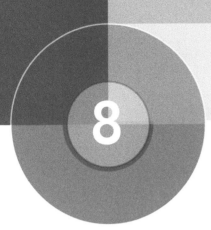

The conjunctiva and sclera

8

This chapter explores some of the more common conditions seen.

THE CONJUNCTIVA

The conjunctiva is a thin, transparent mucous membrane lining the upper and lower lids and covering the globe up to the limbus.

AREAS OF THE CONJUNCTIVA

There are three areas to the conjunctiva:

1. Palpebral conjunctiva – lines the upper and lower lids
2. Bulbar conjunctiva – reflects back to cover the sclera up to the limbus
3. Fornices – the upper and lower fornices are blind sacs, formed where the bulbar and palpebral conjunctiva fold back over each other

LAYERS OF THE CONJUNCTIVA

The epithelial layer contains the goblet cells; the stromal layer contains the blood vessels, nerves and the glands of Krause and Wolfring (in upper part only).

The conjunctiva is connected to Tenon's capsule around the limbus. Elsewhere, it is loosely attached, especially in the fornices where there are folds of the conjunctiva. This allows for easy mobility of the eyeball.

FUNCTIONS OF THE CONJUNCTIVA

- The conjunctiva allows easy movement of the eyeball.
- Goblet cells provide mucin for the tear film.
- The conjunctiva is a protective layer to the eyeball by being a physical barrier and because of its rich blood supply.

BLOOD SUPPLY

There is a rich blood supply, especially in the fornices delivered and drained via the

- Two palpebral arches and the anterior ciliary arteries and veins
- Superior and inferior medial palpebral artery and vein

NERVE SUPPLY

The nerve supply to the conjunctiva is by the long ciliary branch of the nasociliary nerve from the trigeminal nerve.

LYMPHATIC DRAINAGE

Lymphatic drainage is through the preauricular, parotid and submaxillary nodes.

CONDITIONS OF THE CONJUNCTIVA

CONJUNCTIVITIS

Conjunctivitis is inflammation of the conjunctiva, which has several causes:

- Bacterial
- Viral
- Allergic
- Chlamydial
- Fungal
- Parasitic
- Associated with other diseases
- Associated with other ophthalmic conditions
- Caused by other forms of conjunctivitis – contact lens-related conjunctivitis, traumatic conjunctivitis, toxicity following exposure to drugs or noxious chemicals, mechanical conjunctivitis such as trichiasis, sutures, foreign bodies and conjunctival concretions.

BACTERIAL CONJUNCTIVITIS

Bacterial conjunctivitis can be either acute or chronic. Acute conjunctivitis usually lasts less than 3 weeks. It is usually self-limiting and usually settles without treatment within 1–2 weeks (Rose 2007). However, evidence from good-quality trials has shown that treating people with proven bacterial conjunctivitis with a topical ocular antibiotic modestly reduces the severity and duration of conjunctivitis (Everitt, Little, and Smith 2006; Sheikh and Hurwitz 2006; Renouf 2007). The risk of serious complication as a result of untreated acute bacterial conjunctivitis is low.

Condition guideline: Bacterial conjunctivitis

CAUSATIVE ORGANISMS

- Streptococcus
- *Staphylococcus aureus*

- Pneumococcus
- Gonococcus
- Haemolytic streptococcus

SIGNS

Typically, there is conjunctival injection, especially in the fornices where the blood supply is rich. The onset is usually acute, and both eyes are usually affected with one eye being affected first. The fellow eye usually becomes involved within 48 hours. Discharge is variable, but typically is present in the mornings and, on waking, the eye is difficult to open because the eyelids are stuck together with mucopurulent discharge. This is a very important point when taking a history from a patient with suspected conjunctivitis as viral conjunctivitis often presents with a watery sticky discharge instead. The eyelids may be red and inflamed. The condition may be unilateral, but very often it is bilateral. The vision is always unaffected and there is usually no pain. The patient may complain of a gritty or foreign-body sensation, some discomfort and, very occasionally, very mild photophobia. In severe cases, inflammatory membranes may be present in the upper and lower eyelids.

NURSING ACTION

1. Take and record the patient's visual acuity to assess baseline visual acuity and to monitor any improvement or deterioration in visual acuity.
2. Taking conjunctival swabs is only necessary if there is any doubt of the diagnosis or if the condition has not resolved as it is not usually considered useful for people with acute infective conjunctivitis (Marsden 2008).
3. Obtain an accurate history from the patient to determine a correct diagnosis. Sometimes there is a history of close contact with someone who is infected. Questioning of the patient should also include any symptoms of upper respiratory infections to aid diagnosis.
4. Examination of the eye on a slit lamp should be carried out to confirm diagnosis. Enlargement of the preauricular lymph node is also an indicative sign of acute conjunctivitis.
5. Clean the eye(s) and instruct the patient on cleaning it (them), using cooled, boiled water.
6. Give verbal and written instruction on how to instil the eye drops. This is usually G. chloramphenicol, which may be prescribed four times a day for a period of 7–10 days. In severe cases, chloramphenicol drops may be prescribed every 2 hours for 2 days and then four times a day for 7–10 days. If warranted, an ointment can also be prescribed for night-time application. According to the BNF (British National Formulary 2015), the notion that chloramphenicol increases the risk of developing aplastic anaemia is poorly founded. Caution should also be exercised in women who are pregnant, especially in the third trimester. If in doubt, fusidic acid (Fucithalmic) can be prescribed instead. In children, it is wise to prescribe fusidic acid as this only necessitates a twice-daily drop regime.
7. Instruct the patient on how to prevent the spread of infection either to his other eye or to other members of the household:
   a. Wash hands before and after instilling eye medications and after touching the eyes.
   b. Use separate face flannels and towels in the home, as this is the usual method of spread of infection. Change face flannels and towels daily.

  c. Use clean tissues rather than handkerchief to reduce the spread of infection.
  d. Change pillowcases daily.
  8. Store chloramphenicol eye drops in a cool place, preferably in a refrigerator.
  9. Never share drops and ointment with anyone else.
  10. It is important that patients are reminded to complete the prescribed course of treatment.
  11. Warn the patient not to wear a pad over the eye, as it provides a suitable environment for further bacterial growth.
  12. If eye make-up is used, advise the patient to discard it and to buy new cosmetics when the infection has cleared up.
  13. If the patient is a wearer of contact lenses, advise him that the wearing of lenses should stop until all signs and symptoms have been completely resolved. This is because the drug and preservative may be absorbed by the lenses resulting in a toxic reaction. Contact lens wear should only be resumed 24 hours after any treatment has been completed (BNF 2014).

Chronic conjunctivitis

Any bacterial conjunctivitis lasting for more than 4 weeks can be considered chronic and usually has a different aetiology. Chronic conjunctivitis is usually caused by *Staphylococcus* species and is often associated with rosacea, blepharitis and facial seborrhea. Complications of chronic conjunctivitis are

- Conjunctival scarring
- Chronic blepharitis due to upset in the tear film
- Conjunctival ulceration leading to perforation due to decreased conjunctival nutrition
- Marginal corneal ulcer

OPHTHALMIA NEONATORUM

Ophthalmia neonatorum is defined as severe conjunctivitis occurring in a baby less than 28 days old and is no longer a notifiable disease. The disease is acquired from the birth canal during delivery. The organisms are those of sexually transmitted pathogens passed from the mother's genito-urinary tract to the baby at birth. The condition is now on the increase (Fearnley 2014).

This may be caused by gonococcus, streptococcus, or Chlamydia, the latter being the most common cause. According to Yanoff and Duker (2009), an infant whose mother is Chlamydia-positive has a 30%–40% chance of developing conjunctivitis, and a 10%–12% chance of developing pneumonia. Ophthalmia neonatorum is an ophthalmic emergency as if untreated, corneal ulceration and perforation may occur. However, this condition needs to be distinguished from the neonatal conjunctivitis caused by nasolacrimal obstruction with other bacterial infection, trauma and inclusion conjunctivitis agents.

Ophthalmia neonatorum often presents itself between 5 and 19 days after birth and can be associated with marked conjunctival injection. All babies presenting with a sticky eye(s) to the department should have microbiology swabs taken, including chlamydial, even if there are no plans to treat with antibiotics. Formal arrangements must be made to review the results 2–4 days later, ideally with patient recall. All results positive for chlamydia or gonococcus should be reported immediately so that appropriate treatment and follow-up can be arranged.

It is not the role of the eye department to provide counselling for the parents. However, it is the role of the department to instigate the proper management of all concerned, which means prompt referral to the sexual health clinic where follow-up of both parents can take place.

Condition guideline: Ophthalmia neonatorum

SIGNS

- Severe discharge
- Red, swollen eyelids
- Chemosis
- Unilateral or bilateral infection

NURSING ACTION

1. The condition must be clearly and sensitively explained to both parents (or carers). They should be told of the baby's diagnosis and the likelihood of how the baby acquired the infection.
2. Both parents must be screened and examined at the genito-urinary medicine clinic.
3. Instruct the parent as to how to clean the eye and instil the prescribed antibiotics.
4. Topical tetracycline and oral erythromycin is the treatment of choice.
5. This condition can be associated with otitis media and gastrointestinal tract infections, so oral antibiotics are usually prescribed.

Condition guideline: Viral conjunctivitis

CAUSES

- Adenovirus
- Measles
- Varicella
- Herpes simplex
- Chlamydia

SIGNS

- Red/pink eye.
- Chemosis, if severe.
- Follicles may be present on the palpebral conjunctiva.
- Cornea – superficial punctate keratitis.
- Enlarged preauricular nodes, which may be tender.
- Bleeding from conjunctival vessels in severe adenoviral conjunctivitis.

PATIENT'S NEEDS

- Relief of symptoms
  - Watering eye
  - Irritation, which may be present
  - Generally unwell feeling
- Instruction on treatment

NURSING ACTION

1. Treatment is mainly supportive and educative since there is no effective treatment for adenovirus conjunctivitis.
2. Usually no treatment is given as viral infections are self-limiting, running a course of 7–10 days.

3. Artificial lubricant can be prescribed for patient comfort.
4. A full explanation of the condition should be given to increase patient awareness.
5. General advice for hygiene is the same as for bacterial conjunctivitis.
6. Thorough cleaning of slit lamps should be carried out using soap and water.
7. If tonometer prisms are used during the examination, use disposable Tonoshield or Tonosafe where possible. If these are unavailable, then the prism must be wiped clean while moist before the face of the lens is immersed in the disinfection fluid recommended by the manufacturer. Rinsing in saline after removal from the disinfectant and before use is essential.
8. Vigilant handwashing should be carried out by all medical and nursing personnel and by those who come into contact with patients.

Condition Guideline: Allergic conjunctivitis

There are different types of allergic conjunctivitis, including atopic keratoconjunctivitis, seasonal conjunctivitis, vernal conjunctivitis and giant papillary conjunctivitis.

CAUSES

- Hay fever – tends to be seasonal as a result of pollen.
- Exposure to eye medications or, if wearing contact lenses, allergy to the solutions.
- Climate may be a factor, especially for those living in warm and dry climates.

SIGNS

- Severe conjunctival chemosis
- Oedematous eyelids
- Red eye
- Possible presence of papillae on the palpebral conjunctiva

SYMPTOMS

- Irritation of the eye
- Itchy eyes
- Watering eye
- Possible presence of nasal signs of hay fever

TREATMENT

- Antihistamines such as xylometazoline hydrochloride (Otrivine-Antistin) drops can be used four times a day or G. sodium cromoglycate (Opticrom) 2% four times a day.
- Opatanol instilled twice a day is also effective in the management of seasonal conjunctivitis.
- Cold compresses to the eyes can help relieve symptoms.
- Steroids can be used if the condition is severe.

Condition guideline: Vernal conjunctivitis or spring catarrh

Vernal conjunctivitis or spring catarrh is a common seasonal, warm-weather condition, with some patients being affected annually in the spring or early summer. It usually affects the 10- to 14-year-old age group, with boys being more affected than girls.

SIGNS

- Giant papillae on sub-tarsal conjunctiva, called 'cobblestones' (see Chapter 4, Figure 4.3)
- Corneal punctate epithelial erosions
- Thick mucus discharge
- Punctate epithelial staining

SYMPTOMS

The symptoms of vernal conjunctivitis or spring catarrh are irritation, ocular itching or the sensation of having a foreign body in the eye.

TREATMENT

- Treatment involves G. sodium cromoglycate 2%; or steroids if severe.
- Test for allergy and avoid the cause, if possible.

Condition guideline: Eczema

SIGNS

- Redness of eye
- Red, dry, scaly eyelid
- Possible involvement of skin around the eye
- Possible presence of slight discharge
- Fine papillae on palpebral conjunctiva

SYMPTOMS

- Burning sensation
- Photophobia

TREATMENT

- Antibiotic drops to prevent secondary infection
- Steroid cream, e.g. betamethasone, sodium phosphate or hydrocortisone to eyelid and affected skin around the eye

Condition guideline: Trachoma

Trachoma, also known as Egyptian ophthalmia or granular conjunctivitis, is caused by an organism called *Chlamydia trachomatis*, which is a parasite closely related to bacteria. Trachoma is caused by serotypes A, B, Ba and C. It is common in hot, dry climates in which there is a poor standard of hygiene and in which flies are abundant (Wright et al. 2008). The disease runs a long and chronic course. The incubation period is 5–14 days. In a child, the onset is insidious, but it is acute in an adult.

SIGNS AND SYMPTOMS

- Oedematous eyelids
- Discharge
- Pain

- Follicles, especially on the upper lid
- Photophobia
- Repeated attacks, leading to entropion and corneal involvement
- Long term – corneal scarring, leading to severe loss of vision and blindness

The World Health Organization (WHO) classification of trachoma is as follows:

TF	Trachomatous inflammation with follicles
TI	Trachomatous inflammation – intense
TS	Trachomatous scarring
TT	Trachomatous trichiasis
CO	Corneal opacity

TREATMENT

Trachoma must be treated in the early stages with tetracyclines, erythromycin or sulphon-amides, for 4–6 weeks.

COMPLICATIONS

- Conjunctival scarring and fibrosis resulting in
  - Blockage to the drainage of the accessory tear glands and lacrimal gland resulting in a reduced tear film.
  - Reduction in secretion of mucin.
- Both the reduced tear film and the reduction in the secretion of mucin will cause a reduction in lysozyme in the tear film, and therefore the patient will be prone to chronic conjunctivitis.
- Blocked lacrimal ducts from conjunctival scarring, which could cause dacryocystitis.
- Entropion and trichiasis.
- Ptosis, due to scarring under the top lid.
- Scarring of the cornea due to pannus formation, trichiasis and scarred palpebral conjunctiva.

TREATMENT OF COMPLICATIONS

- Scarred conjunctival tissue can be treated by expressing and curetting the follicles. Plastic surgery may be necessary to correct lid deformities.
- A corneal graft can be performed to replace the scarred cornea. This can only be performed once the lid deformities have been corrected so that they will not abrade the grafted cornea.
- Replacement teardrops can be administered to treat the dry eyes.
- Antibiotic drops can be prescribed for chronic bacterial conjunctivitis.
- Antibiotic treatment can be prescribed for dacryocystitis.
- A dacryocystorhinostomy can be performed to correct the blocked nasolacrimal ducts.

FUNGAL CONJUNCTIVITIS

Fungal conjunctivitis is rare and is usually caused by *Candida albicans*. Babies can be affected during birth through an infected birth canal. Fine white plaques are apparent on the conjunctiva. Affected adults have blepharitis. The treatment is normally undertaken in specialist units.

PARASITIC CONJUNCTIVITIS

In hot climates, parasites causing onchocerciasis (river blindness) and schistosomiasis (bilharzia) can induce conjunctivitis.

CONJUNCTIVITIS CAUSED BY OTHER DISEASES

General diseases that cause conjunctivitis are

- Skin diseases – psoriasis, pemphigoid, acne rosacea and pemphigus
- Sjögren's syndrome
- Thyroid disease
- Reiter's syndrome

OPHTHALMIC CONDITIONS CAUSING CONJUNCTIVITIS

Ophthalmic conditions that cause conjunctivitis are

- Dacryocystitis
- Canaliculitis
- Dry eyes

The treatment is that of the general disease or ophthalmic condition.

MECHANICAL CONJUNCTIVITIS

Conjunctivitis can occur after the conjunctiva has been exposed to

- Wind
- Fumes
- Smoke
- Dust
- Dirt particles
- Chemicals

Condition guideline: Subconjunctival haemorrhage

Subconjunctival haemorrhage occurs as a result of a blunt or penetrating injury, but it can also occur spontaneously or as a result of a sudden increase in pressure in the eye, as occurs with violent sneezing or heavy lifting. The subconjunctival blood vessels burst, with the affected area varying in size; in severe cases the haemorrhage can cover the whole of the sclera, causing swelling but usually sparing the superior aspect as it pools inferiorly from gravity (Tarlan and Kiratli 2013). In cases occurring spontaneously, the patients usually have few symptoms apart from a dull ache. It is a condition that looks more severe than it is. It can be a sign of hypertension, vascular disease or a blood-clotting disorder.

PATIENT'S NEEDS

Patients with subconjunctival haemorrhage require identification of the location of the cause, if any, of the spontaneous haemorrhage.

NURSING ACTION

1. Ask the patient if he had exerted any undue pressure before the haemorrhage occurred, e.g. by heavy digging in the garden, sneezing fit, rubbing the eye.
2. Take the blood pressure; if abnormally high, take appropriate action including retaking the blood pressure, if still elevated, write to the GP.
3. Reassure the patient that the haemorrhage will not cover the cornea.
4. Inform the patient that it may spread further before it begins to resolve and that it may take 2–3 weeks to clear completely, similar to a bruise. Usually there is no specific treatment.
5. Check if patients are on aspirin, warfarin or any other relevant medication.
6. Advise the patient to see GP for advice such as INR (international normalized ratio) check if appropriate.
7. If subconjunctival haemorrhage is as a result of trauma, the eye has to be carefully examined under the slit lamp for any other injuries.

PTERYGIUM

A pterygium is a triangular-shaped nodule in the conjunctiva (Figure 8.1), usually occurring on the nasal side, but it can be temporal. It usually occurs in people who live in hot, dry climates or who work in the open air. It is a degenerative process and can encroach on the cornea. If it affects the vision or, if there are cosmetic concerns, it can be removed under local anaesthetic. Lamellar keratoplasty is indicated if the visual axis is involved.

PINGUECULA

A pinguecula is a yellow, triangular nodule found in the conjunctiva of the elderly and in people who work in exposed conditions. It affects the nasal side and later the temporal side. It does not spread to the cornea and no treatment is necessary unless it becomes inflamed, in which case steroid drops will reduce the condition. It can be removed for cosmetic reasons.

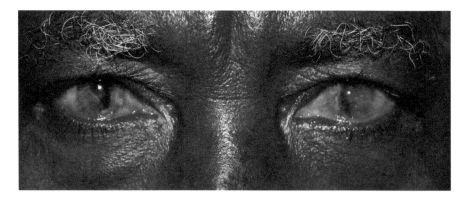

Figure 8.1 Pterygium. (Courtesy of Keith Barton.)

CONCRETIONS

Concretions are white deposits found in the conjunctiva. They are fairly common and usually do not exhibit symptoms. Occasionally, they are large enough to give a foreign-body sensation, in which case they can be removed under local topical anaesthetic using a sterile green needle. If bleeding occurs during this procedure, a pad and bandage should be applied. Topical antibiotic cover may be prescribed.

CONJUNCTIVAL CYSTS

Cysts can occur in the conjunctiva. If they cause symptoms, they are easily punctured under local topical anaesthetic using a sterile green needle. Topical antibiotic cover may be prescribed. This can be a recurrent condition.

THE SCLERA

'Sclera' in Greek means 'hard'. The sclera is the 'white' of the eye, composed of dense, white, non-uniform collagen fibres. It is kept hydrated and is, therefore, opaque. The sclera extends from the cornea (the limbus) to the optic nerve.

The sclera is 0.6–1.00 mm thick, although where the four recti muscles are inserted into it, it is only 0.3 mm thick. It has a protective function.

AREAS OF THE SCLERA

There are four areas to note:

1. *Lamina cibrosa* – A sieve-like structure where a few strands of scleral tissue pass behind the optic disc
2. *Posterior aperture* – Lies around the optic nerve and is the area where the long and short ciliary vessels and nerves penetrate the sclera to travel forward in the eye to supply the choroid and ciliary body
3. *Four middle apertures* – Situated at the 'equator' where the four vortex veins exit through the sclera
4. *Anterior aperture* – Lies 4 mm posterior to the limbus where the anterior ciliary vessels puncture the sclera

THE LIMBUS

The limbus is the transitional zone, 1.2 mm wide between the cornea, conjunctiva and sclera.

THE EPISCLERA

The episclera is a fine elastic tissue covering the surface of the sclera. It has a rich blood supply from the long posterior ciliary arteries to nourish the sclera lying beneath it.

SCLERAL NERVE SUPPLY

The ciliary nerve from the oculomotor nerve provides the nerve supply to the sclera.

CONDITIONS AFFECTING THE SCLERA

EPISCLERITIS

Episcleritis is inflammation of the episclera. It may be unilateral or bilateral and can be associated with rheumatoid arthritis, gout and ulcerative colitis, but the cause is often unknown.

There is a localised area of redness, usually triangular, with the apex pointing towards the limbus. There may or may not be a nodule present in the area of redness. The area is tender and, on examination, the conjunctiva moves freely over the enlarged episcleral blood vessels. Treatment is with non-steroidal anti-inflammatory drugs such as Acular.

SCLERITIS

Scleritis is a rare condition affecting women more than men. In 50% of cases, it is associated with connective tissue diseases, such as rheumatoid arthritis and ankylosing spondylitis. It can also be associated with uveitis, glaucoma and cataract. If it is anterior, the eye will be red, with tenderness over the affected area. If it is posterior, the eye will look white. Pain is the main feature and may be severe. Steroid drops will be used for anterior scleritis and systemic anti-inflammatory drugs, such as ibuprofen, for posterior scleritis.

Quiz

1. What is the conjunctiva lining the sclera called?
2. What is the conjunctiva lining the lids called?
3. What are the different causes of conjunctivitis?
4. What is ophthalmia neonatorum?
5. Your patient has been diagnosed with a subconjunctival hemorrhage. What observations would you undertake?
6. What is the difference between pterygium and pinguecula?

Reflective activity

Consider a patient whom you have seen recently with a condition of the conjunctiva or sclera:

- What were the presenting signs and symptoms?
- Was there any associated systemic disease or diseases?
- What tests and investigations were carried out and why?
- How did you arrive at a diagnosis?
- What was the treatment plan?
- Outline the care and management of the patient.
- If there were any challenges in caring for the patient, what were they?
- Was any other member of the multidisciplinary team involved in the care and what was his or her input?
- Utilising a recognised health-promotion framework, how would you explain the condition and treatment to the patient in order to ensure that the treatment is adhered to?

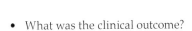

- What was the clinical outcome?
- What local or national policies, guidelines or protocols influenced the care and management of this patient?
- On reflection, would you have done anything differently and, if so, what?

Your completed case study can be used to contribute to your continuing professional development portfolio for Registration and your Knowledge and Skills Framework or appraisal review.

The cornea

9

This chapter provides an overview of the anatomy and physiology of the cornea, as well as an overview of common conditions.

INTRODUCTION

Forming the anterior one-sixth of the eyeball, the cornea is a transparent structure which fits into the surrounding sclera like a watch-glass. It is convex, avascular and highly sensitive. The site where the cornea becomes continuous with the sclera is known as the corneal limbus.

MEASUREMENTS

Measurements of the cornea are as follows: vertical 10.6 mm; horizontal 11.5 mm; and thickness 0.6 mm centrally and 1.0 mm peripherally.

The centre of the cornea measures approximately 0.5–0.6 mm and the periphery of the cornea measures about 0.7 mm. The thinness of the cornea is significant and must be considered when removing central corneal foreign bodies.

FIVE LAYERS OF THE CORNEA

The cornea has five layers from the outermost to the innermost (Wilson and Last 2004), and these are illustrated in Figure 9.1. They are as follows:

- *Epithelium* – There are five to six layers of epithelial cells, which are continuous with the conjunctival epithelium. The basement membrane is the innermost layer of the epithelium. The epithelium is the only layer of the cornea that regenerates following trauma.
- *Bowman's membrane* – This is a layer of connective tissue, which does not regenerate when damaged.
- *Stroma* – This comprises 90% of the cornea, and is composed of parallel connective tissue.
- *Descemet's membrane* – This is a layer of elastic fibres.

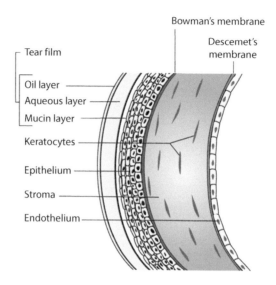

Figure 9.1 The cornea. (Courtesy of Debbie Morley.)

- *Endothelium* – This comprises a single layer of endothelial cells, which are metabolically active, and their primary function is the control of stromal hydration. The endothelium elongates when damaged.
- Recent research by Dua et al. (2013) has discovered an additional layer of the cornea which lies between the stroma and Descemet's layer. This is dubbed as the Dua's layer and is a skinny but tough structure measuring just 15 microns thick. Its recognition will have considerable impact on posterior corneal surgery and the understanding of corneal biomechanics and posterior corneal pathology such as acute hydrops, Descemetocele and pre-Descemet's dystrophies.

FUNCTION OF THE CORNEA

The function of the cornea is to protect the eye, and to enable refraction of light. The convex shape of the cornea allows most of the refraction of light rays within the eye to take place here, approximately 40 dioptres. The cornea must remain transparent to allow light rays to enter the eye and for sight to be clear. Clarity is maintained by

- *Avascularity of the structure* – There are no blood vessels to impede the transmission of light rays.
- *Uniform structure of the stromal layer* – The fibres lie in a parallel fashion; if they are pushed apart, for example by oedema, the structure becomes opaque and blurred vision results.
- *Dehydration* – The cornea is kept semi-dehydrated by the endothelial layer. This is a sodium pump whereby sodium, and therefore water, is pumped out of the cornea to be replaced by potassium. Where this layer is damaged, the pump ceases to work efficiently.

BLOOD SUPPLY

The blood supply and drainage is via the anterior ciliary artery and vein by limbal diffusion which ends at the circumference of the cornea. The cornea itself is avascular. The cornea receives some nourishment from the aqueous humour and capillaries at the edge of the cornea and from the tear film, containing oxygen from the air.

NERVE SUPPLY

The cornea is highly sensitive, receiving its nerve supply from the long ciliary nerve of the naso-ciliary nerve. This is the third branch of the ophthalmic division of the trigeminal nerve. The nerve endings lie under the epithelial layer.

PHYSIOLOGY OF CORNEAL SYMPTOMS

- Pain – Due to many pain fibres being present in the cornea
- Blurred or reduced vision – Due to a lesion obstructing light rays entering and refracting at the cornea
- Watering – Due to irritation of the corneal nerve endings

CONDITIONS OF THE CORNEA

EXPOSURE KERATITIS

Exposure keratitis is an inflammation of the cornea resulting from drying of the cornea because the eyelids cannot protect it adequately. It is potentially a dangerous condition as, without treatment, it can lead to ulceration and perforation of the cornea.

The lids are unable to cover the cornea, either because of proptosis of the eyeball or the inability of the lids to move over the eyeball. Once recognised, this condition must be treated promptly by taking measures to protect the cornea. Bandage contact lenses can be used or a tarsorrhaphy performed, with the use of eye ointment to form a protective layer. Other causes of exposure keratitis include facial nerve palsy and scarring of the eyelids. Certain individuals with no abnormal pathology may be prone to exposure keratitis during sleep.

CORNEAL ULCERS

Corneal ulcers develop as a result of local necrosis of corneal tissue by bacteria, viruses, fungi or *Acanthamoeba*. The most common corneal ulcer is caused by bacteria such as staphylococcus, pseudomonas or streptococcus. Bacterial invasion and infection can be as a result of corneal trauma, corneal foreign body, chronic blepharitis and contact lens wearing. Lid abnormalities such as entropion, trichiasis and corneal exposure due to incomplete eyelid closure – such as Bell's palsy – may also lead to the development of corneal ulcer.

Condition guideline: Corneal ulcers

SIGNS AND SYMPTOMS

- Foreign-body sensation
- Aching

- Pain
- Red eye
- Decreased visual acuity
- Photophobia
- Hypopyon in severe cases
- Lacrimation
- Circumscribed opacity

PATIENT'S NEEDS

- Relief of symptoms (severe pain, foreign-body sensation, lacrimation, photophobia, reduced visual acuity)
- Antibiotic treatment to the eye
- Addressing of psychological needs
- Addressing of sleep deprivation due to frequency of drops

NURSING ACTION

1. Prepare equipment and patient for corneal scrape.
2. If the condition is severe and/or the patient is elderly, admit him to hospital. A clear plan of care must be documented. If admitted to a non-ophthalmic unit, clear instructions on the eye drop regimen must be provided.
3. Give the prescribed antibiotics:
   a. Intensive drops, e.g., G. gentamicin and G. cefuroxime (alternate) every half-hour for the first 24 hours. This means that the patient will be having drops instilled every 15 minutes. The frequency will be reduced according to the response.
   b. Ointment, e.g. Oc. chloramphenicol and gentamicin, may be given at night at a later stage.
   c. Subconjunctival antibiotics may be prescribed.
   d. Oral antibiotics may be given, especially if the ulcer is close to the limbus (Kanski 2007).
   e. If severe, intravenous antibiotics may be given.
4. Give prescribed analgesic drugs as prescribed, monitoring their effectiveness by the use of a pain assessment tool.
5. Instil prescribed topical mydriatics for the prevention of posterior synechiae as a result of secondary anterior synechiae and to reduce pain as a result of ciliary spasm.
6. It is important to recognise signs of sleep deprivation – such as loss of appetite, depression and mood swings – and it is important that this is addressed. It is a good idea to care for these patients in a side ward and to make every effort to minimise the noise level. The room should be darkened and interruptions kept to a minimum. Patients should be offered warm drinks and a light diet. When the patient is well enough, educate him (and, where appropriate, the relatives) in drop instillation technique in preparation for discharge home.
7. It is also important to address any psychological needs of the patient. Good clear explanations at every stage of the management of the corneal ulcer will help to alleviate any anxiety and fear. Where appropriate, involve other agencies such as dietician, district nurses and social worker.
8. If the patient is elderly and is also confused, ensure that a falls risk assessment is carried out and implemented. If appropriate, a Waterlow score should also be carried out and implemented.

9. If the patient is to be treated as an outpatient, instruct him in the instillation of drops and ointment as above. The frequency may be less, e.g. two-hourly. Ensure he has analgesics at home.
10. Advise the patient to wear dark glasses for the photophobia but not to cover the eye with a pad. Explain that the pad could provide an environment in which the infection could thrive.
11. Warn the patient that treatment may be prolonged, perhaps for several weeks until healing is complete.
12. Topical steroids may be introduced once the ulcer begins to heal although this is controversial.
13. It may be necessary to prepare the patient for botulinum injection to induce a ptosis which will cover the cornea.

COMPLICATIONS

- Scarring of the cornea occurs if the ulcer spreads beyond the epithelial layer.
- Uveitis can occur, with its own complications.
- Descemetocele formation – the elastic Descemet's membrane affords some protection against the spreading ulcer. The corneal layers above it have been destroyed and Descemet's membrane herniates through the ulcer. When this happens perforation may occur.
- Perforation of the cornea – this may be a dangerous situation as not only can sight be lost but also the eye itself. If the infection is severe and has spread to the internal structures of the eye, the eye will need to be removed, as no useful vision will be saved and the patient will experience severe pain.

ACANTHAMOEBA KERATITIS

Acanthamoeba keratitis is usually associated with a history of improper cleaning of contact lenses, using homemade sodium chloride solution to clean the lenses, and swimming in fresh water or a swimming pool while contact lenses are worn. Keratitis typically begins with a foreign-body sensation followed by pain, tearing, photophobia, blepharospasm and blurred vision. Patients may have periods of symptom remission with a waxing and waning course. The condition is very painful as the organism has a predilection for the corneal nerves – radial perineuritis and a ring-shaped infiltrate are findings which would strongly suggest *Acanthamoeba* keratitis. Early diagnosis and treatment are paramount for improving outcomes. A high index of suspicion is needed to make the diagnosis, especially in the early stages. The earliest clue to this infection is a dendriform pattern noted on the epithelium of the cornea. Identification of *Acanthamoeba* consist of culture on a buffered charcoal yeast extract or with non-nutrient agar overlaid with organisms such as *Escherichia coli*, polymerase chain reaction of biopsy specimens and scanning confocal corneal microscopy. If corneal specimens are unremarkable, consider culturing the contact lenses and saline solution for *Acanthamoeba* (Kerr 2014).

Medical treatment consists of topical antimicrobial agents, which can achieve high concentration at the site of infection. The cyst form may be highly resistant to therapy, a combination of agents is generally used. Debridement of the corneal epithelium is performed in eye casualty to increase the penetration of drops. Steroids should not be prescribed in eye casualty (Kerr 2014).

CORNEAL ULCERS ASSOCIATED WITH VIRAL INFECTIONS

ADENOVIRUS

Corneal ulcers cause superficial punctate keratitis, which is slightly raised dots on the cornea which show up when stained with G. fluorescein. These conditions have been discussed under viral conjunctivitis.

HERPES SIMPLEX

The herpes simplex virus causes an ulcer on the cornea which has a typical branching pattern and is called a 'dendritic ulcer'. It is usually unilateral. It is imperative that when treating the patient care should be taken with patients who have a history of previous herpitic infection. If topical steroids are to be prescribed in such patients, serious consideration should be given to prescribing topical antivirals as well to protect the cornea. Patients should also be instructed to return before their scheduled appointment if the condition of their eye worsens (Kerr 2014). Patient education is very important in these cases, and patients with previous herpetic infection must be told to always give this history, and also be informed of the possible dangers in using topical steroids in cases of current or past herpetic infection. If management of a patient with a herpetic infection is proving difficult, clinicians of all grades should refer early on to the appropriate specialist.

It is important to remember that other causes of dendritic epithelial defects are common and it is important that patients are not incorrectly labeled as herpes simplex. All previously unconfirmed cases should have a sample of corneal epithelium sent for virology before treatment is started. Corneal sensation is always reduced, and should be tested in both eyes. Bilateral herpes simplex keratitis is rare except in atopic individuals.

Collection of specimens for microscopy and culture

Corneal scrape is performed using a needle or scalpel blade to remove materials from the edge of the ulcer and place on

- Chocolate agar
- Slide for immediate Gram stain and to exclude fungal infection
- Reinforce clostridial medium (RCM) broth
- Blood agar
- Sabouraud agar

A new needle or blade must be used for each of the above. If *Acanthamoeba* is suspected, a larger area of epithelium is removed and placed on *E. Coli*-seeded agar.

Condition guideline: Herpes simplex

SIGNS

- Red eye, usually unilateral
- Dendritic ulcer (Figure 9.2) seen on the cornea once stained with G. fluorescein
- Evidence of herpes simplex lesions around the eye
- Presence of cold sores around the mouth and/or nose

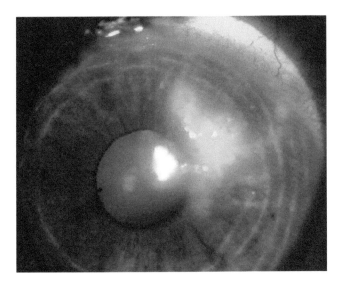

Figure 9.2 Dendritic ulcer. (From Olver, J. and Cassidy, L., *Ophthalmology at a Glance*, Blackwell Publishing, Oxford, 2005, reproduced with permission.)

PATIENT'S NEEDS

- Relief of symptoms:
  - Irritation
  - Watering
  - Photophobia
  - Reduced vision
- Pain may not be a symptom as the cornea may have become anaesthetised by the virus. Monitor pain using a pain assessment tool. Give analgesia as required.
- Treatment for the infection.

NURSING ACTION

1. Take swabs for herpes simplex virus isolation.
2. Instruct the patient on the treatment with antiviral agents: Oc. acyclovir five times a day. Acyclovir resistance is reported, but increasingly rare. If an ulcer fails to respond to treatment it is more likely to be due to something else such as misdiagnosis, neuropathic epithelial defect, stromal necrosis and secondary infections.
3. Treatment is given for 1 week initially, but may need to be continued for longer. Patients are reviewed at approximately 5–10 days (small peripheral ulcers may only need one review). Patients should be warned to attend earlier if there is loss of vision. If the ulcer is healed at 10 days, treatment can be discontinued. The frequency of use does not need to be tailed off. The patient can be discharged, but should be warned that they may get a recurrence and would then need to reattend as an emergency.
4. Steroids are never used for herpes simplex infection because they increase the activity of the virus and introduce the possibility of secondary infection. Perforation of the cornea has been caused by the use of steroids.
5. Acyclovir cream can be applied to affected skin areas. Acyclovir cream for the skin must never be applied to the eye.

COMPLICATIONS

- Amoeboid or geographical ulcer – the dendritic ulcer spreads to take on the appearance of an amoeba or island.
- Disciform keratitis – the stromal layer becomes oedematous and there are folds in Descemet's membrane. The complaint occurs in patients who are immunosuppressed. It is usually a self-limiting condition lasting several weeks but may become chronic, in which case uveitis also occurs. A very low dose of steroids may then be required. G. prednisolone sodium phosphate can then be prescribed in a weak solution, such as 0.003%.
- Corneal scarring can be caused by repeated attacks of herpes simplex keratitis.
- If a corneal graft is performed, the herpes virus can attack the grafted cornea.

HERPES ZOSTER OPHTHALMICUS

Herpes zoster ophthalmicus is caused by the herpes zoster virus attacking the ophthalmic division of the trigeminal nerve. It therefore follows the path of the nerve over the forehead and into the eye (Figure 9.3). It usually affects the elderly and can be debilitating. The disease starts with pain over the forehead and scalp on the affected side. A day or so later, vesicles appear on the same area and may cover the upper lid. These then break down and weep serous fluid before drying up and forming scabs. The patient feels ill, anorexic and nauseated and may be pyrexial, too.

If the nasociliary nerve is affected, the cornea will be involved with white infiltrate and lesions may appear on the side of the nose. This is known as a positive Hutchinson sign.

Condition guideline: Herpes zoster ophthalmicus

PATIENT'S NEEDS

- Relief of symptoms, especially pain
- Admission to hospital if the condition is severe or if the patient is elderly and cannot manage at home
- Instigation of treatment

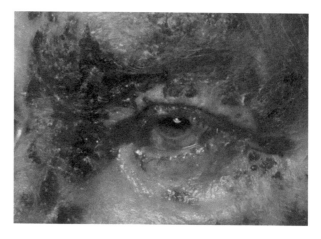

Figure 9.3 Herpes zoster ophthalmicus. (Courtesy of Keith Barton.)

NURSING ACTION

1. Ensure the patient understands the treatment.
2. Provide systemic treatment with either valaciclovir, acyclovir or famciclovir three times a day.
3. Skin lesions:
   a. Acyclovir cream can be applied twice a day to the vesicles.
   b. Hydrocortisone cream can also be used.
4. Corneal involvement:
   a. Antiviral agents can be prescribed, e.g. Oc. acyclovir five times a day.
5. Pain – oral analgesics such as paracetamol can be given regularly 4-hourly. Stronger analgesics such as mefenamic acid or dextropropoxyphene may be necessary. Pain should be monitored using an appropriate pain assessment tool.
6. Anti-inflammatory and anti-epileptic agents have been tried to treat the pain. Night sedation or an antidepressant at night may be required.
7. Advise the patient that he will feel unwell and will require a light diet and plenty of fluids.
8. Warn the patient that although the unaffected eyelid may swell in apparent sympathy, it will not be affected by the virus.

COMPLICATIONS

Fifty percent of patients develop ocular complications:

- Uveitis.
- Glaucoma.
- Cataract.
- Conjunctivitis.
- Keratitis.
- Permanent corneal scarring.
- Anaesthetic cornea due to the nasociliary nerve being damaged by the virus. The cornea is then exposed to damage because the corneal reflex is absent. Bandage contact lenses or protective arms on spectacles can be worn. This may resolve over months or years.
- More rarely, optic neuritis; scleritis; paralysis of the third, fourth and sixth cranial nerves.
- Partial ptosis due to scarring of lid from vesicles.
- Post-herpetic neuralgia is the most debilitating complication which can last intermittently for several years following the initial attack. It is difficult to treat and may require attendance at a pain clinic.

These complications can occur 6–10 years after the initial attack.

INTERSTITIAL KERATITIS

Interstitial keratitis is due to congenital syphilis, manifesting itself when the patient is aged between 5 and 20 years. The disease can also occur as a result of other complications such as leprosy and tuberculosis. Tuberculosis is on the increase in Britain (Public Health England 2015) as the number of immigrants and asylum seekers from countries with a high incidence of tuberculosis rises. Certain viruses, such as the measles virus or the mumps virus, can also cause a type of interstitial keratitis. There is involvement of the deep corneal stromal layer and, if left untreated, the entire cornea develops a ground-glass appearance. The corneal epithelium and endothelium are not involved. There is also invasion of new blood vessels from the limbus.

The patient complains of pain, watering eye, photophobia, blepharospasm and reduced vision. The eye is red and the cornea oedematous. Other signs of congenital syphilis may be present: saddle nose, deafness and notched incisor teeth.

There is no specific treatment. Any treatment given is aimed at preventing uveitis and the formation of posterior synechiae by the use of mydriatics and steroid drops. Wearing dark glasses may help the photophobia. Corneal grafting may be necessary if corneal scarring becomes severe enough to obscure vision.

BULLOUS KERATOPATHY

Bullous keratopathy is prolonged oedema of the cornea resulting in the epithelium being raised into large vesicles or bullae. It is a difficult condition to treat and the bullae may burst periodically causing intense irritating symptoms. It occurs following disturbance to the endothelium when aqueous humour is allowed to percolate into the stroma. This could be as a result of trauma, surgery (especially intraocular lens implants) or long-standing, poorly controlled glaucoma.

Hypertonic (5%) saline eye drops can be prescribed to reduce the corneal oedema and improve vision (Kanski 2007). Grafting may be necessary. Bandage contact lenses make the condition less painful and also flatten the bullae.

CORNEAL DYSTROPHIES

Corneal dystrophies can be categorised according to the corneal layer involved:

- Epithelial/anterior Cogan's, map-dot, recurrent erosions, Reis-Bockler
- Stromal/granular, macular, lattice
- Endothelial/posterior Fuchs' endothelial dystrophy

These dystrophies cause increasing visual loss. Corneal grafting is the main form of treatment, but the dystrophy can recur in the 'new' cornea. Recurrent erosions can be treated with the excimer laser.

Condition guideline: Fuchs' endothelial dystrophy

- Bilateral degenerative disorder of the corneal endothelium with thickened Descemet's membrane
- Late stages, the development of epithelial bullae
- More common in women than men
- Usually seen in the fifth and sixth decade

SIGNS AND SYMPTOMS

- Decreased vision
- Foreign-body sensation
- Pain on waking up

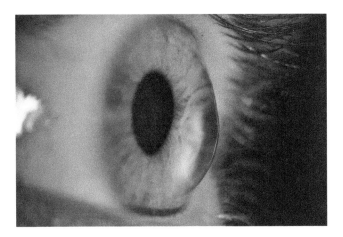

Figure 9.4 Keratoconus. (From Olver, J. and Cassidy, L., *Ophthalmology at a Glance*, Blackwell Publishing, Oxford, 2005, reproduced with permission.)

MEDICAL MANAGEMENT

Medical management varies depending on the severity of the disease:

- Topical hypertonic saline
- Bandage contact lenses
- Surgery – penetrating keratoplasty

KERATOCONUS

Keratoconus or conical cornea is due to a congenital weakness of the cornea, manifesting itself in the early teens. It can be associated with conditions such as eczema, learning disability or blindness as sufferers of these conditions tend to rub their eyes.

Keratoconus is a bilateral condition, one eye usually being affected before the other. The central cornea becomes progressively thinner and more conical in shape (Figure 9.4). The patient complains of blurred vision due to increasing astigmatism of the cornea.

Condition guideline: Keratoconus

SIGNS

- Munson's sign – When the patient looks downward, the conical cornea causes an indentation of the lower lid margin.
- Distorted corneal reflection with Placido's Disc, a keratoscope, a pachymeter or on corneal topography.
- An irregular shadow on retinoscopy.
- Unclear view of fundus because of the corneal distortion.

TREATMENT

Initially the treatment will be with contact lenses to correct the astigmatism and protect the cornea. The astigmatism is too severe to be corrected by spectacles. As the conical shape progresses, an ordinary contact lens becomes useless. Grafting is performed, ideally before the cornea becomes too thin.

COMPLICATIONS

Acute hydrops of the cornea can occur as a result of rupture of Descemet's membrane, usually due to eye rubbing by the patient. Over a period of time, acute hydrops usually clears spontaneously but often leaves scarring.

KERATOPLASTY: CORNEAL GRAFT

The National Institute for Health and Clinical Excellence (NICE) published its guidelines in July 2007 for corneal implants for keratoconus. The guidance from NICE advocated that the current evidence on the safety and efficacy of corneal transplants for keratoconus appears adequate to support this procedure. However, it also advocated that normal arrangements of consenting, audit and clinical governance must be in place to allow for continuous monitoring for safety and efficacy.

Keratoplasty needs to be performed when the cornea is so diseased that the patient's vision is lost (Figure 9.5). It is performed for (in order of occurrence)

1. Keratoconus
2. Bullous keratopathy
3. Scarring/injury
4. Corneal dystrophies
5. Corneal ulcers
6. Dendritic ulcers
7. Failed previous grafts

EYE DONORS

- *Autogenous* – Rarely, a patient requiring a corneal graft has a fellow eye which is blind but with a healthy cornea which can be used for grafting.

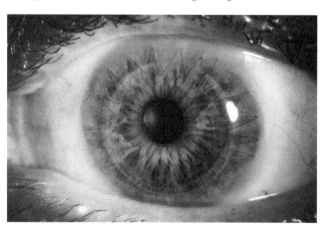

Figure 9.5 Corneal graft. (Courtesy of Debbie Morley.)

- *Live donor* – An enucleated eye with a healthy cornea can be used for grafting onto another patient.
- *Cadavers* – Most of the corneas used for grafting are obtained by this method. They must be removed within 12 hours of death and are stored in media. Organ culture medium permits storage for up to 30 days.

Donor corneas are not used from the following categories:

- Corneal disease
- Anterior segment surgery or disease
- HIV or hepatitis B positive and drug abuse
- Death of unknown cause
- Septicaemia
- Leukaemia, Hodgkin's disease or lymphosarcoma

A culture is taken from the eyes before removal to exclude any infection. Blood is taken to exclude hepatitis B and HIV. Both eyes are taken, including a part of the optic nerve. A suture is fed through the nerve and used to suspend the eye in a sterile jar to prevent the cornea becoming damaged. A prosthesis might be put in each socket or the eyelids are sutured together.

There are national eye donor banks in the United Kingdom in Bristol and Manchester, which store eyes waiting for recipients.

HUMAN AMNIOTIC MEMBRANE TRANSPLANTATION

The first use of amniotic membrane transplantation (AMT) was in 1940 by de Rotth who used this technique in treating symblepharon. In 1946, Sorsby and Symons successfully treated patients with corneal burn following caustic burns. Since then, AMT has been used for persistent corneal epithelial defect (Lee and Tseng 1997), leaking filtering blebs after glaucoma surgery (Budenz et al. 2000), Stevens–Johnson syndrome and many other corneal diseases, including systemic diseases which may cause ocular surface damage.

Human amniotic membrane is believed to be non-immunogenic, which makes it ideal in corneal graft in promoting non-rejection. AMT promotes epithelial healing, reduced inflammation, increased comfort, and decreased severity of vascularisation.

OSTEO-ODONTO-KERAPROSTHESIS SURGERY

Osteo-odonto-keraprosthesis technique is used in treating patients who are not suitable for conventional corneal graft surgery such as severely dry eyes or multiple corneal graft failure. The success of this type of surgery will depend on the lack of any previous ophthalmic history such as retinal disease, glaucoma and optic nerve involvement.

The surgery uses the patient's own tooth root and alveolar bone to act as vital support to an optical cylinder. The patient undergoes a vigorous pre-assessment check including a B-scan, assessment of the retina and optic nerve functioning and, in some cases, electroretinogram and visual-evoked potential. The patient also has an oral assessment by the maxillofacial surgeon and radiography where a decision is made as to which tooth to harvest. The canine tooth is usually harvested and, in the absence of a suitable tooth, a relative's tooth may be used after suitable human leukocyte antigen match. The surgery is usually performed in two stages, which allow the growth of soft tissues around the osteo-odonto lamina and for the reconstruction of the ocular surface, by vascularisation. Potential complications could include buccal mucous ulceration in the early post-operative phase, especially in smokers.

Condition guideline: Eye tissue recipients

PATIENT'S NEEDS

- Admission to hospital
- Pre- and post-operative care

NURSING ACTION

1. The nurse needs to ascertain that the patient understands that he will be receiving a donor cornea, which is most likely to come from a cadaver. The use of the word 'graft' instead of 'transplant' may result in the patient being unaware of the true implications of this type of surgery. The nurse may want to involve the doctor or may discuss this with the patient on her own. Some patients may be distressed at the knowledge. Others, having known for a while, may only face up to the fact at the time of surgery, while some may not have had the opportunity for discussion before. The nurse needs to be aware of those who require further discussion and to talk it through with them.
2. Admit the patient to the ward or day-case unit.
3. Institute pre-operative care. The pupil may be constricted in penetrating keratoplasty to prevent damage to the lens during the operation unless a cataract is to be removed at the same time.
4. Carry out post-operative care. At the first dressing, ensure that the graft is in place, the sutures intact and that the anterior chamber is formed. Aqueous humour may have leaked through the suture line, causing a flat anterior chamber. Instil antibiotic or antibiotic and steroid as well as mydriatic drops.
5. Education of patient must also include having a clear knowledge of the symptoms of graft rejection such as reduced vision, red eye and pain, and an understanding of the relevance of seeking prompt treatment.
6. Following corneal grafting, astigmatism may occur, which will require correction by the wearing of spectacles or contact lenses.

COMPLICATIONS: SHORT TERM

- Damage during the operation to the iris or lens.
- Aqueous humour leak from the graft which has lifted in one area – this will require re-suturing.
- Infection requiring antibiotics.

COMPLICATIONS: LONG TERM

- Neovascularisation around the edge of the graft – No treatment is required unless vision is impaired. Beta rays can be used on the area to destroy the new blood vessels. Regrafting may be necessary.
- Astigmatism caused by excessively tight sutures which may need adjusting – Topography can confirm this.
- Warping of donor graft caused by sutures that are too loose – This may require re-suturing.

- Rejection, which will be treated with steroids – Compared with other transplant operations, keratoplasty does not present the same rejection problems as the cornea does not have a blood supply.

CORNEAL TOPOGRAPHY

Corneal topography is a non-invasive medical imaging technique for mapping the surface curvature of the cornea. The anterior surface of the cornea, with its tear film, is the major refractive element in the eye and, because of this, even minute changes in its shape can reduce vision. Such vision-altering shape changes include irregular astigmatism induced by trauma and surgery, contact lens warpage and tear film irregularities.

The development of computer-assisted corneal topographic analysis was driven by the need for clinicians to know the detailed shape of the cornea as a feedback system that could be used to guide the choice of refractive and optical correction.

The aim of corneal topography is to obtain detailed, accurate data about the corneal contour and to display it in a clinically useful format.

USES OF CORNEAL TOPOGRAPHY

Corneal topography can assist in the diagnosis and treatment of a number of conditions, for example keratoconus. It is also used in planning laser refractive surgery, and can assist in assessing the fit of contact lenses. It can also be used for evaluation of ocular surface abnormalities, such as dry eye, epithelial defects, pterygium and scarring.

PRINCIPLES

Original methods for assessing corneal topography were all based on the principle of reflection but, more recently, techniques using projection have been developed. Instruments which project an image onto the anterior corneal surface directly measure the true shape of the anterior corneal surface in terms of height. From these measurements, slope, curvature and power can be calculated.

DISPLAY

Most maps are displayed as colour coded: steep areas are represented by hot colours (orange, red and black), and flat areas are represented by cool colours (green and blue).

TOPOGRAPHY OF NORMAL CORNEAS

A normal cornea is prolate, which means it is steepest in the centre and flattens towards the periphery. The topography of normal corneas has been classified into five groups: round, oval, symmetrical bow tie, asymmetrical bow tie and irregular. The bow tie appearances occur more commonly in astigmatic corneas, when the red bow lies along the steep meridian. In oblate corneas, for example those flattened by surgery, the bows are blue and lie along the flat meridian.

ARTIFACTS OF CORNEAL TOPOGRAPHY

It is important to be able to recognise when the topographic irregularities are due to external influences, rather than the cornea itself. The acquisition of accurate topography is dependent

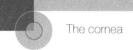

upon the care of the operator and the cooperation of the patient. The patient must maintain fixation of the target and the equipment must be properly centred and focussed. Small errors in alignment can result in an irregular or asymmetric topographic reconstruction. Irregularities of the tear film can also cause topographic errors. Pooling of tears in the lower meniscus produces a focal steepening, and thinning of the tear film by drying shows as a localised flattening of the surface. These artifacts can be reduced by asking the patient to blink immediately before the image is taken.

PRE-OPERATIVE SCREENING

Corneal topography is undertaken for all potential patients presenting for refractive surgery. This will help to exclude conditions such as keratoconus. Keratoconic corneas show greater than normal variation in curvature from the centre to the periphery and generally have irregular astigmatism. In addition, the thinning most commonly occurs just inferior to the corneal centre. Protrusion in this area gives the corneal surface an exaggerated prolate shape. The point of maximum protrusion is the apex of the cone. If the keratoconus is severe, it is difficult to reconstruct the topography, and some data points may be inaccurate or missing.

Topography on moderate and severe cases of keratoconus is usually recognisable, but it can be more difficult to diagnose in subtle cases. To make this easier, many systems have specific corneal indices and detection programmes designed to help the topographic diagnosis of keratoconus. It is also possible to classify keratoconus on the basis of the appearance of colour-coded maps.

With the more widespread use of corneal topography, it has become clear that the condition is more common than previously thought. Topographic features typical of keratoconus have been found in eyes with good spectacle-corrected visual acuity and a normal biomicroscopic appearance.

CONTACT LENS-INDUCED CORNEAL WARPAGE

Corneal topographic changes following contact lens wear are thought to be a result of pressure exerted by the contact lens. The changes are more severe in people who wear hard or rigid gas-permeable contact lenses. Ideally, patients should leave their hard lenses out for 4 weeks or soft lenses out for 1 week, to enable the cornea to return to its original shape. This is not always possible, as keratoconic patients need their lenses to see and cannot manage without them.

CORNEAL SUTURE REMOVAL

In highly irregular corneas, such as after corneal transplantation, corneal topography is more accurate than refraction for determining the accurate position of tight sutures that are causing steepening of the cornea. This is a valuable tool for the medical staff to decide on selective suture removal.

ASTIGMATIC KERATOTOMY

Following removal of all sutures from a corneal transplant, patients can be left with high or irregular astigmatism. This can be corrected by causing compression or relaxation of the cornea. Corneal topography will be required for these patients pre-operatively to assess the degree of astigmatism, as well as refraction. It will also be required post-operatively to assess the correction of the astigmatism.

PACHYMETRY AND SPECULAR PHOTOMICROSCOPY

Pachymeters measure the corneal thickness (normal corneal thickness in the periphery is 1 mm, reducing to 0.58 mm centrally) and are a good indicator for endothelial function. The endothelial cells can be photographed and counted – a procedure known as specular photomicroscopy. This involves a special mounted slit lamp like a camera, which allows the corneal endothelium to be visualised and photographed. The density of the endothelial cells can be counted as well as any endothelial cells deviating from normal (normal endothelial cells are hexagonal in shape). Conditions such as diabetes, anterior segment surgery, glaucoma and contact lens wearing can all contribute to endothelial dysfunction.

MANAGEMENT OF CORNEAL PAIN

Corneal pain is managed using topical non-steroidal anti-inflammatory agents.

The avascular cornea is one of the most sensitive tissues in the body, with the highest density of sensory neurones per millimetre just below the epithelium four to five times greater than in the finger pads (Corbett et al. 1999). Any epithelial loss leads to the exposure of the sub-epithelial plexus nerve endings. Subsequently, the patient's main complaint will be one of pain. The management of corneal pain has often in the past been neglected, and patients are frequently very distressed as their pain can become almost intolerable. Their normal daily activities are often disrupted, including their sleep pattern. In addition to their pain, patients may also be complaining of a red eye, photophobia, foreign body or gritty sensation, lacrimation and a possible decrease in vision.

The most frequent cause of corneal pain, apart from surgery, is corneal abrasion. Traumatic corneal abrasion is one of the commonest causes of attendance in any emergency centre, and these abrasions range from very small to large epithelial defect. Small abrasions usually heal without serious sequelae, but larger and deeper corneal involvement can leave scar formation. Traumatic corneal abrasions can be as a result of any ocular injuries such as from fingernails, twigs and foreign bodies, or work-related injuries such as welding flash and chemical injuries. Other examples of possible causes of corneal abrasion include contact lens wear and epithelial disease such as dry eyes.

During the healing process of the corneal epithelium, the epithelial cells from the corneal limbus flatten and spread across the defect until it is covered completely. At the same time, new cells migrate from the basal layer of the epithelium.

The current management of severe corneal pain associated with a corneal abrasion is to prescribe cycloplegics such as G. mydrilate 0.5%, as well as advising the patient to take oral analgesia. Although cycloplegics have been claimed to reduce ocular pain and inflammation by alleviating ciliary spasm, there are no controlled studies to support this hypothesis (Sabri et al. 1998; Carley and Carley 2001). However, some experts recommend a one-off dose to reduce headache from ciliary muscle spasm.

The use of a topical non-steroidal anti-inflammatory such as Voltarol (diclofenac) or Acular (ketorolac) is not recommended routinely. A review of the ophthalmic literature in the use of non-steroidal anti-inflammatory drugs in controlling corneal pain is well documented.

Jayamanne et al. (1997) report in their study that the use of topical Voltarol significantly reduced pain after traumatic corneal abrasion. Voltarol significantly lowered corneal sensitivity in normal eyes and reduced discomfort, pain and inflammation following photorefractive keratoplasty. In another study Brahma et al. (1996) reports on the use of flurbiprofen as a topical analgesic for superficial corneal injuries and found that it provides more effective pain relief than traditional treatments for superficial corneal injuries. These patients also took less oral analgesia, had normal sleep patterns and took less time off work. McDonald (1998, unpublished paper on the use of ketorolac tromethamine in the treatment of corneal pain, Westbourne Eye Hospital, Bournemouth) examined the use of Acular for relief of corneal pain in 26 patients. It was found to be useful in controlling patients' pain. None of the studies showed any significant adverse effects from the use of topical non-steroidal anti-inflammatory drugs. So far, no evidence exists in the medical literature that the use of non-steroidal anti-inflammatory drugs interferes with the rate of corneal epithelial healing, and this fact is well documented (Hersch et al. 1990; McGarey et al. 1993). This 'risk' is further reduced through limited dose and duration of use.

The routine prescription of a non-steroidal anti-inflammatory must be considered in any patients presenting with corneal pain, following corneal abrasion, on a verbal pain-rating scale of four or more. Caution must be exercised in patients with a history of corneal ulcers, herpes virus infection, corneal dystrophies, post-operative corneal graft or recent ocular surgery within 3 months. In addition, any patients who are asthmatic or who have known allergies to any topical analgesic or non-steroidal anti-inflammatory should also proceed with caution.

Reflective activity

Consider a patient that you have seen recently with a corneal problem:

- What were the presenting signs and symptoms?
- Was there any associated systemic disease or diseases?
- What tests and investigations were carried out and why?
- How did you arrive at a diagnosis?
- What was the treatment plan?
- Outline the care and management of the patient.
- If there were any challenges in caring for the patient, what were they?
- Was any other member of the multidisciplinary team involved in the care and what was his or her input?
- Utilising a recognised health-promotion framework, how would you explain the condition and treatment to the patient in order to ensure that he or she adheres to the treatment?
- What was the clinical outcome?
- What local or national policies, guidelines or protocols influenced the care and management of this patient?
- On reflection, would you have done anything differently, if so, what?

Your completed case study can be used to contribute to your continuing professional development portfolio for Registration and your Knowledge and Skills Framework or appraisal review.

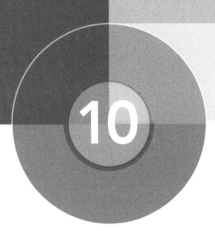

The uveal tract

This chapter looks at the gross anatomy and physiology of the uveal tract and the treatment of uveal tract conditions.

INTRODUCTION

The uveal tract comprises the middle vascular pigmented layer of the eye. It is composed of three areas:

- The choroid, which forms the posterior five-sixths
- The ciliary body
- The iris

These two latter structures (Figure 10.1) together form the anterior one-sixth.

THE CHOROID

The choroid lies between the sclera and retina and extends from the optic nerve forward to the ora serrata where it joins the ciliary body. The choroid is composed of four layers:

- The suprachoroid, containing pigment cells, elastic tissue and collagen.
- The vascular layer, comprising large and small blood vessels, with pigment cells contained in the stroma surrounding the vessels; the large vessels are mainly veins.
- The choriocapillaries, comprising fenestrated capillary vessels.
- Bruch's membrane, which is a barrier with fenestrations which allow nutrients through to the underlying retina; it is also a supportive membrane.

FUNCTIONS OF THE CHOROID

The main functions of the choroid are

- To provide nourishment to the outer layer of the underlying retina
- To enable heat exchange from the retina
- To conduct blood vessels to the anterior portion of the eye
- To prevent reflection

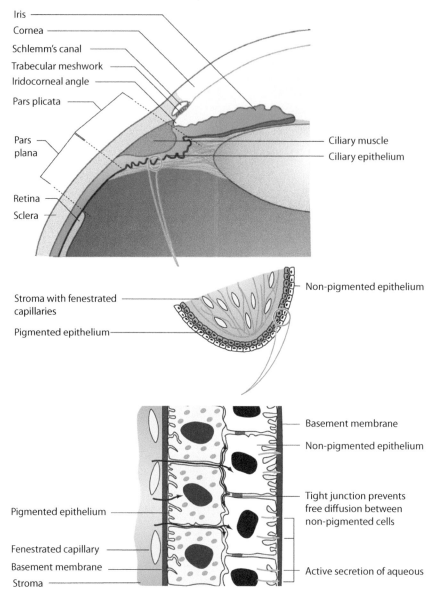

Figure 10.1 The anatomy of the ciliary body. (From James, B. et al., *Lecture Notes*: *Ophthalmology*, Blackwell Publishing, 2007. Reproduced with permission.)

BLOOD SUPPLY TO THE CHOROID

The blood supply to and drainage from the choroid is via the short posterior ciliary artery; and the choroidal and vortex veins.

NERVE SUPPLY TO THE CHOROID

The nerve supply to the choroid is by the long and short ciliary nerves.

THE CILIARY BODY

The ciliary body is a triangular structure lying between the choroid and the iris, being 6 mm wide. It has three areas:

1. The pars plana is the posterior aspect lying next to the ora serrata and is 4 mm wide.
2. The pars plicata is the area which lies between the pars plana and the iris and is 2 mm wide. It contains 70–80 radiating strips – the ciliary processes. Composed of vascular tissue – mainly veins and capillaries – the ciliary processes are 2 mm long and 0.5 mm wide. Their function is to produce and secrete aqueous humour, which fills the posterior chamber and then flows through the pupil into the anterior chamber. The zonular fibres or suspensory ligaments, which hold the lens in place, originate in the valleys formed by the processes.
3. The ciliary muscles lie in the anterior section of the ciliary body, underneath the sclera. Known as the muscles of accommodation, the ciliary muscles contract and relax to change the shape of the lens so that light rays can be brought to a focus on the retina when looking at objects at varying distances. When the ciliary muscles contract, the zonules relax and decrease the tension on the lens capsule. The lens thus becomes more spherical and light rays can be focussed on the retina for near vision. When the ciliary muscles relax, the zonules tighten and there is increased tension on the lens capsule. The lens thus becomes less spherical and light rays are focussed on the retina for distance vision.

FUNCTIONS OF THE CILIARY BODY

The main functions of the ciliary body are

- Accommodation
- Suspension of the crystalline lens
- Production of aqueous humour

BLOOD SUPPLY TO THE CILIARY BODY

The blood supply to and drainage from the ciliary body is via

- Anterior ciliary arteries and veins
- Long posterior ciliary arteries and veins
- Vortex vein

NERVE SUPPLY TO THE CILIARY BODY

The nerve supply to the ciliary body is through the short ciliary nerve from the oculomotor nerve.

THE IRIS

The iris is the coloured circular diaphragm situated behind the cornea and in front of the lens. It is attached at its periphery to the ciliary body. The pupil is the aperture in the middle of the iris.

The iris forms the posterior wall of the anterior chamber and the anterior wall of the posterior chamber. There are two zones:

1. The ciliary zone on the periphery
2. The pupillary zone on the central aspect

THREE LAYERS OF THE IRIS

The iris has three layers:

1. The endothelium
2. The stroma, containing connective tissue, pigment cells, blood vessels, nerves and muscles
3. Pigment epithelium, which is an extension of the pigment epithelium of the retina (note that the epithelium of the iris is situated at the back of the structure)

MUSCLE OF THE IRIS

There are two muscles in the iris, whose actions are either to constrict or dilate the pupil:

1. The sphincter muscle is a circular muscle lying around the pupillary zone. This muscle constricts the pupil. It is served by the short ciliary nerve of the oculomotor nerve.
2. The dilator muscle is a radial muscle lying under the pigmented layer of the iris. As its name indicates, it is the muscle that dilates the pupil and is supplied by the long ciliary nerve from the nasociliary nerve, the third branch of the ophthalmic division of the trigeminal nerve.

The sphincter muscle is more powerful than the dilator muscle so, if both muscles are equally affected by intraocular inflammation, the pupil will tend to constrict. The sphincter muscle and the ciliary muscle both have their nerve supply from the oculomotor nerve, therefore drugs stimulating or paralysing this nerve will affect both dilation and accommodation.

COLOUR OF THE IRIS

The pigment melanin gives the colour to the iris. The colour depends on the amount of pigment laid down in the stroma after birth, and this is genetically determined. The pigment in the pigment epithelium is present at birth and is consistent throughout life. This gives newborn babies light-coloured eyes. After a few days of life, pigment begins to be laid down in the stroma and the baby's eyes become darker. The more melanin is laid down, the darker the eyes become. All babies are therefore born with light-coloured eyes, despite what some doting parents may say. The amount of pigment produced in the stroma can vary during life, so that the colour of eyes can alter. Dark irises with dense pigment cause the pupil to take longer to dilate following instillation of mydriatics.

BLOOD SUPPLY TO THE IRIS

The arterial blood supply to the iris is via the long posterior ciliary arteries. The capillaries from these arteries anastomose with the anterior ciliary arteries to form the arterial circle of the iris. The venous drainage is through the anterior ciliary veins and vortex veins.

NERVE SUPPLY TO THE IRIS

The nerve supply to the iris is via the long and short ciliary nerves.

FUNCTION OF THE IRIS

The main function of the iris is to control the amount of light entering the eye, through the dilation and constriction of the pupil.

CONDITIONS OF THE UVEAL TRACT

ANTERIOR UVEITIS OR IRITIS

Anterior uveitis or iritis is inflammation of the iris, or iris and ciliary body (see Figure 10.2). It is usually a recurring condition in which the cause is unknown in 70% of cases.

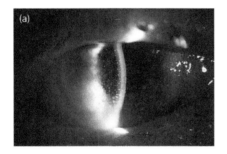

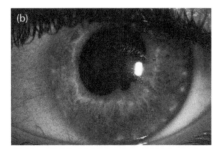

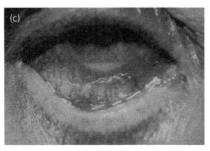

Figure 10.2 Acute iritis. (a) Cells and flare in the anterior chamber. (b) Distorted pupil. (c) Hypopyon. (Courtesy of Keith Barton.)

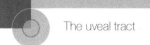

Condition guideline: Anterior uveitis or iritis

CAUSES

Causes of anterior uveitis include

- Ankylosing spondylitis.
- Idiopathic causes.
- Behçet's disease/syndrome.
- Lens-associated causes.
- Still's disease or childhood arthritis.
- Seronegative rheumatoid disease.
- Ophthalmic surgery.
- Trauma – perforating injury, corneal foreign body.
- Corneal ulcer.
- Sarcoid.
- Tuberculosis.
- Syphilis.
- Ulcerative colitis and Crohn's disease.
- Rarely, neovascularisation from diabetes mellitus.
- Also rarely, heterochromic uveitis – patients with different-coloured irises may develop this chronic, progressive condition in which the pigment of the affected eye is dislodged, with the iris becoming gradually paler.

SIGNS AND SYMPTOMS

- The visual acuity may be reduced. Ciliary limbal injection will be observed.
- Cornea is usually clear. Keratic precipitates may be present on the posterior surface of the cornea if the inflammation is severe. These are plaques of precipitates from the inflamed iris. In the case of a patient with tuberculosis or sarcoid, these are particularly marked and are called 'mutton fat' because of their appearance.
- The anterior chamber is of normal depth but 'flare and cells' may be seen in the beam of the slit lamp. Flares are as a result of exudative protein from the inflamed iris and cells are seen as leucocytes. Inflammatory cells may be sufficient in number to settle and form a hypopyon.
- The iris vessels may be dilated. A nodule may be present if the cause is tuberculosis.
- The intraocular pressure may be elevated.
- The pupil is small because the iris muscles are in spasm, and the sphincter muscle is the stronger of the two iris muscles. The pupil will be irregular if posterior synaechiae has occurred when the posterior surface of the swollen iris adheres to the anterior surface of the lens.
- There may be cells in the vitreous humour.
- Macular oedema may be present in severe anterior or intermediate uveitis.

MANAGEMENT OF PATIENTS WITH ACUTE ANTERIOR UVEITIS

It is important to assess and obtain a good and accurate history from the patient. History taking should include

- Age, gender and race
- Symptoms such as redness, pain, photophobia

- Past ophthalmic history, such as previous trauma or ocular history
- Medical history to include any joint pain or any other systemic diseases related to the aetiology of anterior uveitis
- Medication
- Allergies

OCULAR EXAMINATION

Accurate ocular examination forms an important part in the diagnosis of acute anterior uveitis and should include the following:

- Visual acuity – the patient's best corrected visual acuity should be taken and recorded.
- Slit lamp examination of the eye.
- Tonometry to establish intraocular pressure.
- Gonioscopy to determine the presence of any anterior or posterior synaechiae.
- Fundus examination as intermediate or posterior uveitis often results in anterior inflammation.

INVESTIGATIONS

Investigations, e.g. blood samples, may be taken to aid diagnosis, and examples include the following:

- Angiotensin-converting enzyme – This will be raised in cases of sarcoidosis.
- Antinuclear antibody – Positive in patients with autoimmune disease.
- Full blood count (FBC), including with differential, which is useful in identifying any underlying bacterial or viral aetiology.
- Erythrocyte sedimentation rate (ESR) – An elevated ESR can indicate general inflammatory activity.
- Human leukocyte antigen – B27(HLA-B27) – Is positive in Reiter's syndrome and ankylosing spondylitis.
- Serology test for syphilis.
- Chest x-ray (CX-R).
- Urinalysis.

Other possible investigations are skin testing, extraocular tissue biopsy, lumbar puncture or intraocular sampling.

PATIENT'S NEEDS

- Relief of symptoms
  - Pain due to the spasm of the nerves of the iris
  - Photophobia due to irritation of the nerves of the iris
  - Watering eye, again due to irritation of the nerves of the iris
  - Reduced visual acuity due to the presence of 'flare and cells' in the anterior chamber
- Investigation of the cause in recurrent cases, and treatment, if applicable
- Instigation of treatment

NURSING ACTION

1. Dilation of the pupil to prevent posterior synaechiae from forming or to break down any that have formed.

   a. Instil prescribed mydriatic drops, often a 'cocktail' will be used, e.g. G. phenylephrine hydrochloride 10% and G. cyclopentolate 1%. These may need to be repeated if synaechiae are present.

   b. The application of heat by means of eye-pads soaked in hot water and wrung out then placed over, but not on, closed lids will enhance the action of the mydriatics and cause the pupil to dilate more quickly. The heat will also afford some pain relief. Do not apply the hot pads directly onto the closed eyelids.

   c. A subconjunctival injection of mydriatics, e.g. mydricaine, may need to be given. This may be given in conjunction with steroids such as Betnesol.

2. Ensure that the patient understands the treatment to be instilled at home. This will involve
   a. Mydriatic, e.g. G. cyclopentolate 1% twice a day
   b. Steroid, e.g. G. pred forte 1% 2-hourly or four times a day, depending on the severity of the condition.

3. If investigations are to be carried out, ensure that the patient understands where and when to attend for these. These tests will include x-rays – skull, chest and joints to exclude sarcoid, tuberculosis, arthritis and ankylosing spondylitis; blood tests – haemoglobin, full blood count, ESR, serology and autoimmune profile.

4. Advise the patient to wear dark glasses to help counter the photophobia.

5. Advise the patient to shake steroid drops well before use.

6. Ensure that the patient complies with drops tapering (reducing gradually over a given stated period) instructions.

7. Ensure that the patient knows when to return for follow-up treatment, which will probably be in 1 or 2 days.

8. Ensure that the patient is aware that anterior uveitis can reoccur, especially in cases where there is a systemic aetiology. Advice given to the patient must include where and how to seek help and advice if the need arises.

Often the management of patients with uveitis can be complex and time consuming and, according to Jones (2012), the management of these patients must be optimised by early setting of targets for achievement, gaining the patient's understanding and cooperation, and by setting clear plans for management. Ophthalmic nurse practitioners have a significant role to play in achieving these goals.

COMPLICATIONS

- Secondary glaucoma from three causes:
  - Posterior synaechiae, if not broken down, can cause a ring synaechiae when all of the pupillary zone of the iris is bound down to the anterior lens surface. The aqueous humour cannot flow through the pupil, so as the pressure builds up in the posterior chamber, and the iris is pushed forward. This condition is known as iris bombe. Ring synaechiae can be divided surgically if mydriatics do not cause the pupil to dilate and thus break the synaechiae.
  - The peripheral anterior surface of the iris bombe adheres to the peripheral posterior surface of the cornea, causing peripheral anterior synaechiae. These block the drainage angle.
  - Debris from the inflamed iris blocks the drainage angle.
- Cataract formation from impairment of the metabolism of the lens.

- Hypopyon of sterile pus.
- Cystoid macular oedema.
- Band keratopathy in longstanding uveitis.

THE ROLE OF THE UVEITIS NURSE PRACTITIONER

As management of patients with uveitis is often complex and, for some patients, this can be chronic and be for life, it is important that the care and management of a uveitis patient be managed by appropriately trained staff. Such staff could include an ophthalmic trained nurse who has special experience in looking after the physical, emotional and social needs of people suffering from complex uveitis.

In order to maximise the best visual outcome for patients, it is important to gain their full understanding of the disease process and treatment regime (Jones 2012). As the main aim of treatment is to control inflammation, prevent visual loss and minimise the long-term complications of the disease and its treatment, a concordant approach would ensure that both the patient and ophthalmologist form a partnership in the management of the condition, where clear plans are set, implemented and evaluated.

The role of the uveitis nurse is clearly an important aspect in the fulfilment of a successful patient-care pathway in uveitis management. There are many aspects to the role, and patient education is fundamental to the management of patients with uveitis. Patient education commences at the point of diagnosis, and it is important that patient education is seen as a two-way continuous process, with the nurse as a facilitator. Other aspects of the role include the following:

- Help patients to learn about drug treatment and monitoring needs associated with their treatment.
- Provide emotional support.
- Provide telephone support.
- Liaise with the multidisciplinary team.
- Undertake annual health reviews.

EDUCATIONAL SUPPORT

As some types of uveitis can be chronic, patient education is a fundamental aspect of the uveitis nurse practitioner role. For education to be truly effective resulting in a positive change in knowledge, attitudes, belief and behaviour, education must take into account the following:

- Understanding of the patient's experience and condition
- Readiness of the patient to learn, taking into account extrinsic and intrinsic factors that can affect learning
- The educator's knowledge in the subject material and the ability to utilise various strategies to address the needs of patients with different levels of understanding
- The patient's motivation to learn, and the acceptance of the disease

Patient education, regardless of what aspect is being addressed, can result in positive changes in knowledge, health, behaviours, beliefs and attitudes that can, in turn, affect the health status and quality of life of the individual.

As drug treatment plays a key role in the management of uveitis, patients are provided with information before starting steroids and immunosuppressants so that they are fully involved in their treatment. This includes information on

- The benefit of the drug
- How to take the drug
- Side effects and what to do if they occur
- Any special requirements
- Contact telephone number

MONITORING OF PATIENTS ON TREATMENT

Patients on steroids and immunosuppressants are monitored regularly. At each visit, the patient's blood pressure, weight and urinalysis are recorded. Blood tests are carried out at each 6–8 weekly clinic appointment. Blood samples for full blood count, urea and electrolytes, liver function test and lipids and cyclosporine levels are taken every 6 months. The results of this monitoring are documented on a flow chart in the patient's notes. This provides safe and efficient monitoring, allowing us to check at a glance whether the results are within the defined safe limits.

PROVIDING SUPPORT AND EDUCATION TO PATIENTS UNDERGOING INVESTIGATIONS

As uveitis is a complex disease, various investigations are available to support ophthalmologists in arriving at an appropriate diagnosis. As the tests and investigations that are available are often complex, expensive and invasive, it is important that the nurse is familiar with them and the reasons for them being requested, so that she can provide the appropriate explanation and ensure that all tests and investigations are accurately carried out. It is also important that patients are adequately prepared for any invasive tests such as skin biopsy, lumber puncture or intraocular sampling.

PROVIDING EMOTIONAL SUPPORT

The diagnosis of uveitis and associated conditions can lead to a mixture of emotions. These include anger, bewilderment, fear and anxiety. A detailed explanation about what the diagnosis means can reduce anxiety and fear. The uveitis nurse practitioner can listen to a patient's particular concerns and provide information and support. In addition, having uveitis and reduced vision can have a major effect on how the patient feels about himself, his mood, his job and his relationships with other people. The uveitis nurse practitioner can provide help and support by listening, offering advice and referring to other agencies, such as Henshaw's Society for Blind People (specialist charity for visually impaired patients) and uveitis support groups. Telephone support is also available for the patients. This service is seen as invaluable by the patients, as they are able to gain not only easy access to the uveitis nurse, but have the confidence of knowing that the uveitis nurse is aware of who they are and their condition, and that the nurse is familiar with the management of the condition.

LIAISING WITH OTHER HEALTHCARE PROFESSIONALS AND ACTING AS A RESOURCE

The uveitis nurse also often has to liaise with other healthcare professionals such as the TB nurse, GP, dietician, dentist, social worker to discuss the patient's medication regime, and this may have an impact on the well-being of the uveitis patients.

MEDICATION

The management plan for some of the uveitis patients can be complex, with patients potentially having side effects from the medication such as steroids (topical, systemic, periocular) and immunosuppressants. The systemic and ocular side effects of steroids include mood changes, insomnia, elation, depression and psychosis; nausea, dyspepsia, gastritis; Cushingoid state, skin fragility, stretch marks, hirsutism, sweating; raised BP, heart failure, diabetes and susceptibility to infections, e.g. TB, have all been recorded. Ocular side effects such as glaucoma, cataracts and central serous retinopathy have all been noted.

The use of immunosuppressant drugs as an additional, second-line treatment is indicated in patients with severe uveitis, in whom the dose of systemic steroids required to control the inflammation is leading to unacceptable side effects. 'Unacceptable' dose level varies from patient to patient, but few can tolerate more than 20 mg/day in the long term. The most commonly used immunosuppressant drugs are cyclosporine, azathioprine, mycophenolate and methotrexate. Some common side effects are headaches, paraesthesiae/burning, nausea and vomiting, hirsutism, loss of libido, anaemia, bone marrow depression and increased cardiovascular risks.

INTERMEDIATE UVEITIS

Intermediate uveitis is inflammation of the uveal tract which is localised to the vitreous humour and peripheral retina. Intermediate uveitis may be idiopathic or it can be associated with systemic diseases such as multiple sclerosis, sarcoidosis or infections including Lyme disease. It affects predominantly the young. Signs and symptoms are bilateral blurred vision and floaters.

POSTERIOR UVEITIS

Posterior uveitis is inflammation of the choroid and retina and the optic nerve. Some of the causes of posterior uveitis include

- Cells may be seen in the vitreous humour, and inflammatory lesions may be seen on the retina or choroid. They may look yellow when fresh, while older ones have a more distinct edge and a whitish appearance.
- The appearance of fluffy white perivascular deposit may be significant of retinal vasculitis.
- Oedema of the optic nerve may be another feature.

One of the signs and symptoms of posterior uveitis is that patients will complain of painless impairment of vision. Floaters are also common.

INVESTIGATIONS

Depending upon suspected aetiology, the following tests may be performed:

- FBC
- CX-R
- Antinuclear antibody (ANA)
- Angiotensin converting enzyme (ACE) level
- Syphilis serology
- Toxoplasmosis titre
- Toxocara titre
- Titre for CMV, H Simplex, H Zoster
- Borrelia serology
- vitreous biology (e.g. infection, lymphoma)
- Ultrasound B (U/S B) scan
- Fundus fluorescein angiograph (FFA)
- Culture (blood) for infections aetiology

PANUVEITIS

Panuveitis is inflammation of the whole uveal tract. Again the cause is unknown, but some of the possible causes include sarcoidosis, Behçet's disease, lupus, syphilis, Vogt–Koyanagi–Harada syndrome and TB fungal retinitis.

CHOROIDITIS

Choroiditis is a condition manifesting itself as patches of inflammation on the choroid. On examination with an ophthalmoscope, fluffy white patches can be seen through a hazy vitreous humour. When these patches heal, they leave pigmented areas of scar tissue.

Condition guideline: Choroiditis

SYMPTOMS

The patient complains of reduced vision due to infiltrates in the vitreous humour and of an increased number of vitreous humour floaters. In 60% of cases, the cause is unknown. It can be caused by *Toxocara*, toxoplasmosis (see Figure 10.3) or syphilis. If the cause is known, this should be treated. A short course of high-dose steroids is also given.

COMPLICATIONS

- Cataract due to defective nourishment of the lens.
- Optic neuritis and secondary optic atrophy.
- Retinal changes and progressive degeneration, resulting in retinal atrophy – A decrease in the size of the visual field will be noted.
- Cystoid macular oedema.

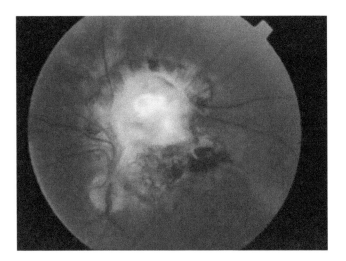

Figure 10.3 Toxoplasmosis.

OPHTHALMIC MANIFESTATIONS OF HIV INFECTION

Patients with HIV may present with ocular manifestations involving the anterior or posterior segment of the eye. Due to recent advances in therapeutic agents for treating such infections, early diagnosis is important. All HIV patients should undergo an ophthalmological review so that prompt treatment can be instigated where appropriate. Anterior segment diseases of HIV include Kaposi's sarcoma of the eyelids, conjunctiva and rarely the orbit. Herpes zoster ophthalmicus, herpes simplex virus and fungal infections can be associated with early clinical manifestations of HIV infection. Uveitis, Reiter's syndrome and syphilis are frequently seen in HIV patients. Posterior segment diseases afflicting HIV sufferers involve the retina, choroid and optic nerve, and are categorised into two: those associated with non-infectious causes and those associated with a variety of infectious disorders. Cytomegalovirus (CMV) retinitis is found in 25%–40% of patients with HIV and is the most common retinal infection. Treatment for CMV includes Ganciclovir or Foscarnet, or a combination of both these agents.

TUMOURS

BENIGN NAEVI

Benign naevi can be present in the uveal tract and must be observed carefully and regularly for malignant changes. They can be removed by laser. Melanomas are the variety of malignant tumour affecting the uveal tract. They are more common in the choroid but can occur in the iris and, more rarely, in the ciliary body where they carry a higher mortality.

MELANOMA OF THE CHOROID

Melanoma of the choroid can occur at any age but is more common over the age of 55 years. It usually occurs in the posterior pole and, as it grows, it pushes the retina forward. A retinal detachment thus caused is often the first sign of a melanoma, so careful differential diagnoses

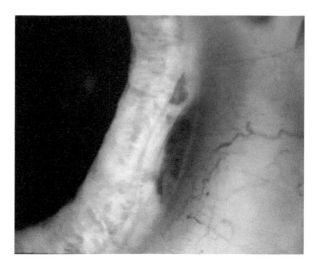

Figure 10.4 Iris melanoma.

must be made between a malignant and a simple retinal detachment. The edge of a malignant detachment is usually smoother than that of a simple detachment. Investigations include trans-illumination, colour fundus photography and ocular ultrasound. Treatment is with ruthenium or iodine plaques, proton beam radiotherapy, trans-scleral or trans-vitreal local resection or laser photocoagulation. The aim is to conserve the eye. Enucleation is reserved for patients who have visual loss, pain and poor cosmetic appearance, and those who are unable to cope with the thought of tumour spread or with prolonged treatment and follow-up. A length of optic nerve must also be removed with the whole eyeball. If the optic nerve is found to be involved on histological examination, radiotherapy should be given to the socket. The 5-year mortality rate varies from 16% for small tumours less than 10 mm in diameter, to 53% for tumours larger than 15 mm. For nursing care following enucleation, see Chapter 6.

MELANOMA OF THE IRIS

Melanoma of the iris is illustrated in Figure 10.4. If a naevus in the iris is noted to be enlarging, local excision should be performed. The prognosis, providing treatment is prompt, is usually good.

Melanoma of the ciliary body

Ciliary body melanoma comprises only 12% of uveal melanoma (Kanski 2007). Due to the location of the ciliary body, small ciliary body melanomas are often fairly difficult to locate, and patients are often asymptomatic. Patients presenting with a large ciliary body melanoma may complain of a painless blurred vision due to secondary lens subluxation or astigmatism. Other secondary complications include hyphaema, cataract, retinal detachment and haemorrhage.

Reflective activity

Consider a patient whom you have seen recently with a uveal tract problem:

- What were the presenting signs and symptoms?
- Was there any associated systemic disease or diseases?

- What tests and investigations were carried out and why?
- How did you arrive at a diagnosis?
- What was the treatment plan?
- Outline the care and management of the patient.
- If there were any challenges in caring for the patient, what were they?
- Was any other member of the multidisciplinary team involved in the care and what was their input?
- Utilising a recognised health-promotion framework, how would you explain the condition and treatment to the patient in order to ensure that he or she adheres to the treatment?
- What was the clinical outcome?
- What local or national policies, guidelines or protocols influenced the care and management of this patient?
- On reflection, would you have done anything differently and, if so, what?

Your completed case study can be used to contribute to your continuing professional development portfolio for Registration and your Knowledge and Skills Framework review or appraisal.

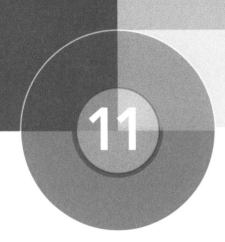

Glaucoma

This chapter explores the assessment, diagnosis and management of glaucomas.

INTRODUCTION

There are numerous types of glaucoma, and each has the potential to cause blindness. In the United Kingdom, it accounts for 10% of blind registrations and partial sight certification (Sparrow 2009). A general characteristic of glaucoma is a rise in the intraocular pressure that is sufficient to cause damage to the optic nerve head. Intraocular pressure is determined by the balance between the rate of production and the rate of drainage of aqueous fluid. Normal intraocular pressure is 15–20 mmHg, but this measurement depends to some extent on which method is used to measure it. In addition, the thickness of the cornea can influence intraocular pressure readings. Thin corneas give rise to artificially low readings, and thicker corneas may give rise to artificially high readings. For this reason, corneal pachymetry is performed.

METHODS OF MEASURING INTRAOCULAR PRESSURE

DIGITAL

The patient looks downward, closing the eye to be examined, and the nurse gently palpates the eyeball with the two index fingers to assess the degree of 'hardness'. This is not an accurate measurement, but an eye with raised pressure will feel harder than one with normal pressure. It is a useful initial method of assessment, especially if none of the specialised equipment needed for measuring intraocular pressure is available, as in the GP's surgery.

GOLDMANN APPLANATION TONOMETER

The tonometer head comprises a double prism. It is attached to a slit lamp. This is a contact method of determining the intraocular pressure, and the eye must be anaesthetised first with anaesthetic drops such as proxymetacaine hydrochloride 0.5%. Fluorescein sodium drops are also instilled to stain the tear film and allow the semicircles in the tonometer head (prism) to be viewed. The dial should be preset between 1 and 2. The cobalt blue light is used, and the prism

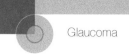
is placed against the cornea and the pressure measurement is read off a dial on the tonometer. The reading on the dial has to be multiplied by 10.

The tonometer should be calibrated on a daily basis to ensure accuracy.

Because of concerns about cross-infection, disposable prism heads or prism sheaths should be used. Where non-disposable prisms are used, they must be properly disinfected after each patient, according to the manufacturer's instructions. In addition, non-disposable prisms should be inspected regularly to ensure that they are not damaged as this could result in corneal irritation or damage to the epithelium.

PERKINS' APPLANATION TONOMETER

The Perkins' applanation tonometer is a hand-held tonometer, working on the principles of the Goldmann tonometer mentioned above. It is useful for patients who are unable to sit at a slit lamp, e.g. those who are in wheelchairs, who are bed-bound or unconscious. The method of use and normal pressure readings are the same as for the Goldmann tonometer.

TONO-PEN

Tono-Pens are small pen-like instruments that measure pressure in a similar fashion to the applanation method. This method is becoming increasingly popular as the operator does not have to have skill in the use of the slit lamp.

NON-CONTACT TONOMETER

Non-contact tonometers, employed by optometrists, use a puff of air blown against the eye. The time required to flatten the cornea is converted into a figure to denote the intraocular pressure.

SCHIOTZ TONOMETRY

Schiotz tonometry is a contact method of measuring intraocular pressure that does not require a power source. This is rarely used but is used more in developed countries.

ANATOMY AND PHYSIOLOGY

ANTERIOR CHAMBER

The anterior chamber is the area between the posterior surface of the cornea and the anterior surface of the iris. The angle of the anterior chamber may be examined using a gonioscope.

POSTERIOR CHAMBER

The posterior chamber is the area between the posterior surface of the iris and the anterior surface of the lens and suspensory ligaments.

AQUEOUS HUMOUR

Both the anterior and posterior chambers are filled with aqueous humour, which is a clear fluid produced by the ciliary processes of the ciliary body. Aqueous humour flows from the ciliary body into the posterior chamber, through the pupil, into the anterior chamber, and drains through the anterior chamber angle at the rate of approximately 2 μL/min.

COMPOSITION OF AQUEOUS HUMOUR

Aqueous humour is similar in constitution to plasma: 99% water and 1% nutrients, e.g. sodium, potassium, chloride, bicarbonate and glucose. Volume is approximately 125 μL.

AQUEOUS HUMOUR CIRCULATION

The aqueous humour circulation is central to intra-ocula pressure balance:

- Produced continuously by the ciliary body (specifically by the ciliary epithelium of the ciliary processes) at a rate of 2–6 mL/min.
- Drained out of the eye via the trabecular meshwork (TM):
  - TM is a sieve-like structure around the periphery of the anterior chamber.
- Fluid then passes into Schlemm's canal and on into collector channels.
- The fluid finally drains into episcleral vessels.

FUNCTIONS OF AQUEOUS FLUID

- To maintain intraocular pressure (IOP)
- To provide a clear medium for refraction
- To provide nourishment to the lens, and to the posterior surface of the cornea

FACTORS WHICH DETERMINE IOP

Intraocular pressure is determined by a number of factors. These are

- Rate of aqueous production.
- Resistance encountered in outflow channels.
- Level of episcleral venous pressure – If increased, the aqueous outflow is decreased as there is no longer a passive gradient from the eye to the collector channels, and into the episcleral vessels.
- Aqueous circulation is dependent on a pressure gradient forcing aqueous out through outflow channels, i.e. the highest pressure should be within the eye and the pressure gradually lowering as you pass through each of the various parts of the drainage mechanism, with the lowest pressure in the episcleral vessels.
- Any disruption to the aqueous flow causes IOP change, i.e. an increase in episcleral venous pressure, a blockage within the TM or Schlemm's canal.

ANGLE OF THE ANTERIOR CHAMBER

The angle of the anterior chamber lies between the limbus (corneal-scleral junction) and the iris, and it surrounds the circumference of the anterior chamber. It is composed of the trabecular meshwork and the canal of Schlemm. The trabecular meshwork is made up of fibrous connective tissue, perforated with oval holes (sieve-like) and lined with endothelium, which is continuous with that of the posterior surface of the cornea. There are three distinct parts:

1. The uveal meshwork, which is innermost extending from the iris root to Schwalbe's line
2. The middle section, which is the corneo-scleral meshwork
3. The largest section; the endothelial meshwork, which communicates directly with Schlemm's canal

Aqueous humour drains via two routes: 90% through the meshwork from the anterior chamber into the canal of Schlemm – an oval-shaped channel lined with endothelium. Between 25 and 30 collector channels leave the canal of Schlemm and anastomose to form the intrascleral plexus. From here, the aqueous humour drains into the aqueous humour veins, the vortex veins and the inferior ophthalmic vein. The uveoscleral route accounts for the remaining 10% of aqueous humour drainage. Aqueous humour flows across the ciliary body to the suprachoroidal space; from here, it enters the venous circulation.

FUNCTION OF THE ANGLE

The anterior chamber angle is for the drainage of aqueous fluid from the eye into the venous circulation.

BLOOD SUPPLY

The blood supply to and drainage from the angle of the anterior chamber is via

- Anterior ciliary arteries
- Aqueous humour vein

RELATED DISORDERS – GLAUCOMA

Glaucoma is a group of conditions that can cause permanent sight loss. There is damage to the optic nerve head that may or may not be the result of a rise in the intraocular pressure. It is the damage to the optic nerve head that results in a visual field loss (see Figure 11.1). The four types of glaucoma, each with a different aetiology, are

1. Primary acute glaucoma
2. Chronic open-angle glaucoma
3. Secondary glaucoma
4. Buphthalmos/childhood glaucoma (ox-eye)

PRIMARY ACUTE GLAUCOMA (ACUTE CLOSED-ANGLE GLAUCOMA)

Primary acute glaucoma affects one person in 1000 over the age of 40. The incidence increases with age and affects women four times more frequently than men. It is also more common in Asians, Inuits and Chinese. It is uncommon in blacks. The condition can be divided into two types:

- Primary pupil block
- Primary irido-trabecular block

PUPIL BLOCK

Some 94% of primary acute glaucoma cases are of the pupil block type. The eye that is predisposed to this type has

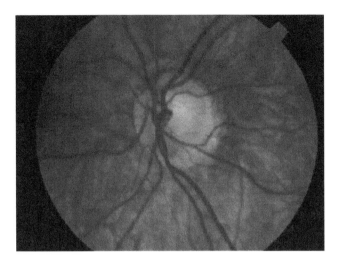

Figure 11.1 Glaucomatous disc changes.

- A dome iris: an iris that is characteristically bowed forward
- Hypermetropia
- A shallow anterior chamber
- A narrow drainage angle
- A large anteriorly placed lens

The pupil becomes blocked by the lens when the pupil is semi-dilated. The aqueous humour cannot flow through the pupil, resulting in a rise in pressure behind the iris. This causes the iris to be pushed forward (iris bombe), and the forward-placed iris blocks the drainage angle. Treatment for this involves the use of miotic drops such as G. pilocarpine 2%, which brings the iris away from the angle, and laser iridotomy which will allow the aqueous humour to pass into the anterior chamber, bypassing the blocked pupil. Beta-blockers such as G. timoptol are used to reduce aqueous humour secretion in the affected eye and as a prophylactic measure in the other eye.

Note: YAG laser iridotomy is performed when the eye has responded to treatment, usually the next day, and the fellow eye is also treated as a prophylactic measure.

IRIDO-TRABECULAR BLOCK

Irido-trabecular block only occurs in 6% of primary acute glaucoma cases. In irido-trabecular block, the eye typically has

- A plateau iris
- Emmetropia
- A deep anterior chamber
- Deeply recessed angles

Pupillary dilation leads to a progressive irido-trabecular blockage. Treatment is by the use of miotic drops to bring the iris away from the angle.

Primary acute glaucoma usually presents unilaterally, but the fellow eye can also be affected, so it must receive prophylactic treatment.

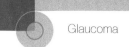

Primary acute glaucoma can be divided into five stages which may overlap but the overlap may not be orderly from one stage to the next:

- Latent – asymptomatic
- Intermittent or subacute
- Acute
- Chronic
- Absolute – end stage

LATENT

As the patients are asymptomatic the condition is diagnosed either at a routine eye examination or when another eye condition is being investigated. These patients must be warned of the prodromal symptoms (see below) in case they progress to the next stage.

INTERMITTENT OR SUB-ACUTE

A rapid closure of parts of the angle (see Gonioscopy section) causes the pressure to rise. This results in certain prodromal symptoms and signs:

- Headache
- Eye pain
- Blurred vision and haloes seen around lights, due to corneal oedema
- Nausea
- General malaise

These prodromal symptoms and signs usually occur at night and improve by the morning when the miosed pupil during sleep has come away from the angle. Patients often think they have a migraine or 'sick headache'. An attack may develop into an acute attack or may bypass this stage. As more of the angle becomes blocked with subsequent attacks, chronic closed-angle glaucoma develops. It is therefore important to diagnose and treat this stage early. Treatment is by laser iridotomy, followed by intensive miotic drops.

INVESTIGATIONS

Provocative tests

Provocative tests are performed on patients with prodromal or latent symptoms to see if the intraocular pressure rises when the eye has been subjected to certain situations. Although rare, they are still in use in some centres.

Non-provocative tests

Utilising gonioscopy, the depth of the patient's anterior chamber angle can be assessed. The gonioscope is a large contact lens with either two or three mirrors placed at differing angles to each other (Figure 11.2), enabling the angle of the anterior chamber to be viewed when used with the slit lamp. The patient's eye is anaesthetised with anaesthetic drops such as G. proxymetacaine hydrochloride 0.5%. A lubricant such as methylcellulose is applied to the surface of the lens, which is placed against the cornea. This lubricates the lens and fills the space between the lens and the cornea. The degree to which the angle is open is graded using a

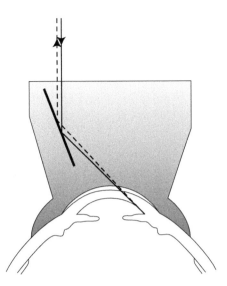

Figure 11.2 Optical systems of Goldmann contact lens used in gonioscopy.

grading system such as Shaffer. The Shaffer system records the degree to which the angle is open on a scale from 0 to 4; 0 being closed and 4 being fully open. Grades 1 and 2 demonstrate that angle closure is probable/possible. The circumference of the angle usually has variable degrees of closure.

ACUTE GLAUCOMA

Acute glaucoma is an ophthalmic emergency as the acute raise in intraocular pressure can damage the optic nerve irreversibly.

Condition guideline: Acute glaucoma

SIGNS AND SYMPTOMS
- A sudden rise in intraocular pressure due either to pupil block or angle closure causes congestion and oedema of the structures involved.
- Lids may be red and swollen.
- Periocular pain may be experienced.
- Conjunctiva may show dusky red injection and may be chemosed.
- Hazy cornea may be observed.
- Iris may appear 'muddy' and swollen with loss of its usual clear pattern.
- Pupil may be fixed, semi-dilated and oval in shape.
- Shallow anterior chamber may be observed.
- Raised intraocular pressure (can be as high as 70 mmHg or more) may be recorded.
- Rapidly reduced visual acuity may be experienced.
- Patient may suffer from nausea and vomiting in severe cases.
- Patient generally feels unwell.

PATIENT'S NEEDS

- Relief of symptoms: severe headache; pain in the eye; nausea; vomiting; abdominal pain; generally feeling unwell. These symptoms can sometimes be confused with other conditions such as acute abdomen and, with the dilated pupil, neurological conditions.
- Reassurance and explanation.
- Possible admission to hospital.
- Preparation for laser treatment.
- Instructions on discharge from hospital.

NURSING PRIORITIES

- Inform medical staff at once. Immediate treatment will bring relief of symptoms and prevent complications occurring.
- Prepare medication and commence instillation of drops as soon as possible after they have been prescribed.

IMMEDIATE NURSING ACTION

Test visual acuity, if the patient is fit enough:

1. Explain that treatment to the eye will relieve general symptoms.
2. Lay the patient on a couch in a quiet, darkened area.
3. Provide the patient with a vomit bowl and tissues.
4. The patient may appreciate a cold compress on the forehead.
5. Acetazolamide 500 mg is prescribed to be given intravenously to reduce the production of aqueous humour.
6. Commence the instillation of G. pilocarpine 4% four times per day to the affected eye once it has been prescribed. Intensive miotics are not effective in pulling away the iris from the angle as the sphincter muscle is usually ischaemic if the pressure is above 30 mmHg (Kanski 2007).
7. Commence G. pilocarpine one to two times a day to unaffected eye.
8. Commence a beta-blocker (e.g. G. levobunolol hydrochloride [Betagan]) to the affected eye.
9. Commence steroid eye drops, e.g. G. prednisolone acetate (Pred Forte), to the affected eye as there is usually an associated inflammation.
10. Give analgesics and/or anti-emetics if headache, nausea and vomiting continue despite treatment. Monitor pain and the effect of treatment using an appropriate pain assessment tool.
11. Offer mouthwash if vomiting to freshen the mouth and breath.
12. Prepare further treatment, if necessary, to reduce the intraocular pressure if initial treatment has failed to bring it down:
    a. Intravenous mannitol 20% – 200 mL given over 1–2 hours.
    b. Care for intravenous rate of flow and the site of the cannula, as leakage into the surrounding tissues (extravasation) which causes phlebitis.
    c. When required, assist the patient to the toilet or give a urinal or bedpan, as mannitol has a diuretic effect.
    d. Glycerol (1–5 mg/kg body weight) orally, in orange juice to disguise the taste. This in itself may induce nausea and vomiting.

The patient may resent the frequent attention he requires in the initial stages of treatment of this condition and may just want to be left alone. Handle the patient sympathetically and show understanding of his feelings.

FURTHER NURSING ACTION

Prepare the patient for laser iridotomy to both eyes (prophylactically to the fellow eye). Such preparation is restricted to explanation of the procedure and ensuring that the patient has his pain assessed and appropriate analgesia provided before he attends for the laser treatment. If the patient is still nauseous, anti-emetics should also be given as prescribed.

CHRONIC

Often referred to as 'creeping angle closure', this is when repeated attacks of either intermittent or untreated acute episodes cause further adhesions of the peripheral iris to the posterior surface of the cornea (peripheral anterior synaechiae), thus closing the angle. The signs and symptoms are similar to chronic open-angle glaucoma (see below).

ABSOLUTE

This is the end stage of primary acute, chronic and secondary (see below) glaucoma when treatment has failed. Cataracts are usually present and occur due to the medical or surgical treatment rather than to the disease process (Kuppens et al. 1995).

Blind, painful eyes which occur at this stage are best treated by enucleation. Alternatively, periodic retrobulbar or facial nerve injections can be administered. Phthisis bulbi, or shrinkage of the eye, occurs as it atrophies when enucleation is the most appropriate course of action.

NICE has published guidelines relating to the diagnosis and subsequent management of chronic open-angle glaucoma and ocular hypertension (Sparrow 2009).

CHRONIC OPEN-ANGLE GLAUCOMA (COAG)

Glaucoma is a major health problem worldwide, and the global prevalence of glaucoma was estimated at 67 million people in 2001 and, by 2020, it is predicted to be 79.6 million (Quigley 2006, Quigley and Broman 2006) and 111.8 million by 2040 (Tham et al. 2014). In the United Kingdom, it is the leading cause of preventable blindness, accounting for 10% of blind registrations in England (Sparrow 2009). Despite increasing public health awareness of the condition and the availability of highly trained community opticians and sophisticated equipment, a high proportion of suspected glaucoma cases remained undiagnosed. The number of patients with undetected glaucoma is set to rise as the elderly population are living longer. Early detection of glaucoma is essential if we are to not only maximise the benefits of treatment but also to minimise the impact of the disease on patients and their carers.

Chronic open-angle glaucoma occurs in patients of either sex over the age of 45 years with symptoms usually occurring after the age of 65 if the disease is undetected. This is not to be confused with the chronic form of primary acute glaucoma, which has an insidious onset and is slowly progressive. The patient does not usually notice symptoms of chronic open-angle glaucoma until the disease has progressed so far as to result in marked visual field loss. This is because it is the nasal visual field that is lost initially; the fellow eye compensates for the vision loss. It is a bilateral condition, with one eye often being involved earlier and more severely than the other. The patient usually first notices that he cannot see so well in his peripheral vision and

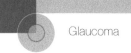

has started bumping into things. He often thinks it is just old age or something a new pair of glasses will correct. Hence, it is optometrists who often refer these patients to ophthalmologists.

Certain optometrists, orthoptists and ophthalmic nurses have received additional training in the care and management of patients with glaucoma. Glaucoma suspects are referred to them either by fellow optometrists or from GPs. These highly trained healthcare professionals undertake a thorough examination and assessment of the patient and treat the patient according to protocols; they only refer on to an ophthalmologist those people with glaucoma – who therefore fall outside the protocol. This allows some patients – those who do not actually have glaucoma – to be reassured that they are in the clear, and allows them to be discharged. It is thought that without such schemes, as many as 20% of referrals to hospitals would be false positives. Patients who have stable glaucoma are also managed by this group of healthcare professionals. Providing education to patients and their carers, and ensuring that patients comply with their treatment plan, are also important aspects to the role. It must be noted, however, that NICE guidelines (Sparrow 2009) indicate that all patients with an intraocular pressure of >21 mmHg on more than one occasion must be referred to an ophthalmologist for diagnosis.

COAG is a chronic, progressive disease of the optic nerve with characteristic features (Sparrow 2009):

- Optic nerve head cupping and atrophy (common to other types of glaucoma).
- Typical patterns of visual field loss (common to other types of glaucoma).
- COAG usually has a raised intraocular pressure >21 mmHg.
- COAG has open and normal appearing drainage angles, nothing else to be seen on gonioscopy.

OTHER FEATURES OF COAG

- Usually bilateral, may be asymmetrical in terms of the amount of damage and field loss – only one eye may appear affected on diagnosis, usually at some point both eyes are affected.
- Adult onset.
- No secondary causes of raised IOP – no sign in the angle of any pigment, pseudoexfoliated material with an open and healthy-looking angle.
- Usually insidious onset, slowly progressive but painless.
- Often a positive family history of COAG (not the case with most other types of glaucoma).

COAG STATISTICS

- Chronic open-angle glaucoma is the most prevalent of all glaucomas.
- It affects 1 in 200 of the general population over age 40 years.
- Incidence increases with age.
- When considering male versus female, there is equal gender distribution.
- It is responsible for approximately 12% of blind registrations in the United Kingdom and the United States.
- It is usually treatable and manageable, but it is not always possible to prevent vision loss.

ETHNIC VARIATIONS

COAG has ethnic variations in both its incidence and how it behaves:

- COAG is four to five times more common in black populations than white populations.

- Often COAG appears to be more aggressive in African and African-Caribbean people or other black populations.
- Surgery is more often required to control IOP in black populations (medical treatment is often not enough), but it carries a greater risk of failure in this ethnic group. This is concerning because there is no adequate way of treating COAG any differently at this moment in time – the management is the same with all ethnicities.
- Blindness from glaucoma is four to eight times more common in black Americans than in white Americans.

INHERITANCE

It is always useful to ask about a family history of COAG on the first clinic visit:

- COAG is often associated with a family history of the disease.
- There is a 3.7 times increase in risk of developing glaucoma for individuals with a sibling who has COAG (Baltimore Eye Study).
- Probably multifactor inheritance pattern, i.e. not everybody with a COAG family member will develop the disease.
- Therefore it is important that everyone with positive family history (particularly a first-degree relative – parent, sibling) should undergo an annual IOP check as part of their sight test.

OTHER RISK FACTORS FOR COAG

No one really knows what the exact mechanism of developing COAG is, so the following risk factors that are statistically more often present in people with COAG are

- Raised IOP.
- Myopia – A greater risk with higher myopia, no hard evidence for the mechanism responsible, just a statistical fact.
- Diabetes mellitus – This may be related to the fact that diabetes damages small blood vessels, these are the type of vessels which provide nutrition to the optic nerve – predisposing an individual to developing further damage to the optic nerve.
- Untreated hypertension – While there is no hard evidence, there may be a similar mechanism to diabetes as it also damages small blood vessels.
- Retinal vein occlusion – Glaucoma may coexist at presentation with retinal changes. The raised IOP usually present in COAG actually causes the retinal vein occlusion, so diagnosis of glaucoma often occurs at the time of the occlusion. It is not the case that developing a later retinal vein occlusion puts the patient at risk of COAG, it puts them at risk of developing other types of glaucoma, i.e. rubeotic glaucoma.
- Retinitis pigmentosa – There is a possible 5% increased risk of developing COAG.

INTRAOCULAR PRESSURE (IOP)

Previously it was thought that COAG was direct damage to the optic nerve caused by a high IOP, it is less clear cut now, because it is known that IOP is usually raised in COAG – however the cause-and-effect relationship is unclear.

- The 'normal' range of IOP is 10–21 mmHg (two standard deviations [SD] from the mean IOP in the population of 16 mmHg). Although the majority of people do fall within this range, not everybody does, but this has been the classic way to diagnose glaucoma.
- There is a wide variation in IOP in the population.
- IOP is not static – individual people have IOP fluctuations based on daily rhythms, heart rate and blood pressure.
- The levels of these normal IOP fluctuations are increased in COAG – A change of 15 mmHg may occur within 24 hours in untreated cases and so causes great difficulty in making a diagnosis based on IOP.
- Raised IOP is now considered a risk factor for glaucoma, not a cause, though usually present in COAG.

PATHOPHYSIOLOGY

- Raised IOP previously thought to be the direct cause of optic nerve and visual field (VF) damage.
- It is now believed that several contributory factors are likely including
  - Ischaemia of the optic nerve – which explains the risk to diabetic and hypertensive patients.
  - Abnormalities of axonal or ganglion cell metabolism – degenerative products damaging the optic nerve.
  - Disorders of the extracellular matrix of the lamina cribrosa, i.e. the scaffold of the sclera at the lamina cribrosa where the optic nerve enters the eye.
  - It should be noted that it is possible to have all or any of the above glaucomatous damage to the VF and optic nerve without a raised IOP above 21 mmHg.

PATIENT ASSESSMENT IN SUSPECTED GLAUCOMA

Usually patients are asymptomatic at presentation – they do not notice any change in their vision and it requires a great deal of education to help them understand the condition and how the treatment may halt its progress. This is essential if we are to improve adherence with treatment. Suspicious features will probably have been detected by the optometrist at a routine eye examination.

HOW TO ASSESS THE PATIENT

- Measure the IOP – On several occasions, to find their highest IOP, enabling us to classify the glaucoma and allowing us to monitor the effect of treatment. Day phasing is useful, IOP checks are repeated every couple of hours, sometimes revealing a spike in IOP that we are not otherwise picking up in clinic.
- Irrespective of a high or low IOP, to make the diagnosis as to whether or not glaucoma is present we need to look at the better signs:
  - Optic nerve appearance and visual field defects now the defining features in COAG.
  - Gonioscopy – in order to ascertain the reason for this patient's glaucoma – open, narrow or closed angle?
  - Examine for other causes of glaucoma.

OPTIC DISC CHANGES IN GLAUCOMA

Patients with glaucoma may present with the following changes in their optic disc:

- Asymmetry of the neuro-retinal rim (NRR) of nerve fibres or cupping, strictly speaking anything greater than a 0.3 cup-disc ratio (CDR) should be considered as potentially abnormal.
- Asymmetry of CDR between the two eyes, the eye with a healthier optic nerve acts as the control, as both eyes probably used to look like that.
- Localised thinning or notching of the NRR, quite subtle to determine. The use of the ISNT (Inferior, Superior, Nasal, Temporal) rule helps with this – NRR should be thickest inferiorly (viewed as the superior part of the image when using the Superfield), the inferior NRR is often the part which gets damaged first in glaucoma, if it looks thinner then it is damaged.
- Optic disc haemorrhage – usually flame/splinter shaped. A sign of imminent damage to the optic nerve head – suspicious sign of glaucomatous changes.
- Bayoneting of blood vessels – where they briefly disappear under the NRR and reappear further round. If the depth of the cup (i.e. a large cup due to thinner NRR) is considerably enlarged due to glaucomatous damage, the blood vessels as they emerge from the optic nerve, have to go down and across the optic nerve to make their way onto the retina, usually they would just pass across the top of the optic nerve and straight out. This is a sign of glaucomatous change.
- 'Lamellar dot' sign – pores of lamina cribrosa are visible to the periphery of disc cup – can be normal, in a damaged nerve the dots become lines and more obvious.

VISUAL FIELD DEFECTS

If the signs above are seen in the optic nerve, it is probable that the eye has glaucoma, irrespective of how high or low the IOP is. Always compare the two eyes and look at the VF analysis, the abnormal appearance of the optic nerve should be mirrored in the VF defects if there is glaucoma.

VF defects correspond to the loss of the nerve fibre layer of the retina (and optic disc changes). If the nerve fibres are damaged within the optic nerve they will no longer be able to provide that little bit of vision and it will result in classic VF defects:

- Nasal scotoma.
- Paracentral scotoma.
- Arcuate scotoma.
- Ring scotoma – defects in both halves of field coalesce, present with quite a large amount of glaucomatous loss.
- Eventually only a small central field is left (tunnel vision).

Usually the temporal wedge of the VF will go before the central field, but everyone is different, this group of patients are usually old, there could be macular degeneration occurring as well, damaging their central field.

MAKING THE DIAGNOSIS

Making a diagnosis on the first presentation is not always easy; however, the ophthalmologist will make the diagnosis if

- Elevated IOP on more than one occasion, in conjunction with
  - Glaucomatous optic nerve changes.

- Typical field defects.
- May only affect one eye initially.
- Evidence of progressive change in disc or field appearance may be awaited before making the diagnosis – it is important to monitor your patient.

OTHER CONSIDERATIONS TO COAG

- The glaucoma suspect with only one suspicious feature, they should be followed up, but they may never develop glaucoma.
- Ocular hypertension with raised IOP but no evidence of disc or field changes. Some patients may previously have been labelled as having glaucoma purely on the basis of their IOP. However, some will still require treatment if they have an IOP over 30 mmHg because they are at risk of developing retinal vein occlusion.
- Normal tension glaucoma with a normal IOP, never measured as high, but there are typical optic disc and visual field changes. This is difficult to treat as the only course of action is to lower the IOP but this is already low. Often the patient requires surgery to lower the IOP in order to limit the damage to his vision. These patients tend to be elderly, and it is likely that a vascular profusion problem is probably a large part of why they have glaucoma in the first place.
- Secondary open-angle glaucoma because of pseudo-exfoliation, pigment dispersion syndrome, red blood cells.
- Angle-closure glaucoma, which may be easily missed if it is chronic and asymptomatic, where a patient has a narrow angle, threatening angle closure but no acute episodes, the patient has a limit to the aqueous drainage so the IOP rises but the real problem is that the angle is compromised by the iris. This emphasizes the importance of performing gonioscopy on all new patients. Treatment is a peripheral iridotomy to lower the IOP without any other treatment. This is unlike the typical acute angle closure, which has a very high IOP and pain associated with it.
- If there is a history of ischaemic heart disease, hypertension, migraines, peripheral vascular disease, Raynaud's phenomenon or the patient is taking beta-blockers (can give an artificially low IOP), it is probably more likely that the glaucoma the patient has is normal tension glaucoma.

EVIDENCE FOR TREATMENT

- Numerous studies have shown a beneficial effect from lowering the IOP in open-angle glaucoma patients, though not the cause. It must be a contributory part of the damage to the optic nerve, and we can limit further progression in glaucomatous changes.
- Effective treatment reduces the risk of further loss of visual field (Garway-Heath et al. 2015).

MANAGEMENT

- If there are optic disc changes and typical visual field defects are present, begin treatment for glaucoma. We are going to titrate how well the patient is responding by examining the IOP and the progression of the disease.

- If there is insufficient information to diagnose COAG – repeat assessment for signs of progression before treating.
- In glaucoma suspects or ocular hypertensives it is important to repeat assessment.

TREATMENT (SUMMARY)

1. Topical eye medication, e.g.
   a. Beta-blockers
   b. Prostaglandin analogues
   c. Carbonic anhydrase inhibitors
2. Argon laser trabeculoplasty while not common, is useful in lowering IOP for a limited period of time, approximately 5 years.
3. Selective laser trabeculoplasty (SLT). SLT differs from conventional argon laser in that it protects the trabecular meshwork against thermal or coagulative effects by selectively targeting only the pigmented cells and preserving surrounding tissue.

   SLT can be an effective adjunct to medication therapy or used as a primary treatment to reduce or eliminate the need for topical glaucoma medications, along with their common systemic side effects.
4. Trabeculectomy – main surgical procedure, with or without cytotoxic agents to limit the scarring.
5. Viscocanalostomy. Canulate the Schlemm's canal, on order to improve the aqueous outflow without going right into the eye, a possible lower risk to the eye than a trabeculectomy, but does not work quite as well in lowering the IOP. This is not a common procedure at the moment in the United Kingdom.

FOLLOW-UP

It is important that any patient diagnosed with COAG is followed-up regularly for life. At each clinic visit, assessment of visual acuity, IOP and optic discs assessment should be undertaken. Visual fields should be performed every 12–18 months or more often if changes are suspected, if IOP is poorly uncontrolled or progression is evident within the optic disc.

Gonioscopy should be carried out if there is a rise in IOP or change in depth of the anterior chamber. It should be noted that the appearance of the angle can change with time. Angle closure patients have the added problem that their lens is becoming bigger and bigger with age compromising the anterior chamber.

PATIENT OUTLOOK

- Patients require help with understanding the diagnosis and need for treatment.
- Repeated explanations may be necessary to reinforce the importance of the drop therapy.
- Patient adherence with treatment must always be considered – especially if the IOP seems uncontrolled. For example, some patients only put their drops in on the morning of the clinic, other people deliberately do not put in their drops for their clinic visit.
- Changes in treatment may be required and it must be considered if this is still the best treatment for the individual patient.
- Good patient rapport greatly helps. The patient will be a regular visitor.

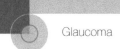

Condition guideline: Chronic open-angle glaucoma

PATIENT'S NEEDS

- An understanding of the condition, treatment and prognosis
- Someone to listen and explain procedures
- Advice about work/recreation/lifestyle changes
- Guidance/help with mobility because of visual impairment, such registration as sight impaired, including advice on the UK Driver and Vehicle Licensing Agency regulations
- Information in a format that the patient can read and understand
- Assistance with investigations, especially perimetry
- Instruction in instillation of drops and taking of oral medication, and the impact they have on the disease process
- Preparation for laser treatment or surgery

NURSING ACTION

Guide/help patient while he is at the hospital. His degree of visual impairment will depend on the amount of glaucomatous damage. If he has peripheral field loss, he will tend to knock into furniture, doors, etc. and will need to be escorted to the varying departments during his visit. McBride (2000, 2002) found that hospitals were not meeting the needs of people with visual impairment; while this is a dated study, it remains relevant. Patients need people to respect them as human beings and not just to view them as another case. Nurses should be proactive in ensuring that the environment is conducive to the needs of people with visual impairment.

Assist the patient with or perform perimetry. These tests require concentration on the part of the patient. As many patients are elderly, concentration is not always easy to maintain, and therefore the patient needs encouragement and assistance during these tests.

Provide the patient with information on his treatment and treatment options which will be either medical or surgical.

INVESTIGATIONS

Perimetry, posterior-segment examination and applanation tonometry are carried out to diagnose and monitor the disease. Corneal pachymetry is also performed to determine the thickness of the cornea.

Perimetry

These tests are performed to assess the degree of peripheral and central visual loss. They are used to detect the disease and follow its progress. There are several different types of test, but they all use the same principle. The patient, with one eye covered, stares at a white spot or light. Without moving his eye from this spot or light, he indicates verbally or by pressing a buzzer as soon as he sees another spot or light entering his peripheral vision from any angle in the 360° circle. Most machines these days are computerised.

Posterior-segment examination

Examination of the optic disc can be made using a slit lamp and handheld magnifying lenses, such as 60D, 78D, 90D, to assess the degree of cupping, the state of the neuro-retinal rim and any changes to the retinal vasculature, e.g. bayoneting or flame haemorrhages.

Laser scanning tomography

Laser scanning tomography is a more sophisticated investigation of the optic disc which quantifies the areas of neural tissue at the optic disc, by taking sections through the nerve head in a similar manner to a CT scan.

Tonometry

Measurement of the intraocular pressure is recorded. The pressure is not always markedly raised, especially early in the disease.

Gonioscopy

Gonioscopy will be carried out to assess the degree to which the angle is open. Patients may have narrow angles as well as chronic glaucoma.

Phasing

The patient normally attends as a day case to see if the intraocular pressure is raised at various times of the day. There is a normal diurnal pattern to intraocular pressure, with the pressure being higher in the mornings. The intraocular pressure is normally recorded every 4–6 hours, ideally by the same operator and with the same equipment.

Heidelberg retinal topograph

The Heidelberg retinal topograph (HRT) takes three-dimensional topographic measurements of the optic disc and retina. This allows the analysis of any glaucomatous optic nerve head, macula holes and macula oedema and any nerve fibre layer damage.

Optical coherence tomography

Optical coherence tomography (OCT) is a non-contact, non-invasive imaging technique used to produce and obtain high-resolution cross-sectional images of the retina. As a result of the high resolution, OCT is particularly suitable for measuring retinal thickness and, in so doing, detecting retinal pathologies. In addition, OCT has the capability of measuring retinal fibre thickness in glaucoma and other diseases of the optic nerve. The images presented on the OCT are shown either as cross-sectional images or as topographic maps. It is patient and user friendly, and dilation of the pupil is not essential.

Conditions affecting the retina that are suitable for OCT include the following:

- Glaucoma – In glaucoma, the OCT measures the retinal nerve fibre thickness at standardised locations around the optic nerve head. A circular scan produces a cylindrical cross section of the retina from which the nerve fibre layer can be analysed. In addition, radial scans through the optic nerve head are used to evaluate cupping and juxtapapillary nerve fibre thickness. Early progression of the disease and early diagnosis of glaucoma can be made using the OCT.
- Diabetic macular oedema – OCT is particularly useful in assessing the presence and area of retinal thickening, the amount of thickening at the centre, the proximity of retinal thickening to the centre, the presence or absence of cyst information and, most importantly, the presence or absence of clinically significant macula oedema.
- Cystoid macular oedema from a variety of disorders including cataract extraction, uveitis and venous occlusions – The use of OCT as a means of measuring cystoid macula oedema is a useful diagnostic tool.

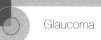

- Age-related macular degeneration – OCT is used to image subretinal fluid, intraretinal thickening and choroidal neovascularisation in the assessment prior to treatment.

MEDICAL TREATMENT

As mentioned earlier, the model for the management and treatment of people with chronic open-angle glaucoma is increasingly a shared responsibility. Nurses, orthoptists and optometrists have expanded their roles to include managing caseloads of patients with stable glaucoma. Protocols and guidelines following risk assessment support such roles.

As adherence can be a particular problem in this chronic condition, there is a need to emphasise the importance of instilling the drops in order to control the intraocular pressure, with a view to preventing further visual field loss. Following clinical examination and interpretation of results, discussion with the patient should be about explaining findings, ensuring that he has an understanding of what has been said. Any queries the patient may have should be answered. A target intraocular pressure will be set, usually a 30% reduction from the baseline measurement (Sparrow 2009). When setting the target pressure, factors relating to the patient's quality of life should be taken into account, such as the patient's level of anxiety relative to the chronic nature of the condition, current level of vision loss, cost, inconvenience and side effects of treatment.

Instruct the patient about his drops and any other medication; the patient needs to be aware of the effects and side effects. Then one, or perhaps two, of the following medications may be instigated:

- Prostaglandin analogues, e.g. latanoprost 0.005% or travoprost 0.004% nocte or tafluprost 15 µg/mL once a day.
- Beta-blocker, e.g. timolol maleate (Timoptol) twice a day or betaxolol 0.25% twice a day.
- Acetazolamide tablets 250–500 mg four times a day, or slow-release twice a day.
- With drop instillation, there is a need to prevent systemic absorption. This can be achieved by asking the patient to close his eye gently after instilling the drop and to count slowly to 60 before opening it again.
- Combined topical preparations, e.g. Cosopt (dorzolamide 2% and timolol 0.5%) or Xalacom (latanoprost 0.005% and timolol 0.5%).

Where topical medication proves to be ineffective, consideration may be given to changing the medication before adding additional medication, unless the patient's preference is a surgical option (Sparrow 2009).

IMPROVING ADHERENCE WITH MEDICATION

Non-adherence with glaucoma medication is a problem and is set to continue unless all healthcare professionals, together with the patient, take a joint approach to glaucoma management. Non-adherence is particularly high in patients with chronic glaucoma because of the following reasons:

- Glaucoma is asymptomatic in the early stages.
- Glaucoma is a chronic condition.

- The treatment is perceived as being worse than the disease, i.e. the side effects of the drops.
- There is no obvious improvement.
- The condition is lifelong.
- The majority of patients are elderly with other systemic problems.

Various studies (Olthoff and Schoutan 2005; Sleat et al. 2006) have examined the reasons for non-adherence and these are summarised below:

- Cognitive impairment (up to 20% of the elderly) or a simple lack of understanding/ knowledge, failing memory
- Language barriers
- Inadequate knowledge of the condition and treatment
- Type and number of medications prescribed for systemic and ocular conditions
- Unsuitable type of container, e.g. minims eye drops
- Route of administration
- Frequency of administration
- Inadequate advice about importance of adherence and motivation
- Physical difficulties/dexterity and poor coordination, such as arthritis, Parkinson's
- Mental disabilities such as learning disabilities
- Having to cope with other systemic conditions such as diabetes, hypertension, cerebral vascular accident
- Living alone with lack of support
- Work factors such as shift worker
- Eye drops regarded as unpleasant
- Perceptions of side effects
- Specific difficulty associated with the diverse range of bottle sizes and shapes, and difficulty in aiming and squeezing the bottle and fear of poking the eye with tip of dropper bottle
- Reflex blinking
- Poor eyesight and associated problems

OTHER ISSUES WHICH AFFECT NON-ADHERENCE/NON-ADHERENCE IN GLAUCOMA

- Time pressures placed on busy ophthalmology departments, thereby affecting the amount of time allocated to teaching and education.
- Patient's beliefs and denial problem exists.
- Patient not feeling in control of what is happening.
- Lack of communication:
  - In a pressurised environment, communication skills can be the first to go.
  - Non-adherence is directly related to the duration of therapy.

The problems associated with non-adherence are

- Possibility of reduced therapeutic benefit and associated increase in morbidity, such as declining ocular health resulting in more outpatient attendance
- Significant incidental costs to the Health Service arise from non-adherence, resulting in admission to hospital for surgery or re-admission

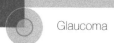

SOME WAYS TO IMPROVE ADHERENCE

- Tailor treatment to the individual needs and wishes.
- Appropriate clinic staff should talk with the patient at each visit about how he is managing his treatment.
- Practice should be supervised, on as many visits as necessary.
- Reduce the number of medications – use combination products or long-acting preparations.
- Establish realistic drop times.
- Encourage the use of drop aids – devices for dropping and opening.
- Use written and verbal instructions.
- Consider the use of letter or colour coding on drop boxes or bottles.

Condition guideline: Chronic open-angle glaucoma

LASER TREATMENT

Prepare the patient for laser trabeculoplasty. This procedure involves bombarding the trabecular meshwork with the laser. It is thought that scarring of the tissue stretches the meshwork and opens it up.

SURGICAL TREATMENT

Admit patient to the day unit:

- Prepare patient for the operation, which is usually performed under a local anaesthetic unless there are indications for general anaesthetic.
- Trabeculectomy is the commonest type of drainage operation performed. This operation involves making a scleral flap and removing a strip of trabecular meshwork below this flap. The scleral flap is sutured back into place but, as this does not heal properly, it causes a fistula through which the aqueous fluid can drain into the scleral vessels. The bulge over the scleral flap, lying under the conjunctiva, is called a 'bleb'. Sparrow (2009) recommend the use of MMC (mitomycin C) or 5-FU (5-fluorouracil) to prevent the bleb from healing.
- Give post-operative care:
  - Eye dressing:
    - Remove and discard the Cartella shield.
    - Bleb should be noted under the conjunctiva.
    - The anterior chamber will be shallow but should not be flat. If it is flat, the bleb is probably draining too much aqueous fluid. A firm pad and bandage should be applied to seal the bleb. The medical staff should be notified.
  - Instillation of eye drops:
    - Antibiotic.
    - Steroid.
    - Mydriatic.
- Discharge of patient. If he is receiving antagonistic drops to each eye, he must be warned of the danger of a mix-up. The operated eye may be receiving a mydriatic, and the unoperated eye may be receiving a miotic as treatment for chronic glaucoma. He may need to be reminded to continue to take the medication to the unoperated eye.

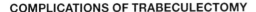

COMPLICATIONS OF TRABECULECTOMY

EARLY

- Over-drainage
- Under-drainage
- Hyphaema
- Aqueous humour misdirection into posterior segment of eye

LATE

- Subconjunctival fibrosis – patients who have had long-term medical treatment prior to their surgery are more prone to fibrosis (Kanski 2007). Cytotoxic agents, such as 5-fluorouracil or mitomycin, given at the time of surgery or a few days post-operatively, can prevent this occurring (Kanski 2007). Care must be taken when handling cytotoxic agents. Wear protective gloves, goggles, face mask and apron when drawing it up. Ensure correct disposal of used syringes, needles and other equipment used in an appropriately labelled container.
- Cataract formation due to surgical intervention.
- Infection as the bleb/fistula is only covered by conjunctiva.

OCULAR HYPERTENSION

Intraocular pressure is higher than normal, over 21 mmHg on more than one occasion, and yet there is no damage to the optic disc and no visual field loss. The condition may never progress to open-angle glaucoma. NICE (Sparrow 2009) recommendation is to measure central cornel thickness (pachtmetry) and have based their ocular hypertension pathway on this, along with age and untreated intraocular pressure measurement at presentation.

Risk factors

- Age – increasing age
- Race – African-Caribbeans and mixed race
- Gender – affects women more than men
- Type II diabetes
- Systemic hypertension
- Family history of glaucoma
- Corticosteroid treatments

NORMAL-TENSION GLAUCOMA

Normal-tension glaucoma is sometimes referred to as low-tension glaucoma.

Risk factors

Risk factors include age, as it affects the elderly, and sex, as women are affected more than men. It is seen more often in Japan than in Europe or the United States.

Clinical presentation other than intraocular pressure is similar to open-angle glaucoma and treatment is also the same. Blood pressure is monitored and dips in systemic blood pressure, especially at night, should be noted. Any anti-hypertensive medication should be avoided at night.

Condition guideline: Secondary glaucoma

CAUSES

Secondary glaucoma can be due to any of the following causes:

- *Conditions of the lens:*
  - Dislocation. The dislocated lens falls into the drainage angle or into the posterior chamber blocking the pupil.
  - Cataract formation.
    - The enlarged lens pushes forward, blocking the pupil or angle. This is called *intumescence of the lens.*
    - Lens material oozes out through the lens capsule clogging the angle. This is called *phacolytic glaucoma.*
- *Conditions of the uveal tract:*
  - Uveitis.
    - Debris from the inflammation of the uveal tract may clog the drainage angle.
    - Pupil block caused by posterior synaechiae.
    - Permanent peripheral anterior synaechiae may develop from repeated attacks of uveitis.
  - Tumours. Melanomas in the uveal tract cause raised intraocular pressure by volume replacement, encroachment on the angle or by blocking the vortex veins.
- *Trauma:*
  - Haemorrhage (hyphaema) into the anterior chamber. The blood in the anterior chamber clots in the angle, effectively obstructing aqueous humour outflow.
  - Angle recession.
  - Corneal or limbal laceration. The anterior chamber is flattened and the angle closed by adherence of the anterior surface of the iris onto the posterior surface of the cornea.
- *Post-operative causes:*
  - Flat anterior chamber – Following intraocular surgery, aqueous humour may escape through the wound, causing a flat anterior chamber. If this persists, permanent anterior and posterior synaechiae may develop.
  - Post-operative hyphaema – Blood clotting in the angle blocks the drainage channels.
- *Rubeosis iridis* – In diabetes mellitus and following occlusion of the central retinal vein, small blood vessels grow into the anterior surface of the iris (neovascularisation) and into the angle of the anterior chamber where they may block the drainage channels (thrombotic glaucoma). The new vessels may also cause a spontaneous hyphaema. Currently eyes with iris neovascularisation are treated with panretinal photocoagulation in order to reduce the production of vascular endothelial growth factor (VEGF) by destroying peripheral retinal tissue. However, pilot studies suggest that anti-VEGF Avastin may be effective for treating neovascular glaucoma (Chalam 2007).
- *Steroids* – It is not clearly understood why long-term treatment with topical steroids causes a rise in intraocular pressure. Care must be taken in the use of topical steroids

in patients with a family history of chronic glaucoma. Regular checks of intraocular pressure in these patients and in long-term users of topical and, in some cases, systemic, steroids must be undertaken.

- *Thyroid eye disease* – Infiltration of the orbital fat and extraocular muscles pushes the globe forward, causing pressure on the globe with a subsequent increase in intraocular pressure.

PATIENT'S NEEDS

The patient's needs are similar to those of primary acute glaucoma. A careful history must be taken because of the similarity in presenting signs and symptoms to primary acute glaucoma, and the other eye must be examined for depth of the anterior chamber.

NURSING ACTION

The cause of the secondary glaucoma, once diagnosed, is treated first.

Therefore the nursing action will be that of the cause.

The intraocular pressure is reduced by medical treatment initially. Surgical intervention may be required if medical treatment fails to keep the intraocular pressure within normal limits. Nursing action will therefore be instruction of the patient on instillation of drops and taking medication, and administration of pre- and post-operative care when surgery is performed.

GLAUCOMA SCREENING, SOME DISCUSSION

Glaucoma is a leading cause of incurable visual disability and blindness. It is generally acknowledged that the population are living longer, the number of people affected by glaucoma is likely to increase from 60 to about 80 million people worldwide in the course of the present decade. As glaucoma is largely asymptomatic, early detection, treatment and education of patients are key strategies in preventing glaucoma associated blindness and low vision.

At present, according to Bettin and Matteo (2013), the predictive power of the available screening techniques is still insufficient, and no single test can discriminate glaucoma from normality accurately enough to be effective as a mass screening tool. However, there is growing evidence to support the argument that screening programmes targeting specific at risk groups such as age group, risk factors, ethnicities and 'at risk' families may be more efficient. Much hope also rests on genetic screening, which is likely to be a future tool for detecting glaucoma in general or in selected populations much earlier than is possible by clinical methods (Bettin and Matteo 2013).

BUPHTHALMOS/CHILDHOOD GLAUCOMA (OX-EYE)

Buphthalmos is a rare congenital condition affecting one in 10,000 births and resulting in increased intraocular pressure caused by a defect or blockage of the drainage angle by an embryonic membrane. Occasionally, the canal of Schlemm is absent. Forty percent have raised intraocular pressures in utero, 50% manifest in the first year of life, and 10% manifest between the first and third year of life.

Buphthalmos is usually a bilateral condition, boys being more commonly affected than girls.

Condition guideline: Buphthalmos/childhood glaucoma (ox-eye)

SIGNS

- Large bulging eyes (Figure 11.3). In childhood, the sclera is more elastic than in the adult eye and the ever-increasing intraocular pressure stretches the sclera. It becomes thinned and appears bluish due to the pigment of the uveal tract showing through. The cornea also stretches. The enlargement of these two structures gives the child's eye the appearance of an ox-eye.
- Deep anterior chamber. The lens is pushed backwards by the increased pressure, thus forming a deep anterior chamber.
- Large cornea. As the cornea is stretched, its diameter increases from a normal 9.0–11.5 to 12–14 mm. Tears may appear in Descemet's membrane.
- Deep cupping of the optic disc due to the raised intraocular pressure.
- The intraocular pressure will be between 25 and 45 mmHg.

PATIENT'S NEEDS

- Relief of symptoms:
  - Lacrimation – Child always appears to have running eyes and nose.
  - Photophobia – Child often puts his arm over his eyes to shield them from the light.
  - Irritability – Child is generally irritable.
- Admission to hospital.
- General care of the child in hospital.

NURSING ACTION

1. Admit the child to the paediatric ward.
2. Give an explanation and reassurance to the parents or guardians. Involve them in as much of the child's care as possible.
3. Prepare the patient for examination under anaesthetic. The following investigations are carried out. These investigations are performed initially to diagnose the disease and thereafter at periodic intervals to assess the success of treatment or the progression of the disease:
   a. Measurement of intraocular pressure.
   b. Gonioscopy.

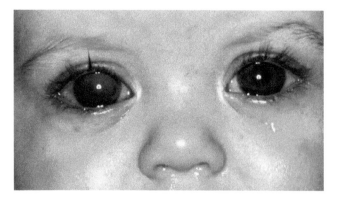

Figure 11.3 Buphthalmos.

    c. Ophthalmoscopy of optic disc.

    d. Measurement of corneal diameter.

4. Give post-anaesthetic care following examination under anaesthesia.

5. Administer pre-operative care if surgery is to be performed:

    a. A goniotomy will be performed to open up the drainage channels by sweeping a goniotomy knife around the whole of the anterior chamber angle.

    b. A drainage operation, such as a trabeculectomy, will be performed where the canal of Schlemm is absent or if the goniotomy fails to keep the intraocular pressure within normal limits.

6. Give post-operative care:

    a. Monitor for pain and give prescribed analgesia.

    b. Instil antibiotic and/or steroid drops – a mydriatic may be used.

    c. Observe the 'bleb' and depth of anterior chamber following trabeculectomy.

If the glaucoma is unilateral, amblyopia must be prevented in that eye. Patching of the unaffected eye will be instituted to encourage the child to use the glaucomatous eye.

PROGNOSIS

The prognosis depends on when the disease became manifest (see above). The earlier the disease is present, the worse is the prognosis, and visual impairment may be severe.

COMPLICATIONS

- Corneal/scleral perforation may be present due to the thinning of those structures. Perforation may occur with the least trauma.
- Exposure keratitis is a possible complication due to the lids being unable to lubricate the enlarged cornea adequately.

A bandage contact lens can be used to prevent and treat both these conditions.

JUVENILE GLAUCOMA

Juvenile glaucoma is associated with neurofibromatosis, Sturge–Weber syndrome, rubella and aniridia. It presents later than buphthalmos and behaves like chronic open-angle glaucoma. Hence care of the patient is similar.

Reflective activity

Consider a patient whom you have seen recently with glaucoma:

- What were the presenting signs and symptoms?
- Was there any associated systemic disease or diseases?
- What tests and investigations were carried out and why?
- How did you arrive at a diagnosis?
- What was the treatment plan?
- Outline the care and management of the patient.
- If there were any challenges in caring for the patient, what were they?
- Was any other member of the multidisciplinary team involved in the care and what was his or her input?

- Utilising a recognised health-promotion framework, how would you explain the condition and treatment to the patient in order to ensure that he or she adheres to the treatment?
- What was the clinical outcome?
- What local or national policies, guidelines or protocols influenced the care and management of this patient?
- On reflection, would you have done anything differently and, if so, what?

Your completed case study can be used to contribute to your continuing professional development portfolio for Registration and your Knowledge and Skills Framework review or appraisal.

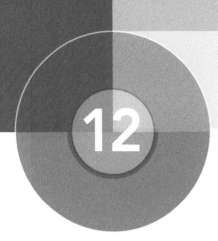

The crystalline lens

This chapter examines the anatomy and physiology of the lens and the common conditions affecting the function of the lens, including the treatment and management.

INTRODUCTION

STRUCTURE OF THE LENS

The lens is a biconvex, transparent, avascular structure with no nerve supply (Figure 12.1). It measures 9 mm by 4 mm in diameter and lies behind the iris and in front of the vitreous humour. It is supported by the zonules or suspensory ligaments, which attach it to the ciliary processes.

The lens has an elastic capsule, which enables it to change shape during accommodation. This capsule is semi-permeable to water and electrolytes. The lens receives its nourishment from the aqueous humour.

The anterior surface has a single layer of epithelial cells. The anterior pole is less convex than the posterior pole.

The cortex of the lens is composed of a gelatinous substance and lamella fibres, which are arranged in layers, like an onion, and originate from the anterior epithelial layer. These fibres are continually being produced so that the lens enlarges slowly throughout life, compressing towards the centre. Where the lamella fibres meet end-to-end, suture lines are formed. In the nucleus these are Y-shaped and, when viewed with the slit lamp, can be seen to be erect anteriorly, i.e. Y, and inverted posteriorly, i.e. λ.

The nucleus is composed of sclerosed lens fibres, which are old cortical fibres that cannot be cast off and are therefore massed together in the centre as the nucleus. The nucleus grows in size and is harder than the cortex.

COMPOSITION OF THE LENS

The lens comprises 65% water and 35% protein. In addition, there are trace minerals, the most important being sodium, potassium and calcium.

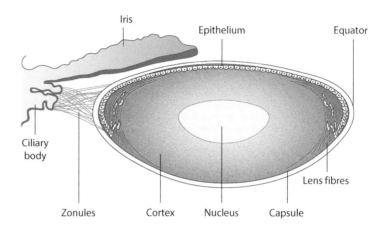

Figure 12.1 The anatomy of the lens. (From Marsden, J., *Ophthalmic Care*. Wiley, Chichester, 2006, reproduced with permission.)

FUNCTION OF THE CRYSTALLINE LENS

The function of the lens is to focus light rays on the retina by 'accommodation'. The lens has a power of approximately 21 dioptres (21 D). After the age of 45 years, the lens becomes so solid that it gradually loses its ability to change shape. This means that the lens cannot accommodate for near vision, a condition called presbyopia. Spectacles are therefore needed for reading and close work. The presbyopia slowly progresses until about the age of 70 years, with those affected requiring increasingly stronger lenses for reading and fine work.

CATARACT

A cataract is an opacity of the crystalline lens. See Figure 12.2. The lens is a delicate structure, and any insult on it causes the absorption of water, resulting in the lens becoming opaque. Cataracts can be defined according to their type, location and degree:

TYPES OF CATARACT

- Congenital
- Age-related
- Familial
- Traumatic
- Toxic
- Secondary to existing eye disease
- Associated with systemic disease

LOCATION OF THE OPACITY

Cataracts can occur in different parts of the lens:

- Anterior pole cataract
- Posterior pole cataract

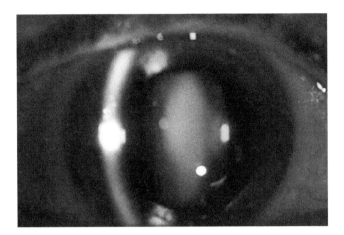

Figure 12.2 Cataractus lens. (Courtesy of Keith Barton.)

- Nuclear cataract
- Cortical cataract
- Lamellar cataract

DEGREES OF CATARACT

- Immature cataract – Part of the lens is opaque.
- Mature cataract – The whole lens is opaque and may be swollen (intumescent).
- Hypermature cataract – The lens becomes dehydrated because water has escaped from the lens, leaving an opaque lens and wrinkled capsule.
- Phacolytic lens – Lens matter leaks out, causing uveitis and secondary glaucoma. Cataracts should be extracted before this situation arises.

The mature and hypermature cataracts can be viewed through the pupil. An immature cataract can be seen when viewed with a slit lamp.

CONGENITAL CATARACT

CAUSES

- Rubella or malnutrition in the first trimester of pregnancy results in a lamellar cataract in the baby.
- Abnormal development of the eye in the foetus causes pressure on the anterior pole, resulting in an anterior pole cataract.
- A tag of hyaloid membrane remaining from foetal life can result in a posterior pole cataract. (The hyaloid artery runs from the retina to the lens during foetal life.)
- A metabolic disturbance such as galactosaemia results in a nuclear cataract.

SIGNS OF A CATARACT IN A BABY OR CHILD

- A white pupil may be noted by the parents or health visitor. It may be unilateral or bilateral. The cause of the white pupil must be diagnosed to differentiate it from the more serious condition of retinoblastoma.

- The parents may notice that the child does not see well. They may also notice changes in the child's behaviour, such as a loss of concentration, as he cannot follow words or pictures, or the inability to catch a ball because of loss of depth perception.
- A squint will indicate that there is a lesion in the visual pathway, preventing the sight from developing. The cause again must be differentiated from a retinoblastoma.
- It is important that cataracts are removed as soon as possible to prevent amblyopia. This is especially important if the cataracts are bilateral and dense, in which case extraction should be carried out before the baby is 2 months old.
- The rule of thumb is that if the fundus can be seen, then light must be reaching the retina. Amblyopia will therefore not develop. Removal of the lens will itself cause amblyopia as the light rays are not directed onto the retina by the lens. Compliance with aphakic correction is therefore very important in these children.

FAMILIAL CATARACT

Familial cataracts can occur, but they are rare, affecting the 30- to 40-year age group.

AGE-RELATED CATARACT

Age-related cataracts occur in patients over the age of 60 years. They result from sclerosis of the lens due to a degenerative process. The rate of progression varies. It is usually a bilateral condition, one eye being affected before the other.

The cataract is either nuclear or cortical.

A nuclear cataract affects the central lens and takes on a brown colour. In this instance, the patient sees better in dim light when the pupil is dilated and the light rays can enter the eye around the central opacity. Mydriatics can be given to dilate the pupil and give some vision around the cataract.

A cortical cataract affects the periphery of the lens and looks white. This type of cataract can produce a uni-ocular diplopia as the opacity splits the light rays. Vision is usually better in bright light when the pupil constricts and so reduces the peripheral distortion.

TRAUMATIC CATARACT

A discussion of traumatic cataract can be seen in Chapter 15, which is devoted to ophthalmic trauma.

TOXIC CATARACT

Toxic substances can affect the metabolism of the lens and cause opacity formation. Radiation and drugs such as topical steroids have this effect.

CATARACTS SECONDARY TO EXISTING EYE DISEASES

Glaucoma, retinitis pigmentosa, retinal detachments, retinopathies, choroiditis and uveitis upset the metabolism of the lens, causing cataract formation. The opacities form in the posterior subcapsular area, eventually involving the entire lens.

CATARACTS ASSOCIATED WITH SYSTEMIC DISEASE

Some systemic diseases cause an upset in the metabolism of the lens, causing, in the main, posterior subcapsular opacities:

- *Diabetes mellitus, type 1 and type 2* – The increased glucose level in the aqueous humour is taken up by the lens disturbing its metabolism. Cataracts can occur with rapid onset in juvenile diabetics, the lens becoming completely opaque within several weeks. In older diabetic patients, the opacities are nuclear, posterior subcapsular or cortical in nature and take longer to develop.
- *Hypoparathyroidism* – Cataract formation from this cause is usually seen after the removal of the parathyroid glands during thyroid gland removal. It can be idiopathic. Low calcium levels disturb the lens metabolism.
- *Atopic disease* – Dermatological conditions such as eczema and scleroderma can, when severe and widespread, cause cataract formation.

EFFECTS OF A CATARACT ON VISION

Patients with cataracts complain of gradually fading vision, often reporting that their vision is 'misty'. Other visual disturbances include distortion of images, changes in colour vision and contrast sensitivity. Depending on the site of the cataract, as mentioned above, they may be able to see better in dim or bright conditions. Some complain of dazzling bright lights due to irregular refraction of rays through the opacities in the lens. Some patients experience monocular diplopia. Posterior capsular opacities cause difficulty in near vision, leaving distance vision unaffected.

PATIENT'S NEEDS

Patient's needs are many and varied but include information on the following:

- Knowledge of the condition
- How the cataract will be treated and whether they will have an artificial lens implanted
- Type of anaesthetic (especially important as there are several possibilities ranging from topical to general anaesthetic)
- Informed consent to the surgery
- When they can have the surgery
- How long they will be at the hospital or treatment centre
- How their vision will be after the operation and how long before they can get new glasses
- How to manage their post-operative eye drops
- How to clean their eye
- Wearing the Cartella shield at night-time (usually at night for 1–2 weeks only)
- Recognising and managing post-operative complications
- Resuming normal activities
- Written information/advice sheets
- Detail of any follow-up appointment
- How soon the other eye can be operated on (if needed)

Cataract extraction is normally performed as a day case, unless there are factors that require inpatient admission. The waiting times for cataract surgery are generally short, some centres having no waiting list at all.

PRE-ASSESSMENT

Most centres now have cataract pathway management documents to guide the process from first visit to discharge. These may be accessed electronically or as hard copy. They are designed to streamline care from the multidisciplinary team. The patient may be seen by optometrists and nurses for the pre-operative and post-operative management phase of care, only seeing the doctor for the surgical procedure itself.

Special needs should be identified at or before the pre-assessment visit – such as the need for an interpreter, whether transport is needed, etc.

PRE-OPERATIVE INVESTIGATIONS

Pre-operative investigations include keratometry and biometry.

'B' SCAN

The 'B' Scan is an ultrasound scan used before cataract extractions. It gives a three-dimensional picture of the eye, showing up any abnormality in the media, such as a retinal detachment or tumour. This examination is necessary because the ophthalmologist is unable to examine the fundus through an opaque lens. If a tumour or retinal detachment were noted, the lens extraction might not take place, as no improvement in vision would occur.

Visual potential may need to be assessed because, for example, a patient may not have good post-operative visual acuity due to undiagnosed, age-related macular degeneration. Optical coherence tomography is an example of a diagnostic tool.

Procedure guideline: Pre- and post-operative care

NURSING ACTION

1. Prepare the patient for a local, topical or general anaesthetic. The surgeon will mark the eye to be operated on to comply with correct site surgery best practice. Probably, the most frequently used local anaesthetic method now is sub-Tenon's as it has fewer complications/risks than more traditional methods. Some ophthalmic surgeons advocate the use of topical local anaesthetic agents. The pupil will be dilated before surgery so that the surgeon can see and access the cataract during the procedure.
2. Give post-operative care.
3. Eye care:
   a. On examination with a good pen-torch or slit lamp, the conjunctiva will be mildly injected:
      i. The cornea should be clear.
      ii. The anterior chamber should be deep and quiet.
      iii. The pupil should be central – it may still be dilated from the effects of the pre-operative mydriatics and slightly eccentric initially.
   b. If a posterior chamber intraocular lens is *in situ*, its reflection may be noted through the pupil.
   c. A combined antibiotic and steroid drop will be instilled.
   d. Cataract surgery is usually considered relatively pain free. Paracetamol can be taken for the mild pain or dull ache that is sometimes experienced.

e. A post-operative information leaflet must be given. This provides information on what to look for in the event of post-operative complications, together with contact numbers.

The patient should be advised to contact the unit if he experiences an increase in peri-ocular pain or reduced vision, or complains of flashes and floaters.

COMPLICATIONS OF CATARACT EXTRACTION

Modern cataract surgery gives good visual results and is a relatively safe procedure. However, complications do occur (Kanski 2007).

EARLY

- Zonular/posterior capsule rupture
- Lens dislocation into vitreous humour
- Vitreous humour loss
- Wound gape/iris prolapse
- Hyphaema
- Vitreous humour/choroidal haemorrhage
- Hypopyon
- Endophthalmitis

LATE

- Posterior capsular opacification, though occurs less frequently with the newer lenses
- Uveitis
- Cystoid macular oedema
- Raised intraocular pressure
- Dislocated/malpositioned intraocular lens
- Retinal detachment
- Bullous keratopathy

Phacoemulsification requires less stringent post-operative restrictions, swimming and driving being the two main activities to be avoided until advised otherwise, usually at the first post-operative outpatient visit. This is because swimming could cause irritation and an eye-rubbing response; and vision may be insufficient to meet the Driver and Vehicle Licensing Agency (DVLA) guidelines until the patient gets corrective spectacles.

The patient may be seen and discharged by a health professional other than a doctor. This is usually a specially trained nurse or optometrist.

Patients will normally be advised to visit their optician at 2–4 weeks after surgery for refraction and, should they require glasses, the prescription will be given.

Listing for the second eye (if there is cataract) should be done as appropriate, often the assessment being undertaken over the telephone.

CATARACT OPERATIONS

The approach is via a limbal incision under a conjunctival flap or via a peripheral corneal incision.

PHACOEMULSIFICATION

Phacoemulsification is the most frequently used method with cataract in the adult patient. With phacoemulsification, the lens is broken down by ultrasonic vibrations. This technique is the most popular as it reduces the risk of expulsive haemorrhage and post-operative astigmatism, as the incision is smaller (as small as 3 mm in some cases) than that used in the operations described above. Suturing the wound is not required if it is properly sealed. A foldable intraocular lens is positioned in the posterior chamber. Alternatively, the wound is enlarged to accommodate a non-foldable lens implant.

COOL LASER

The cool laser procedure is similar to phacoemulsification but uses 'cool laser' shock waves to fragment the lens. The fragments are aspirated. There are fewer intraoperative complications. As with the phacoemulsification technique, a lens implant is inserted (O'hEineachain 2002).

NEEDLING OR LENS ASPIRATION

Needling or lens aspiration is performed on an infant or child under the age of 15 years. The cortex and nucleus of the lens are irrigated out through an incision in the anterior lens capsule, leaving the posterior capsule behind in order to prevent vitreous humour prolapse. At this age, the lens matter is soft enough to be aspirated.

The posterior lens capsule left behind may sclerose, causing visual impairment, and necessitating a capsulotomy to be performed using the YAG laser.

'LENSECTOMY' (PHACOFRAGMENTATION)

Lensectomy involves removing the entire lens and capsule and an anterior segment of the vitreous humour using specialised equipment. It is used for congenital cataracts and has the advantage of not requiring future capsulotomies.

INTRACAPSULAR LENS EXTRACTION

In an intracapsular lens extraction, the entire lens plus its capsule is removed. An enzyme, chymotrypsin, is introduced into the eye to dissolve the zonular fibres. The lens is then free of its attachments and can be removed from the eye by forceps or the cryoprobe. An anterior chamber intraocular lens will be implanted (see below). This procedure is rarely employed nowadays, but the nurse may encounter patients having had this type of surgery in the past.

EXTRACAPSULAR LENS EXTRACTION

In an extracapsular lens extraction, the anterior lens capsule, the cortex and nucleus are removed, leaving the posterior lens capsule in place. The type of incision made in the anterior lens capsule may vary, e.g. endocapsular or capsulorrhexis. Following this type of surgery, cortical matter may proliferate on the intact posterior capsule, a condition requiring capsulotomy (see above). A posterior chamber intraocular lens will be implanted.

APHAKIA

CORRECTION OF APHAKIA

Aphakia is the absence of the lens. Without the lens, the eye becomes very hypermetropic, requiring some kind of lens replacement to enable the patient to see adequately. The only people who do not require correction of the aphakia are those who are very myopic, in whom the absence of the lens causes the light rays to focus on the retina.

Aphakia causes loss of accommodation, so patients will need correction for both near and distance vision. Following surgery, a degree of astigmatism will result, requiring correction as well.

Aphakia can be corrected using glasses, contact lenses or intraocular lenses.

APHAKIC GLASSES

Aphakia glasses are rarely used nowadays. If they are worn, the patient needs to be made aware of the 'Jack-in-the box' effect they have on vision, when objects appear to be jumping into the field of vision. They may be used in babies when contact lenses are unsuitable.

CONTACT LENSES

Contact lenses are increasingly being superseded by intraocular lenses (see below), but nurses may meet patients who have had earlier surgery and wear contact lenses to correct their aphakia. Contact lenses may be used in unilateral or bilateral aphakia.

The advantages of using contact lenses for the correction of aphakia are as follows:

- Contact lenses can be used for unilateral aphakia.
- Contact lenses give a full field of vision.
- Contact lenses can be used in babies and children.
- Contact lenses only cause 7% magnification.

The disadvantages of using contact lenses for the correction of aphakia are as follows (see also Appendix 2):

- Patients have to become accustomed to wearing contact lenses; some may find them intolerable.
- Corneal abrasions and infections can result from contact lens wearing and from unclean lenses.
- Patients with arthritis cannot manipulate contact lenses, but extended-wear lenses overcome this problem.
- The lenses are easily lost.
- Contact lenses need scrupulous cleaning, especially soft contact lenses. People with bilateral aphakia may find difficulty in putting the first lens in because of poor sight in the other eye. Again, extended-wear lenses can overcome this.
- Contact lenses are expensive for those who are not eligible to have them supplied by the NHS.
- Contact lenses may not be suitable to be worn in some occupations, e.g. when working in a dusty environment.

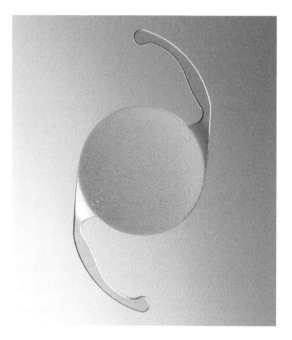

Figure 12.3 An intraocular lens. (Courtesy of Alcon.)

INTRAOCULAR LENSES

An intraocular lens is shown in Figure 12.3. Intraocular lenses can be used for the correction of unilateral and bilateral aphakia.

Many different types of intraocular lens are made by a number of companies. The following are examples of what is available on the market.

Lenses are either rigid or foldable and come in a variety of materials, including polymethylmethacrylate and acrylic. Some foldable lenses can be injected into the lens capsule. Where needed, multifocal and varifocal lenses can be used.

- The lenses are designed specifically for either the anterior chamber or the posterior chamber.
- Intraocular lenses for the anterior chamber, while they are rarely used now, are used following an intracapsular extraction or if the posterior capsule ruptures during surgery.
- Posterior chamber lenses are inserted into the posterior chamber of the eye following an extracapsular extraction, fitting into the posterior lens capsule which has been left behind. Newer lenses are being manufactured with 'laser ridges' to keep the lens away from the capsule to prevent the lens being damaged by the laser beam during a capsulotomy.
- Folding lenses, e.g. AcrySof, are used with phacoemulsification and are placed in the posterior capsule. They require a much smaller incision. Some are designed so that they can be injected into the capsule.

Selection of intraocular lens

The choice of type and power of the intraocular lens is determined by the surgeon who will take into account the needs of the patient. Such needs include the anatomy and physiology of the eye, whether the patient is myopic or hypermetropic. When the patient is having both eyes treated, there may be an opportunity to alter focal length.

Advantages of intraocular lenses

- Full field of vision is attained 24 hours a day.
- Intraocular lenses can be inserted at any time after the initial cataract extraction.
- No manual dexterity or manipulation is required by the wearer.
- Intraocular lenses are suitable for workers in industry or those in a humid environment/occupation.
- Vision is good even without glasses. Bifocal intraocular lenses are available and are increasingly being used.
- Posterior chamber intraocular lenses have been successfully implanted in children.
- Heparin-coated lenses can be used in patients with diabetes and also those who have repeated attacks of uveitis.

Disadvantages of intraocular lenses

- Intraocular lenses can cause uveitis and glaucoma.
- Intraocular lenses can dislocate.
- Anterior chamber lenses may cause bullous keratopathy.

DISLOCATED LENS

A total dislocation of the lens or a partial dislocation (subluxation) can occur.

A dislocated lens can be a result of trauma, it may be hereditary, or it may be associated with certain syndromes such as Marfan's syndrome. Vision will be blurred, but the degree of visual disturbance depends on the degree of dislocation. A partially dislocated lens can usually be seen through the pupil. A cataract may develop in the lens. A dislocated lens can cause uveitis or glaucoma by blocking either the posterior or anterior chambers.

If no complications occur, dislocated lenses are best left untreated. If complications do occur, treatment should be given to the complications before cataract extraction is attempted, as surgery in these instances is difficult.

Reflective activity

Consider a patient whom you have seen recently with a problem associated with the crystalline lens:

- What were the presenting signs and symptoms?
- Was there any associated systemic disease or diseases?
- What tests and investigations were carried out and why?
- How did you arrive at a diagnosis?
- What was the treatment plan?
- Outline the care and management of the patient.
- If there were any challenges in caring for the patient, what were they?
- Was any other member of the multidisciplinary team involved in the care and what was his or her input?

- Utilising a recognised health-promotion framework, how would you explain the condition and treatment to the patient in order to ensure that he or she adheres to the treatment?
- What was the clinical outcome?
- What local or national policies, guidelines or protocols influenced the care and management of this patient?
- On reflection, would you have done anything differently and, if so, what?

Your completed case study can be used to contribute to your continuing professional development portfolio for Registration and your Knowledge and Skills Framework or appraisal review.

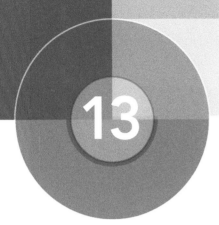

The retina, optic nerve and vitreous humour

13

This chapter examines conditions and treatment of these structures.

THE RETINA

The retina is composed of 10 layers: one epithelial layer and nine neural layers. There is a potential space between the epithelial layer and the neural layers, which is significant in retinal detachment. The retina extends from the ora serrata anteriorly to the optic disc posteriorly, where the nerve fibres leave the eye as the optic nerve.

TEN LAYERS OF THE RETINA

The 10 layers of the retina are illustrated in Figure 13.1:

1. The epithelial layer lies at the posterior of the structure beneath the choroid and contains varying amounts of melanin pigment. It absorbs light that is not picked up by the rods and cones.
2. The receptor layer contains the rods and cones, which are the two main types of nerve endings in the retina. The rods, numbering about 120 million in each eye, are situated mainly at the periphery of the retina. They function in dim light. The cones, numbering around 7 million in each eye, are situated at the centre of the retina and are concentrated, in particular, in the fovea of the macula. They function in bright light, pick up colours and make detailed vision possible.
3. The external limiting membrane is like a sheet of wire netting and has a supportive function.
4. The outer nuclear layer contains the nuclei of the rods and cones.
5. The outer plexiform layer contains the axons of the rods and cones and the dendrites of the bipolar cells.
6. The inner nuclear layer contains the nuclei of the bipolar cells.
7. The inner plexiform layer contains the axons of bipolar cells and the dendrites of the ganglion cells.
8. The ganglion cell layer contains the nuclei of the ganglion cells.

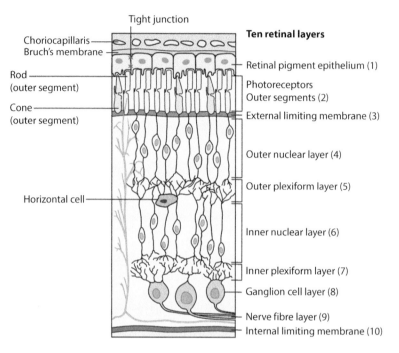

Figure 13.1 Ten retinal layers. (From Olver, J., and Cassidy, J. *Ophthalmology at a Glance*, Blackwell Publishing, 2005. reproduced with permission.)

9. The nerve fibre layer contains the axons of the ganglion cells which pass through the optic disc and lamina cribrosa to become continuous with the optic nerve.
10. The internal limiting membrane has a supportive function.

Layers 2–10 are known as the 'neural layers'.

AREAS OF THE RETINA

ORA SERRATA

The ora serrata is the anterior termination of the retina where the retinal pigment epithelial layer continues forward to become the ciliary epithelium. The neural layer of the retina ends at the ora serrata.

MACULA

The macula (Figure 13.2) is an area of the retina 1.5 mm in diameter situated 3 mm to the temporal side of the optic disc. It contains a high concentration of cones. In its centre is the fovea centralis, a slight depression where only cones are present. The other layers of the retina are absent here, causing a depression and making it thinner than the rest of the retina. The macula is the region of the retina where central precise vision takes place. It is not completely developed until 6 months after birth. No blood vessels cross the macula, and it receives its blood supply entirely from the choriocapillaries.

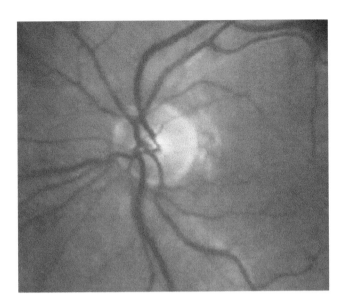

Figure 13.2 Ophthalmoscopy of normal fundus. (Courtesy of Keith Barton.)

OPTIC DISC

The optic disc (Figure 13.2) is the area of the retina where the axons of the ganglion cells leave the eye through the lamina cribrosa to become continuous with the optic nerve. It therefore contains no nerve cells, so that vision cannot take place here. This is known as the 'blind spot'. The central retinal artery and vein pass through the optic disc. Its blood supply is from the posterior ciliary artery, a branch of the temporal artery.

BLOOD SUPPLY TO THE RETINA

The outer layers of the retina are supplied by the choriocapillaries of the choroid. The inner layers of the retina are supplied by the central retinal artery. The central retinal vein drains the venous blood.

FUNCTION OF THE RETINA

The retinal nerve cells pick up and transmit impulses from light rays reaching the retina. These impulses then travel via the optic pathways to the visual cortex where they are interpreted as sight (see Figure 13.3). As light rays travel in straight lines, they will fall on the diagonally opposite area of the retina from the object in view; for example, the light rays from an object viewed superiorly will fall on the inferior area of the retina. The same happens on the horizontal plane. The brain converts the image so that it appears the right way up.

OPTIC NERVE

The optic nerve runs from the optic disc through the optic foramen to the optic chiasma where it becomes the optic tract. It is 5 cm in length and is surrounded by pia mater, arachnoid mater and dura mater. Its blood supply is via the ophthalmic artery and vein.

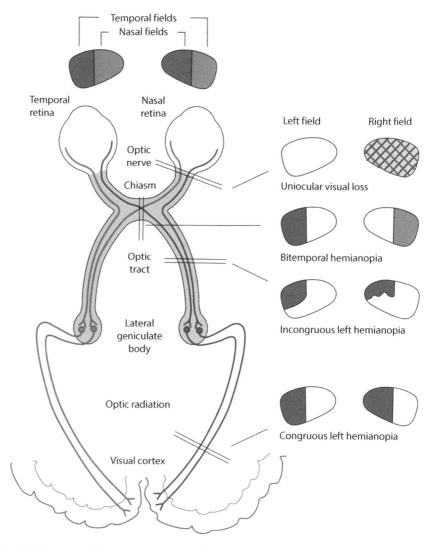

Figure 13.3 Anatomy of the optic pathway and the field defects produced by lesions at different sites. (From James, B. et al., *Lecture Notes*: *Ophthalmology*, Blackwell Publishing, 2007, reproduced with permission.)

OPTIC PATHWAYS

The optic pathways are illustrated in Figure 13.3. The optic nerve leaves each eye, passing through the optic foramen to the optic chiasma. From there, the fibres from the left-hand side of each eye travel in the left-hand side of the brain, and the right-hand fibres travel in the right-hand side of the brain. Thus the nasal fibres in the left eye cross at the chiasma to travel on the right side, and the nasal fibres of the right eye cross to travel on the left side. The temporal fibres of each eye stay on their respective side. From the optic chiasma, the fibres travel in the optic tracts to the lateral geniculate bodies where they pass into the optic radiations. From there, the fibres pass to the visual area of the occipital cortex where sight is interpreted.

THE VITREOUS HUMOUR

The vitreous humour fills the vitreous chamber which is the posterior segment of the eye lying between the lens and the retina (not to be confused with the posterior chamber).

The vitreous humour is a semi-gelatinous, transparent substance having no blood or nerve supply. The composition of the vitreous humour is 98%–99% water; and 1%–2% hyaluronic acid and collagen fibres.

ATTACHMENTS

The vitreous humour is attached more firmly to the underlying retina at the ora serrata and around the optic disc. Elsewhere, it lies loosely against the retina. Sometimes it attaches itself to blood vessels, which could bleed if the vitreous humour pulled on them.

FUNCTIONS OF THE VITREOUS HUMOUR

The function of the vitreous humour is the refraction of light: light rays travel in a converged manner through the vitreous humour towards the retina.

The vitreous humour also maintains the shape of the eye; if it were lost, the eye would collapse. Vitreous humour cannot be replaced naturally by the eye.

COLOUR VISION

The cones in the retina can be divided into three types: red, blue and green. Each of these types is sensitive to different light rays. The red cones absorb long waves; the green cones absorb mid-length waves; and the blue cones absorb short waves. These differing wavelengths – or a combination of them – are interpreted as colour.

RHODOPSIN

Rhodopsin is a photosensitive chemical present in the rods in the retina. In low-intensity light, rhodopsin breaks down, taking a few moments to work and enabling the eye to adapt to dim light. When changing from low-intensity light to bright light, it takes a few seconds to bleach the rhodopsin and enable the eye to adapt to bright light. Vitamin A is necessary for rhodopsin to function; thus a deficiency of vitamin A can lead to night-blindness.

CONDITIONS OF THE RETINA

RETINAL DETACHMENT

Retinal detachment is a misnomer, because it is not a detachment of the retina from the underlying choroid. It is, in fact, a separation of the epithelial layer from the neural layers of the retina. Because of the potential space between the first layer and the rest of the retina, it can become separated as a result of disease or trauma.

Condition guideline: Retinal detachment

CAUSES

The neural retina can be either pulled, pushed or floated off the underlying epithelial layer.

- *Pulled off* – The neural retina is pulled off the epithelial layer by vitreous traction. Vitreous traction occurs when new blood vessels have grown into the vitreous humour. The fragile vessels bleed and fibrous tissue forms in the healing process. These fibrous bands contract, pulling the neural layer away. Conditions causing this type of detachment are diabetes mellitus, retinopathy of prematurity, retinal haemorrhage and vitreous haemorrhage (see Figures 13.4 and 13.5).

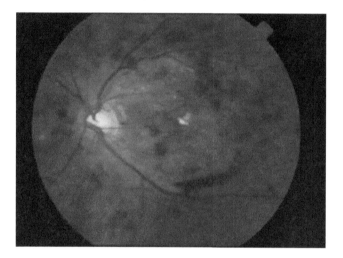

Figure 13.4 Proliferative diabetic retinopathy.

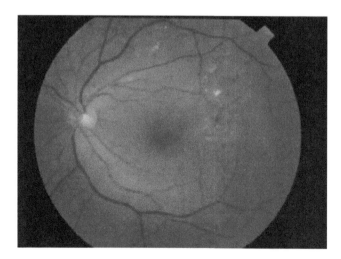

Figure 13.5 Background retinopathy.

- *Pushed off* – A lesion behind the retina pushes the retina forward, causing fluid or exudate to separate the layers of the retina. Conditions causing this type of detachment are choroidal tumours, choroidal haemorrhage, choroiditis and retinopathies.
- *Floated off* – If a tear or hole appears in the retina, subretinal fluid or vitreous fluid enters the hole, floating the neural layers off the epithelial layer. Tears in the retina occur following trauma, in high myopes, retinal degeneration and aphakia. The tears usually occur in the periphery or equator of the retina.

PATIENT'S NEEDS

- Relief of symptoms:
  - Flashing lights (photopsia) – Caused by the separating layers of the retina stimulating the rods and cones – are experienced.
  - Floaters – A sudden increase in the number of floaters in the vision, or a shower of floaters, occurs. These are small haemorrhages, usually from retinal vessels.
  - Field loss – As the retina separates, the affected part causes loss of vision in the corresponding visual field. It must be remembered that the visual field loss is opposite to the detachment; for example, if the upper half of the retina is detached, the visual loss would be the lower half of the visual field. It is important to prevent the macula from detaching, as the visual prognosis following this occurrence is not good. The separated macula will be denied its blood supply from the choriocapillaries and will therefore become anoxic. Unfortunately, the most common site for a detachment is in the superior temporal area causing an inferior nasal visual field loss. This area of the visual field is occluded to some extent by the nose, the vision in the other eye compensating for it. Therefore, field loss in this area is not noticed as quickly as field loss in another area. Also, a superior detachment can progress more rapidly due to gravity, and the danger of a macular detachment is therefore greater.
  - Relief of anxiety – An explanation of the management of the condition and reassurance are needed.
- Admission to hospital for bed rest and pre- and post-operative care is required.
- Surgery should be carried out to reattach the retina.

NURSING ACTION

1. Take an accurate history.
2. Inform the doctor of the patient's history and type of visual loss.
3. Instil prescribed mydriatic drops as prescribed or as per Patient Group Direction (PGD), for ophthalmoscopic examination of the fundus.
4. Admit patient to the ward or instruct them to bed rest either at home or ward if same-day surgery.
5. Give pre-operative care:
   a. Bed rest, to prevent further detachment occurring, though the patient is likely to have surgery sooner rather than later.
   b. Dependent positioning – this is decided, to some extent, by the doctor's wishes and the site of the detachment. The rationale is to position the patient so that the detachment lies dependently against its underlying epithelial layer, encouraging the subretinal fluid to be absorbed and reattachment to occur.

c. Instil prescribed mydriatic drops regularly to maintain mydriasis so that a good fundal examination can be carried out. This is performed using an indirect ophthalmoscope and a 20-dioptre lens to obtain an accurate diagram of the retina, including tears, holes, detached and attached areas, and the presence of subretinal fluid. This helps the surgeon at the time of the operation. The other eye is also dilated and inspected. Retinopathies, degenerations and myopia can affect both eyes. Problems in the other eye must be noted and treated if present, often using laser or cryotherapy prophylactically.

6. Give post-operative care:

    a. Eye care:

        i. The lids and conjunctiva are usually swollen following retinal detachment because of the amount of movement of the eye that is necessary during the operation.

        ii. In the rare event that a scleral band has been used, the cornea must be noted for its clarity; if it is cloudy, this could indicate ischaemia of the anterior segment of the eye caused by the encirclement band being too tight.

        iii. The pupil will remain dilated.

        iv. Antibiotic, mydriatic and steroid drops, non-steroidal anti-inflammatory drops may be prescribed.

    b. General care: the patient may be nursed in a dependent position following surgery. This is especially important following vitrectomy, when the injected gas or air bubble must be uppermost to put pressure on the detached retina (see below). Analgesia will need to be given regularly as ocular pain will be experienced by most patients. It must be ascertained that the cause of pain is not raised pressure due to anterior segment ischaemia (see above).

    c. Cryotherapy or laser photocoagulation is performed to seal holes or tears by setting up a local inflammatory reaction and thereby preventing fluid seeping between the retinal layers. Holes and tears, if present, must be sealed during detachment operations for this surgery to be successful (see Figure 13.6).

    d. Plombage or scleral buckling – a silastic sponge or 'plomb' (a small square of inert material) is sutured onto the sclera over the site of the hole, causing an indentation and bringing the separated layers of the retina together.

    e. Encirclement (rarely used but mentioned here as may be seen in some centres) – a silicone band is positioned around the globe, underneath the extraocular muscles. This enables greater indentation to occur and is used where there is a large area of detachment or multiple holes.

Drainage of subretinal fluid must be performed at the time of each of the above surgical procedures to allow the separated layers to realign.

Vitrectomy may be performed in certain circumstances (see below).

COMPLICATIONS

- Early
  - Subretinal fluid may continue to accumulate between the layers of the retina. This must be removed if spontaneous reabsorption does not occur in order to prevent further detachment occurring and to aid reattachment.
  - Ischaemia of the anterior segment of the eye following encirclement if the band is too tight.

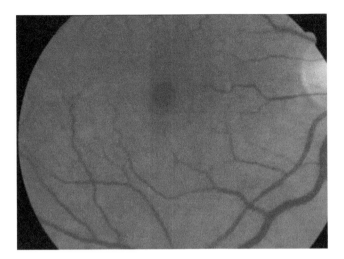

Figure 13.6 Macular hole.

- Late
    - Infection of the plomb or band, in which case removal is necessary.
    - Extrusion of the plomb – the plomb may become loose and work its way to the surface under the conjunctiva.
    - Distortion of visual acuity (VA).

VITRECTOMY

Vitrectomy is performed for the following conditions:

- Giant tears
- Retinal detachment with scar formation
- Macula hole
- To remove vitreous opacities
- Fibrovascular tissue in diabetic retinopathy
- Epiretinal membrane (see Figure 13.7)
- Dislocated lens (subluxation – see Figure 13.8)
- Foreign body in posterior segment
- Penetrating injury with resulting intraocular foreign body
- Endophthalmitis
- Dislocated lens fragment
- Vitreous tap for microscopy

Vitreous humour cannot be replaced naturally. One of the following substances is used as replacement material:

- Gas, e.g. SF_6 (sulphur hexafluoride), C_3F_8 (perfluoropropane) – The patient cannot see through the gas until it has been absorbed, and this takes 2–3 weeks.
- Silicone oil – The patient can see through the oil but it makes the eye hypermetropic. Silicone oil is not absorbed and is removed later.
- Air – This is absorbed within 24–36 hours.
- Gas and air mixture can be used.
- $C_{10}F_{18}$ (perfluorodecalin) – This is a heavy liquid which is not absorbed.

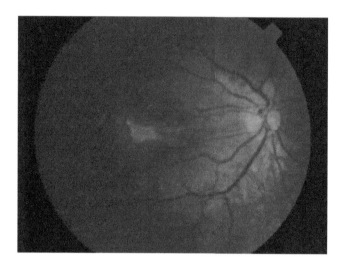

Figure 13.7 Epiretinal membrane.

Aqueous humour will gradually fill the vitreous chamber to replace the above substances as they are absorbed (except the oil and $C_{10}F_{18}$).

In order to carry out a vitrectomy, the vitreous chamber/posterior segment is approached via three entry ports at the ora serrata (pars plana) to prevent damage to the retina. The vitreous humour is broken up and aspirated out of the eye. All instruments entering the vitreous chamber are normally 23 g. Up to 90% of the vitreous humour can be removed. The surgery may be sutureless or with suture.

COMPLICATIONS OF VITRECTOMY SURGERY

- Corneal epithelial defect
- Corneal edema
- Hemorrhage
- Infection

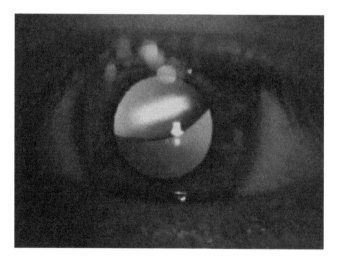

Figure 13.8 Subluxation of the lens.

- Cataract formation
- Raised intraocular pressure
- Oil in the anterior segment
- Emulsified oil in the anterior chamber or between the main bubble and the retina
- Retinal re-detachment – usually occurs when the gas bubble has been absorbed (3–6 weeks post-operatively) or after removal of silicone oil

The bubble will expand when flying. Patients are advised not to fly if the bubble is more than 10% of the volume of the eye.

ADDITIONAL POST-OPERATIVE NURSING CARE

- Eye care – Observe the entry sites in the sclera for bleeding and gaping.
- Post-operative positioning – The head must be positioned so that the gas, air or oil is lying against the hole/detachment. If a macular hole has been repaired, it is especially important that the patient is positioned face down usually for first 24 hours only and if the size of the gas bubble is more than 70%. Avoid lying on the back unless if the macular hole was large then posture sitting upright up to 5 days (Dhawahir-Scala et al. 2008).
- During this time, the patient is at risk of the complications of immobility, including pressure sores. The patient can have 5–10 minutes 'relief from positioning every hour', depending on the surgeon's wishes.

CENTRAL RETINAL ARTERY OCCLUSION

Central retinal artery occlusion is considered an ophthalmic emergency because instituting treatment within 2 hours of occurrence may restore the vision which would otherwise be permanently lost. This condition occurs suddenly, without warning, causing painless loss of vision. It is rare, usually only affecting one eye. It is caused by an embolus or thrombus due to arteriosclerosis, mitral stenosis, carotid insufficiency or temporal arteritis and as a complication of thyroid eye disease.

Condition guideline: Central retinal artery occlusion

SIGNS AND SYMPTOMS

- There will be a sudden acute loss of vision.
- The eye will look white.
- Visual acuity will be reduced to counting fingers, watching hand movements or a perception of light only.
- The fundus looks pale due to oedema obliterating the normal red reflex. The macula stands out as a 'cherry red spot', this area being unaffected by the oedema as the retina here is thinner and no blood vessels cross it. The red reflex from the underlying choroid can therefore be seen. The retinal arteries are small, containing segmented columns of blood called 'cattle tracking'. The retinal veins appear normal.

PATIENT'S NEEDS

- Prompt medical attention for diagnosis to be made and treatment commenced
- Investigation into the cause and relevant treatment given if necessary

NURSING PRIORITIES

- Inform the medical staff immediately of the patient's visual acuity and sudden onset of symptoms.
- Prepare equipment for treatment (see below).

NURSING ACTION

1. Instil prescribed mydriatic for ophthalmoscopic examination of the retina, so that the diagnosis can be established.
2. Take blood for erythrocyte sedimentation rate.
3. Prepare the patient and the equipment that the doctor may require to try to restore vision. The following methods can be employed, the aim of the treatment being to dislodge the embolus or thrombus or increase the oxygen supply to the retina. However, the nurse should not institute any of these measures without instructions from the doctor, as the diagnosis of sudden visual loss must be differentiated from that of a retinal detachment, temporal arteritis or central retinal vein occlusion (see below).
   a. An anterior chamber paracentesis – a needle is introduced into the anterior chamber to reduce the intraocular pressure suddenly.
   b. Give 500 mg of acetazolamide intravenously to reduce the intraocular pressure.
   c. Massage over the globe.
   d. Ask the patient to blow into a paper bag to raise the carbon dioxide levels in the blood which, in turn, will stimulate more oxygen to be produced.
   e. Vasodilators may be prescribed.
4. Measure blood pressure and test a specimen of urine.

If sight is not restored by any of these methods, there is no other treatment available. If sight is already poor in the other eye, the patient will need help and advice from the social services department.

CENTRAL RETINAL VEIN OCCLUSION

Central retinal vein occlusion is a more common occurrence than retinal artery occlusion. It also affects one eye, the visual loss being sudden but usually less devastating. It is caused by hypertension, diabetes mellitus, arteriosclerosis, glaucoma and thyroid eye disease.

Condition guideline: Central retinal vein occlusion

SIGNS

- The eye will be white.
- The visual acuity will have dropped to 6/36 or less.
- The fundus will be red and swollen, with dilated and tortuous veins. Retinal haemorrhages will be present.

PATIENT'S NEEDS

- Prompt medical attention is essential, so that a diagnosis can be made and treatment commenced.

- Investigation into the cause is required, so that appropriate treatment can be given if necessary.

NURSING PRIORITY

Inform medical staff immediately of the patient's visual acuity and history of sudden onset.

NURSING ACTION

1. Instil the prescribed mydriatic drop so that the fundus can be examined and a diagnosis made.
2. Measure blood pressure and test a specimen of urine.
3. Ensure that the patient understands the instructions for the investigations.
4. Ensure that the patient understands the treatment, which may be one of the following:
   a. Oral steroids.
   b. Dipyridamole and aspirin to prevent the 'stickiness' of the platelets.
   c. Photocoagulation or laser treatment to coagulate bleeding retinal vessels.

PROGNOSIS

Vision may recover spontaneously over several weeks, or it may remain unchanged.

COMPLICATIONS

1. Vitreous haemorrhage from new blood vessels growing in the ischaemic retina which bleed. This could cause a retinal detachment.
2. Thrombotic glaucoma – neovascularisation from the ischaemic retina occurs in the iris and anterior chamber angle, blocking the drainage angle.
3. Atrophy of the retina and optic nerve from ischaemia of these structures can occur.
4. Cystoid macular oedema can arise, in which case an intravitreal injection is given.
5. Currently the most effective treatments for retinal vein occlusion (RVO) are injections administered into the eye. There are two types of injections:
   a. Anti-VEGF (vascular endothelial growth factor) injections – Aflibercept (Eylea) and Ranibizumab (Lucentis).
   b. Steroid injection – Dexamethasone (Ozurdex).
6. Aflibercept (Eylea) and Ranibizumab (Lucentis) are given by injection into the eye and act to slow or stop the growth of the abnormal blood vessels and leakage. These drugs act, broadly speaking, in similar ways by blocking the effects of the chemical VEGF, which causes these blood vessels to form and grow.
7. Steroid injections (Ozurdex) are another option which act to reduce the inflammation in the retina caused by the RVO. The doctor who sees the patient will discuss pros and cons of the various options.
8. Most patients' vision will stabilise after treatment and some patients may regain some vision. Drug injections may not restore vision that has already been lost, and will not always prevent further loss of vision caused by the disease.

RETINAL HAEMORRHAGE

Retinal haemorrhage can occur in any layer of the retina, appearing as flame-shaped areas or as round blots. It can collect in the preretinal space between the retina and the vitreous humour.

Condition guideline: Retinal haemorrhage

CAUSES

- Vascular conditions, e.g. arteriosclerosis and hypertension (see below)
- Blood diseases such as anaemia, leukaemia and sickle-cell anaemia
- Trauma
- Retinopathies due to diabetes, hypertension, nephritis and toxaemia of pregnancy (see below)

The treatment is that of the cause, and bed rest to settle the haemorrhage. Vitrectomy may be required.

RETINOPATHIES

Retinopathies are caused by diabetes mellitus, hypertension, renal disease and toxaemia of pregnancy. The result is a combination of retinal degeneration and inflammation.

DIABETIC RETINOPATHY

Diabetic retinopathy is the leading cause of blindness in the Western world in the under-65-year-olds. The National Service Framework for Diabetes (2002) states that diabetes is the leading cause of blindness in people of working age. Diabetes, being essentially a vascular disease, affects the blood vessels of the retina. Until recently, it was thought that diabetic retinopathy occurred after 20 years or so regardless of the diabetic control. Recent research (The Diabetes Control and Complications Trial Research Group 1995) indicates strongly that good control does prevent ocular and other diabetic complications. Puberty adversely affects the onset and subsequent development of retinopathy (Jose et al. 1994). Other risk factors associated with the development of diabetic retinopathy are blood pressure and serum lipid control. Tight blood pressure control has proved to lead to a 37% reduction in the risk of microvascular disease (UK Prospective Diabetic Study Group 1998). Similarly, the Wisconsin Epidemiologic Study of Diabetic Retinopathy (Klein et al. 1991) and the Early Treatment Diabetic Retinopathy Study (Fong et al. 2000) have demonstrated that elevated serum lipids increase the severity of diabetic retinopathy and retinal hard exudates.

The complications of diabetes such as renal impairment, vascular complications such as strokes and coronary heart disease, and amputation can have a devastating effect on the patients and their families. Effects such as the physical, psychological and material well-being have all been cited in the National Service Framework for Diabetes (2002). Diabetes also has a major impact on the health and social services. Five percent of the total NHS resources have been used for the care of diabetic patients (National Service Framework for Diabetes 2002).

To halt the progression of diabetic retinopathy, it is extremely important that any sight-threatening diabetic retinopathy is detected early and that all patients with diabetes should be screened and, where appropriate, laser treatment instituted. Patients suffering from visual impairment should be supported through the use of low-vision aids, psychological support, financial support and support from voluntary organisations such as the Royal National Institute of the Blind and diabetic retinopathy self-help groups.

There are five stages of diabetic retinopathy:

- Background retinopathy (see Figure 13.5)
- Maculopathy
- Pre-proliferative retinopathy
- Proliferative retinopathy (see Figure 13.4)
- Advanced retinopathy

BACKGROUND RETINOPATHY

Background retinopathy occurs in most diabetics about 20 years after the onset of the disease and therefore can affect all age groups from late teens onward. It usually gives no symptoms to the patient until the macula is involved, with resulting impairment of central vision. The patient may complain of glare due to the light rays being scattered by the oedematous retina.

Condition guideline: Background retinopathy

SIGNS

The fundus has a typical picture of dots, blots and hard waxy exudates. The dots are micro-aneurysms. The blots are small haemorrhages. The hard waxy exudates are leakages of lipids from the haemorrhaging blood vessels. A ring of exudates around the macula suggests maculopathy (see below).

PATIENT'S NEEDS

- The patient should have annual medical ophthalmic check-ups to assess the degree of retinopathy.
- The patient may gain control of cholesterol levels by taking clofibrate tablets, 500 mg three times a day.
- The patient may require advice on his treatment and diet from a diabetic clinic.

NURSING ACTION

1. Care for the patient in the outpatient department when attending for check-ups.
2. Ensure the patient maintains a tight glycaemic (HBA1c) control.

MACULOPATHY

Maculopathy is the main cause of visual impairment in non-insulin-dependent diabetics. There are five types of maculopathy:

1. *Focal/exudative* – Characterised by leaking areas of hard exudates which are well-circumscribed. This can be treated by laser.
2. *Cystoid/diffuse* – Generalised leaking by dilated capillaries with diffuse retinal thickening. In severe cases, in may be difficult to treat with laser due to difficulty in locating the fovea.
3. *Ischaemic* – Reduction in visual acuity with haemorrhages and exudates located elsewhere in the fundus. This cannot be treated with laser.
4. *Mixed* – Contains the characteristics of both diffuse macular oedema and ischaemia. This can be treated by laser.

5. *Significant macular oedema* – Consisting of the following features: retinal oedema that is within one disc diameter of the centre of the fovea, hard exudates and retinal oedema within 55 μm of the centre of the fovea. This must be treated with either direct or grid laser treatment.

Condition guideline: Maculopathy

PATIENT'S NEEDS

- Diagnosis of which type of maculopathy is present
- Preparation for intravitreal injection
- Treatment with the argon laser as appropriate
- Relief from central visual impairment

NURSING ACTION

1. Prepare the patient for fundal fluorescein angiography.
2. Prepare the patient for laser treatment. Laser treatment seals the leaking blood vessels around the macula, thereby reducing the production of hard exudates. The laser beam is directed at the macula but must avoid the fovea itself, as loss of central vision would result if this was hit by the beam.

It should be noted that it is less common for laser to be used to improve vision and more recently new treatments which require intravitreal injection into the eye are being recommended for diabetic macular oedema (DMO).

1. Lucentis (Ranibizumab) – The retinal damage in diabetes releases a chemical called VEGF. VEGF causes leakage of fluid from the retinal vessels.
2. Lucentis blocks the action of VEGF and therefore helps to reduce further leakage.
3. Iluvien is an anti-inflammatory drug used for the treatment of DMO. It is a type of steroid called fluocinolone acetonide and is contained within a long-lasting implant that is injected directly inside the eye. It releases the drug over a period of 3 years.
4. Triamcinolone injection. Triesence (triamcinolone acetonide) is a steroid suspension used to treat inflammation in DMO.

Complications of the intravitreal injection include

- Haemorrhage
- Endophthalmitis
- Cataract
- Retinal detachment
- Raised intraocular pressure

Any of these complications may lead to severe, permanent loss of vision or blindness. In the clinical trials these complications occurred at a rate of less than 0.1% (1 in 1000) of injections. The overall risk over the long-term course of treatment is estimated at about 1% (1 in 100) or less.

More common side effects include

- Periocular pain
- Conjunctival haemorrhage

- Vitreous floaters
- Irregularity or swelling of the cornea
- Inflammation

Other complications of lucentis

There may be an increased risk of experiencing blood clots (which may cause heart attack or stroke) after intravitreal injection of medicines such as Lucentis.

Chance risks

When medications are used in a large number of patients, it is inevitable that other complications may occur that have no connection to the treatment. For example, patients with high blood pressure or those who are smokers are already at increased risk of heart attacks and strokes. If one of these patients is being treated with Lucentis and has a heart attack or stroke, it may not be caused by the Lucentis itself.

PRE-PROLIFERATIVE RETINOPATHY

Pre-proliferative retinopathy may develop in eyes with background retinopathy only.

Condition guideline: Pre-proliferative retinopathy

SIGNS

The retina is ischaemic which causes

- Cotton wool spots – ischaemic nerve fibre layer
- Dilation, beading, looping of blood vessels
- Arteriole narrowing
- Large dark blot haemorrhages
- Intraretinal microvascular abnormalities

NURSING ACTION

There is no specific treatment unless the eye is the only eye with the capability for vision, in which case laser treatment is applied.

There are no symptoms but the patient's eyes need careful observation as they are prone to develop proliferative retinopathy.

Patients will need to be closely monitored as a significant number of these patients will go on to develop proliferative diabetic retinopathy.

PROLIFERATIVE RETINOPATHY

Proliferative retinopathy is the main cause of visual impairment in insulin-dependent diabetics. It occurs sooner, after diagnosis of the disease, in non-insulin-dependent diabetics, possibly because the disease has gone on for longer undetected. The body's natural response to the ischaemic retina is to liberate a vasoprolific factor which stimulates the formation of new blood vessels to try to overcome the lack of oxygen to the structures involved.

The problem with newly formed blood vessels is that they are fragile and bleed easily. In proliferative retinopathy, these blood vessels grow into the vitreous humour and they bleed, causing vitreous haemorrhage. Eventually, traction bands of fibrous tissue form, which pull on the retina causing a retinal detachment. These new vessels can be seen easily on ophthalmoscopy and angiography.

The aim of the treatment is to prevent neovascularisation occurring. The laser beam is applied to the retina. Dead retina will not encourage new vessel growth. Thus the retina is peppered with small areas of scotomas from laser treatment. These scotomas appear to cause little visual impairment to the patient. Vitrectomy will remove the haemorrhage as well as the scaffold that the new vessels grow into.

Condition guideline: Proliferative retinopathy

PATIENT'S NEEDS

- Treatment of proliferative retinopathy by the laser to prevent further deterioration
- Treatment of the vitreous haemorrhage
- Guidance around the hospital if visual acuity is poor

NURSING ACTION

1. Prepare the patient for laser treatment.
2. Admit the patient to hospital and prepare for vitrectomy.
3. Assist the severely visually handicapped patient.

ADVANCED RETINOPATHY

Advanced retinopathy is the end result of uncontrolled proliferative retinopathy and results in blindness.

Condition guideline: Advanced retinopathy

SIGNS

- Persistent vitreous haemorrhage
- Retinal detachment
- 'Burnt-out stage' when no new vessels are stimulated to grow because the retina has become anoxic due to there being more fibrous than vascular tissue
- Neovascular or thrombotic glaucoma due to new vessels growing in the anterior chamber angle obstructing the outflow of aqueous humour

PATIENT'S NEEDS

- Vitrectomy if not performed previously
- Treatment of neovascular glaucoma
- Management of visual impairment

NURSING ACTION

1. Prepare the patient for vitrectomy.
2. Assist in the treatment of glaucoma.
3. Instruct the patient to instil beta-blockers, e.g. Betoptic, twice a day and to take acetazolamide, 250 mg four times a day.

4. Prepare the patient for laser treatment to new vessels in angle and/or for trabeculoplasty.
5. Prepare the patient for trabeculectomy or insertion of a filtering tube, e.g. Molteno, if the above measures have failed.
6. Inform the patient about services available and refer to social worker and low-vision aid clinic as appropriate.

HYPERTENSIVE RETINOPATHY (INCLUDING RENAL DISEASE AND TOXAEMIA OF PREGNANCY)

Hypertensive retinopathy is caused by primary hypertension and hypertension secondary to renal disease and toxaemia of pregnancy. Patients usually have no symptoms until the haemorrhages and exudates affect the macula, with resulting central-field involvement. There are four stages, graded according to their severity:

- *Grade I* – There is generalised arterial constriction which gives the fundal picture of 'silver' or 'copper wiring' due to increased light reflex from the thickened arterial walls.
- *Grade II* – There is arteriovenous 'nipping' due to arteriosclerosis. The thickened arterial wall obscures the vein lying beneath it.
- *Grade III* – In grade III, haemorrhages and exudates appear. Flame-shaped haemorrhages follow the nerve fibres and are superficial. Round haemorrhages lie deeper in the retinal layers. Exudates are not in fact exudates as such but are white 'fluffy' areas of infarcted nerve fibres due to ischaemia.
- *Grade IV* – All the above signs are present plus papilloedema. Renal failure will probably have occurred and vision is grossly impaired. Characteristically, in renal retinopathy, there is a well-defined star appearance of exudates at the macula.

Condition guideline: Hypertensive retinopathy

PATIENT'S NEEDS

- Regular ophthalmic check-ups should be carried out, including fundal fluorescein angiography to document any changes in the retinal blood vessels.
- Treatment of the underlying cause. Referral to a physician may be necessary. If the toxaemia of pregnancy is severe, the pregnancy may need to be terminated to save the mother's sight and life.

NURSING ACTION

1. Assist the patient in the outpatient department.
2. Measure blood pressure and test urine specimen.
3. Prepare the patient for a fundal fluorescein angiography.

PROGNOSIS

If the underlying cause is kept under control, visual prognosis is reasonably good. Once the macular area becomes involved, vision deteriorates. A severe retinopathy results in poor visual acuity and an accompanying poor prognosis. A complication of toxaemic retinopathy is retinal detachment.

RETINAL DEGENERATIONS

Degenerations of the retina occur around its periphery. Some are significant in that they may cause retinal detachment. These are lattice and snail-track degeneration and acquired retinoschisis. Other degenerations—such as snowflake, paving stone and honeycomb—are insignificant, causing no ophthalmic complications.

RETINITIS PIGMENTOSA

Retinitis pigmentosa is a hereditary degeneration of the retinal nerve cells affecting one in 2500. The hereditary aspect is variable, resulting in varying degrees of severity. The autosomal and X-linked recessive forms are severe, with symptoms starting in teenage years. The autosomal dominant form is less severe, with symptoms occurring in later adult life. The rods are slowly destroyed, initially affecting the peripheral retina causing night-blindness. Eventually, the whole retina is affected when tunnel vision results.

An electroretinogram is performed to diagnose the condition. Later, colour vision is affected. Eventually, even the macula may be involved, causing total blindness. Cataracts may develop.

On ophthalmoscopy, the retina is peppered with black pigment. There is no known treatment. Management is aimed at improving visual impairment with low-vision aids, pinhole spectacles and eye shields.

Couples should receive genetic counselling before starting a family if one of them is affected.

RETINOPATHY OF PREMATURITY

The development of retinal blood vessels is not complete until the month after birth. Therefore, a baby born prematurely will have an incompletely developed retinal blood supply. If the baby is given a high concentration of oxygen in an incubator, the stimulus for the continuing development of the retinal vessels is withdrawn. When the baby is removed from the oxygen supply, the retina is receiving insufficient oxygen and it becomes anoxic, resulting in proliferation of new vessels.

Although the oxygen now delivered to incubators is monitored closely, and must continue to be so, the condition is still occurring. It is thought to be due more to the prematurity or low birth weight of the baby than to the concentration of oxygen (Duker and Tolentino 1991). O'Conner and Glasper (1995) suggest it is a multifactorial condition.

There are five stages of the disease. Stages 1 and 2 generally regress without treatment. The other stages are treated by laser to decrease the proliferation. Visual prognosis tends to be poor. Screening of premature and low birth weight babies is essential at approximately 6–9 weeks after birth.

RETINAL TUMOUR: RETINOBLASTOMA

A retinoblastoma is a retinal tumour occurring in children under the age of 5 years. It is rare but highly malignant, occurring in one in 20,000 live births. It usually only affects one eye, but in 30% of cases is bilateral, both growths being primary tumours. There may be a family history of retinoblastoma.

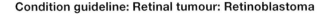

Condition guideline: Retinal tumour: Retinoblastoma

SIGNS

- A white pupil is noted, the tumour showing through the pupil instead of the normal red choroidal reflex. A white pupil may also be a sign of a cataract.
- The child may have a squint because he will not be using the affected eye for seeing and it will deviate inwards.

TREATMENT

The eye will be enucleated, unless the tumour is small, in which case photocoagulation, cryotherapy, laser or radiotherapy treatment will be used, preserving the eye and maybe some sight. External beam radiation providing a lens-sparing technique results in less damage to the eye than whole-eye radiation (Toma et al. 1995). If the child presents with bilateral tumours, the sight of one eye will be preserved as far as possible without endangering the child's life. The eye with the smallest tumour will be treated by one of the methods mentioned.

Careful watch must be kept on an unaffected fellow eye. If a tumour occurs in it, it must be treated promptly as above to destroy the tumour and preserve as much sight as possible.

Siblings must be checked for the presence of a retinoblastoma, and children of surviving sufferers must be examined at birth and observed until the age of 5 years.

PROGNOSIS

The earlier the diagnosis is made and treatment instigated, the higher is the chance of preventing metastases. An untreated tumour spreads within the eye, causing it to become glaucomatous. From the eye, malignant cells track back into the orbit and brain via the optic nerve and can metastasise into the liver and elsewhere in the body. A late diagnosis will result in a poorer prognosis for the child's life.

CYTOMEGALOVIRUS RETINITIS

Cytomegalovirus (CMV) is a common member of the herpes virus family, usually remaining dormant unless the person is immunocompromised. CMV retinitis is the commonest opportunistic infection in people with AIDS, affecting 20%–30% of sufferers (Engstrom and Holland 1995). As it is a progressive disease, it can result in severe visual impairment. Recurrence of the disease heralds a particularly poor visual prognosis.

Condition guideline: CMV retinitis

SIGNS

Retinal haemorrhages and exudates are present which progress to become necrotic, eventually involving the optic disc. Retinal detachment can occur as can cataracts.

PATIENT'S NEEDS

- Diagnosis of the disease
- Medical or surgical treatment as appropriate

- Professional counselling/referral if diagnosis of AIDS is made in the ophthalmic department

NURSING ACTION

1. Assist in diagnostic tests – ophthalmoscopy, fundal photography.
2. Explain the different treatment modalities:
   a. Ganciclovir (dihydroxypropoxymethyl guanine) – Induction: 5 mg/kg body weight intravenously twice a day for 2–3 weeks.
   b. Maintenance – Single daily dose of 5 mg/kg body weight intravenously every day; or 6 mg/kg body weight intravenously for 5 days a week; or 3 g/day oral ganciclovir.
   c. Foscarnet (trisodium phosphonoformate) – Induction: 60 mg/kg body weight three times a day for 2–3 weeks. Maintenance: 90–120 mg/kg body weight intravenously daily indefinitely.
   d. Maintenance treatment has to be given indefinitely as the virus lies dormant. Despite maintenance, recurrences are common. Ganciclovir and foscarnet treat the CMV retinitis but have no effect on the AIDS itself. Drugs that treat the AIDS, e.g. AZT, cannot be given concurrently with ganciclovir as the combined drugs are too toxic to bone marrow. Drugs similar to AZT are on trial that cause less bone marrow toxicity. Ganciclovir implants in the vitreous humour are being tried (Martin et al. 1994).
3. Prepare the patient for retinal detachment surgery/vitrectomy.
4. Refer the patient to counselling/AIDS service as appropriate.
5. Employ infection-control procedures according to local policies. It must be remembered that the HIV virus is very weak and does not survive outside the body. Although it has been isolated in tears, large quantities are required for transmission of the virus.

PROGNOSIS

Patients being treated for CMV retinitis in one eye rarely get it in the fellow eye, whereas untreated patients have an incidence of 60% occurrence in the fellow eye. Thus, if one eye is blind from CMV retinitis, treatment will continue to protect the other eye.

TOXOPLASMOSIS

Toxoplasmosis is caused by a protozoan parasite known as *Toxoplasma gondii* which are found in humans, mammals and birds.

Condition guideline: Toxoplasmosis

CAUSES

Toxoplasmosis is contracted in the following ways:

- Failure to wash one's hands after handling cat's litter
- Eating undercooked meat from infected animals
- Congenital infection

TYPES

In humans, the disease takes the following forms:

- Congenital toxoplasmosis – Transmitted via the placenta to the foetus when a pregnant woman contracts the acute form.
- Acute acquired systemic toxoplasmosis – Usually asymptomatic in an otherwise healthy person. In patients who are immunocompromised, such as AIDS patients, it is potentially a life-threatening disease.
- Toxoplasma retinitis – Features of iridocyclitis, superficial necrotising retinitis and papillitis. Treatment: clindamycin, 300 mg qds for 4 weeks; sulphonamides, 1 g qds for 4 weeks; or co-trimoxazole.

TOXOCARIASIS

Toxocariasis is an infection caused by worms found in the intestines of dogs and cats. The eggs from the worms are found in the faeces, and humans can contract these worms through eating unwashed vegetables that are contaminated with soil containing the eggs.

Toxocariasis types

There are three forms of toxocariasis:

1. Covert toxocariasis – Most common, with mild symptoms or no symptoms at all.
2. Visceral larva migrans – Develops as a result of severe or repeated toxocariasis infection, causing swelling of the central nervous system or body organs.
3. Ocular larva migrans – The worm enters the eye, causing a reduction in visual acuity and, in some cases, causing blindness.

CONDITIONS OF THE MACULA

AGE-RELATED MACULAR DEGENERATION

Age-related macular degeneration is a bilateral condition affecting the cones in the macular region, in old age (see Figure 13.9). There are two types of age-related macular degeneration – dry and wet. It is thought that there might be a hereditary element and that myopia may be a predisposing factor. There is gradual loss of central vision, but peripheral vision is retained so that the patient will always be able to retain his 'navigational' vision. The loss of central vision causes much distress to the patients: they are unable to recognise people because they cannot see their faces clearly; they cannot see bus numbers, sign for their pensions, watch television clearly or read. They need continual reassurance that they will not go completely blind.

DRY (ATROPHIC OR NON-NEOVASCULAR) MACULAR DEGENERATION

The dry form of macular degeneration is more common than the wet macular degeneration, accounting for 85%–90% of all age-related macular degeneration. It is associated with small,

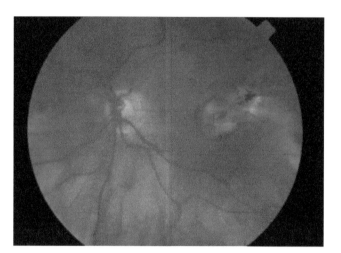

Figure 13.9 Macular degeneration.

round, white-yellow lesions in the macula, called drusen. There is currently no treatment for dry macular degeneration.

WET (CHOROIDAL NEOVASCULARISATION) MACULAR DEGENERATION

Wet, age-related macular degeneration accounts for 10%–15% of all age-related macular degeneration and is characterised by the development of abnormal blood vessels beneath the retinal pigment epithelium layer of the retina. Significant central visual loss is also much greater than with the dry form of macular degeneration. Many studies have been carried out to identify the risk factors for age-related macular degeneration such as age (usually over the age of 50), race (more prevalent in white women), smoking, hypertension, genetics and menopause. The role of vitamins and antioxidants in the prevention of macular degeneration is a much-debated issue.

The current treatment strategies for neovascular age-related macular degeneration are summarised below:

- NICE recommendations.
- Conventional laser photocoagulation – This was the first therapy for age-related macular degeneration and was originally introduced in the 1980s. However, it is now no longer recommended as a first-line treatment in subfoveal or juxtafoveal lesions (Fuchsjager-Mayrl and Schmidt-Erfurth 2007).
- Photodynamic therapy – Using verteporfin as an intravenous infused photosensitising dye.
- Photodynamic therapy combined with intravitreal triamcinolone has a beneficial additive effect on visual acuity, rate of recurrence, retreatment frequency, reduction of lesion size and foveal thickness.
- Anti-angiogenic treatments such as pegaptanib (Macugen), ranibizumab (Lucentis) or bevacizumab (Avastin). These drugs eliminate the pathological stimulus of subfoveal choroidal neovascularisation.
- Combination therapy of anti-angiogenic treatment and photodynamic therapy – The potential benefit of a combined treatment is the reduction in required retreatments, thereby providing a less time- and cost-intensive therapy.

PATIENT'S NEEDS

- Investigations into type of degeneration, OCT/fundus fluorecein angiography (FFA)
- Photodynamic therapy (laser treatment) if applicable
- Psychological needs and social effects, including ability to empathise with patients and an understanding of the grieving process
- Where appropriate, low-vision aids to improve vision and quality of life

NURSING ACTION

1. Prepare the patient for fundal fluorescein angiography and indocyanine green if requested.
2. Prepare the patient for photodynamic therapy.
3. Prepare patient for intravitreal treatment.

PROVIDING PSYCHOLOGICAL SUPPORT

Treatment of age-related macular degeneration is often a bewildering time for both patient and carer, and quality time must be allocated to provide help and support. It is important to remember that each individual patient has differing needs and would require different levels of help and support. Holistic assessment of patients is a key to providing support, and effective communication is vital to ensure that appropriate support is offered in a timely manner. According to the Nursing and Midwifery Council (2015), respecting patient individuality and valuing personal experiences are also important elements in helping patients come to terms with their sight loss. It is therefore important to ensure that patients and relatives receive the following:

- Quality time for explanation and discussion of treatment options and aftercare.
- Streamlining the therapy service to minimise visits and provide a more effective service to ensure that urgent referrals are processed more efficiently and that patients' anxiety is reduced.
- Having the appropriate healthcare professionals with the relevant training and expertise, such as counselling skills, to manage these groups of patients.
- Referral to appropriate services such as the Low Vision Service, which offers social services in a timely fashion so that independence can be maintained and that patients are empowered in their own care and management.
- According to NICE (2002), the two most important aspects of visual loss are related to activities for daily living and reading ability.
- Visual rehabilitation such as eccentric viewing techniques and appliances to help maintain independent living such as the use of cooking aids, telling the time and mobility training.
- Educational advice in the post-treatment stage such as the need to avoid bright lights during the restricted periods and the need to maintain an identity bracelet detailing treatment and contact numbers in case of the need of any emergency interventions.
- After-care advice to include what to do in the event of any visual loss and disturbance, a follow-up appointment and the need to check the fellow eye for any deterioration of vision.
- Nutritional advice such as eating a balanced diet, paying particular attention to vegetables and fruits that are rich in carotenoids and limiting the intake of saturated fats and cholesterol as these fats produce free radicals which can damage macular tissue.

- Reduce or stop smoking to minimise damage to the other eye and reduce other systemic complications.

LOW-VISION AID

Assist the patient with explanations and demonstrations in the available aids. These include low-vision aids which are obtained from the optician and which may be one or more of the following, depending on the individual's needs:

- Magnifying glasses – These can be hand-held in varying shapes and sizes or made with stands to sit on the page and be moved along the line of print.
- Telescopic lenses – These lenses are attached to spectacles, and the item to be read must be held close to the eye. This takes time to become accustomed to and can prove very awkward for the patient. Some telescopes are illuminated with a battery.
- A good light from an anglepoise-type lamp positioned correctly over the shoulder can make a lot of difference to central vision.
- Special aids are available to assist in signing pension books, etc. These are cardboard cut-outs which can be placed over the area to be written on, guiding the patient to sign in the correct place.
- Magnification using computer screens may be useful.

Remember to keep reassuring the patient that peripheral navigation vision will not be lost. He may wish to be registered as sight impaired or severely sight impaired.

CENTRAL SEROUS RETINOPATHY

Central serous retinopathy is a maculopathy affecting a younger age group than age-related macular degeneration. The cause is unknown and occurs in the 25- to 40-year age group, affecting men more than women. The sufferers tend to have an anxious disposition. The patients complain of a sudden painless loss of central vision, for example down to 6/18 with a central blur. The macula is elevated with a diagnostic light reflex around the macula.

The patient will be asked to read the Amsler grid to assess the size and position of the central blur. A fundal fluorescein angiogram will highlight the leaking of serous fluid from the choriocapillaries through the defect in the pigment epithelium. Laser treatment can be applied to seal the leaking vessels. The condition usually resolves itself within 2–4 months.

CYSTOID MACULAR OEDEMA/DEGENERATION

Cystoid macular oedema/degeneration is a rare condition causing loss of central vision. The oedema results from leakages of fluid from the retinal capillaries which infiltrate the retinal layers around the macula. It occurs gradually and can be caused by diabetic retinopathy, retinal vein occlusion, uveitis and following intraocular surgery when the exact causative mechanism is unknown. A fundal fluorescein angiogram shows the leaking vessels forming a petal appearance around the macula. The condition usually regresses spontaneously but there may be permanent visual loss, especially following cataract extraction. Patients who experience slow visual deterioration following intraocular surgery may have this condition.

CONDITIONS OF THE OPTIC NERVE

OPTIC NEURITIS

Optic neuritis is an inflammation, degeneration or demyelinisation of the optic nerve at the optic disc, causing sudden loss of vision.

CAUSES

- Demyelinising diseases such as multiple sclerosis.
- Systemic infections. Viral infections such as poliomyelitis, influenza, mumps and measles.
- Leber's disease is a hereditary inflammation of the optic nerve affecting men aged between 20 and 30 years. Vision is not totally lost but there is no known treatment.
- Local extension of inflammatory disease such as sinusitis, meningitis, orbital cellulitis.
- Toxic amblyopia is caused by a high intake of tobacco, alcohol, quinine and chloroquine.
- It is possible that, on occasion, no cause may be discovered.

SIGNS

- The optic disc is pale and oedematous with blurred disc margins.
- The large retinal veins are distended.

PATIENT'S NEEDS

- Diagnosis of the cause of the optic neuritis
- Instigation of treatment

NURSING PRIORITY

The ophthalmic nurse must inform the medical staff of the patient's sudden loss of vision.

NURSING ACTION

1. Measure blood pressure and test a specimen of urine.
2. Instil prescribed mydriatic, as per prescription or PGD for ophthalmoscopic examination.
3. Ensure the patient understands the blood tests and x-rays necessary to determine the cause.

TREATMENT

- The underlying cause must be treated if possible. Toxic amblyopia is treated by total abstinence of the offending toxin. Patients receiving chloroquine as treatment for rheumatoid arthritis or systemic lupus erythematosus must have regular ophthalmic examinations.
- Systemic steroids.

PROGNOSIS

The visual loss is usually maximal within several days of onset. It will then begin to improve 2–3 weeks afterwards, and a gradual recovery occurs over several months. Recurrent attacks can eventually cause permanent damage.

RETROBULBAR NEURITIS

Retrobulbar neuritis is inflammation of the optic nerve occurring behind the optic disc. This means that changes in the nerve cannot be seen with the ophthalmoscope. The patient's vision suddenly diminishes. It has been said that retrobulbar neuritis is a condition where the patient sees nothing out of the eye and the doctor sees nothing (abnormal) in the eye.

The causes are similar to those of optic neuritis. The treatment is that of the cause plus systemic and maybe retrobulbar steroids.

OPTIC NERVE ATROPHY

Atrophy of the optic nerve can result from any of a number of causes:

- Vascular – central retinal artery and vein occlusion
- Degeneration and resulting atrophy from retinal diseases, such as retinitis pigmentosa, and systemic diseases, such as multiple sclerosis
- Papilloedema
- Optic and retrobulbar neuritis
- Pressure on the optic nerve from aneurysms, glaucoma, tumours and orbital disease
- Toxic conditions, such as toxic amblyopia
- Metabolic disease, such as diabetes mellitus
- Trauma

The signs of optic atrophy are a pale optic disc and loss of pupillary reaction to light.

The visual loss is gradual, resulting in varying degrees from complete blindness to scotoma, depending on the cause. The cause must be elicited so that it can be treated.

The prognosis is usually poor. Optic atrophy caused by pressure may improve once the pressure has been relieved.

CONDITIONS OF THE VITREOUS HUMOUR

VITREOUS FLOATERS

Vitreous floaters are small opacities in the vitreous humour that can stimulate the retina by casting a shadow on it. The mind projects the corresponding dark form onto the appropriate field of vision. Most people experience a mild degree of vitreous floaters. When looking at a uniform background, they will see minute specks in their field of vision. As long as these specks move with eye movement, they are not potentially dangerous.

However, an increase in the number of floaters occurs as one grows older and the vitreous gel degenerates, a condition known as *syneresis*. Myopes are also prone to an increase in the number of their floaters. There is no treatment, and people often learn to live with the floaters which they may refer to as their 'friends'.

Vitreous floaters become significant in the following circumstances.

- A sudden onset of 'cobweb' or 'spider' in the vision indicates that the vitreous attachment at the optic disc has become detached, resulting in a vitreous detachment (see below).
- Flashes of light indicate that the liquefied vitreous humour, swirling around on eye movement, is putting traction on the retina. This could progress to a retinal detachment.
- A sudden crop of black floaters indicates the presence of a retinal tear with an associated vitreous haemorrhage. This may progress to a vitreous detachment followed by a retinal detachment.

Thus it can be seen that vitreous floaters may indicate further vitreous humour and retinal conditions.

POSTERIOR VITREOUS DETACHMENT

Posterior vitreous detachment occurs with the degeneration of the vitreous humour. The vitreous humour detaches from its attachment around the optic disc. A 'spider's web' or 'cobweb' is noticed in the vision and a sudden increase in vitreous floaters occurs. Flashing lights may also be seen as the detaching vitreous humour stimulates the rods and cones.

Vitreous detachment may cause vitreous haemorrhage, retinal tears and retinal detachment and should be investigated.

Patients are often very concerned about these symptoms. Information about this condition should be given to them.

VITREOUS HAEMORRHAGE

Vitreous haemorrhage may vary in degree from minimal bleeding, in which case the patient notices a few more floaters, to a massive bleed obscuring sight suddenly so the patient can only see light.

CAUSES

- Trauma
- Vascular disorders such as hypertension, leukaemia and neovascularisation, especially in diabetic retinopathy, and following a central retinal vein occlusion
- Vitreous detachment

SIGNS

The fundal picture will vary according to the size of the haemorrhage, from small opacities floating in the vitreous humour to a total haemorrhage obscuring the fundus.

PATIENT'S NEEDS

- Diagnosis of the cause of the haemorrhage in order that treatment can be instigated
- Bed rest to assist absorption of haemorrhage
- Preparation for vitrectomy

NURSING ACTION

1. If visual loss has occurred suddenly, the medical staff should be informed immediately.
2. Instil prescribed mydriatic drops for ophthalmoscopy.
3. Admit the patient to the ward if the haemorrhage is severe enough to warrant bed rest in hospital.
4. Give pre-operative care if vitrectomy is to be performed.
5. If the patient is not to be admitted, ensure that he understands the importance of resting at home.
6. Give post-vitrectomy care.

Reflective activity

Consider a patient whom you have seen recently with a retinal or vitreal problem:

- What were the presenting signs and symptoms?
- Was there any associated systemic disease or diseases?
- What tests and investigations were carried out and why?
- How did you arrive at a diagnosis?
- What was the treatment plan?
- Outline the care and management of the patient.
- If there were any challenges in caring for the patient, what were they?
- Was any other member of the multidisciplinary team involved in the care and what was his or her input?
- Utilising a recognised health-promotion framework, how would you explain the condition and treatment to the patient in order to ensure that he or she adheres to the treatment?
- What was the clinical outcome?
- What local or national policies, guidelines or protocols influenced the care and management of this patient?
- On reflection, would you have done anything differently, and if so, what?

Your completed case study can be used to contribute to your continuing professional development portfolio for Registration and your Knowledge and Skills Framework or appraisal review.

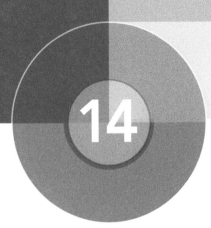

The extraocular muscles

This chapter examines some of the conditions affecting the extraocular muscles.

INTRODUCTION

There are six extraocular muscles which move the eye in the directions of gaze. There are four rectus muscles and two oblique muscles (Figure 14.1):

- The medial rectus muscle originates in the medial aspect annulus of Zinn, a tendinous ring that is continuous with the dura and peri-orbita. The medial rectus projects directly anteriorly running parallel with the medial wall of the orbit. It then attaches approximately at the equator to the anterior, medial sclera 5.5 mm from the limbus. Due to its pathway and insertion angle it acts as a pure adductor, used especially in contralateral lateral gaze, i.e., the right medial rectus is used in left gaze and also when converging. It is supplied by the oculomotor (IIIrd) nerve and by the inferior muscular branch of ophthalmic artery and two anterior ciliary arteries.
- The lateral rectus muscle originates in the lateral aspect of the annulus of Zinn and projects along the lateral wall of the orbit, approaching from the rear of the eye before wrapping around and attaching around the equator of the anterior, lateral sclera 7 mm from the limbus. Its acts purely as an abductor, used especially in ipsilateral lateral gaze and when diverging (looking in the distance). It is supplied by the abducens (VIth) nerve and only the lacrimal artery.
- The superior rectus muscle originates in the superior portion of the annulus of Zinn. The superior rectus projects forward, passing over the superior oblique and approaching the eye at an angle, attaching to the anterior, superior sclera approximately 7.5 mm from the limbus. Due to its angle of insertion it not only elevates the eye but also abducts and intorts the eye. Its action is most prominent in ipsilateral elevated gaze. It is supplied by the oculomotor nerve and ophthalmic artery along with two anterior ciliary arteries.
- The inferior rectus muscle originates in the inferior portion of the annulus of Zinn. The inferior rectus projects forward, passing along the floor of the orbit and approaching the eye at an angle, like the superior oblique attaching to the anterior, inferior sclera approximately 6.5 mm from the limbus. Due to its angle of insertion it not only depresses the eye but also abducts and intorts the eye. Its action is most prominent in ipsilateral elevated gaze. The inferior oblique muscle is often the first affected muscle in thyroid eye disease (TED). It is supplied by the oculomotor nerve and ophthalmic artery along with two anterior ciliary arteries.

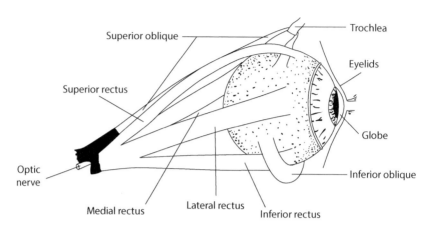

Figure 14.1 The extraocular muscles.

- The lateral rectus muscle originates in the lateral portion of the annulus of Zinn and is supplied by the abducens (VIth) nerve. The muscle projects forward, passing along the side of the orbital wall and approaches the eye directly. It attaches on the lateral sclera approximately 7 mm from the limbus. Due to its angle of insertion it is a pure abductor. Its most prominent action is abduction.
- The superior oblique muscle originates in the superior portion of the annulus of Zinn. The superior oblique projects forward, passing under the superior oblique and passes through the trochlea (a small pulley located on the medial aspect of the frontal bone). Here it reflects backwards, approaching the eye at an angle, attaching to a point just inferior to the superior rectus muscle. Due to its angle of insertion it not only intorts the eye but also depresses and abducts the eye. Its action is most prominent in contralateral depressed gaze. Because of the tortuous journey that the IV nerve takes out of the back of the brain stem, IV palsies are especially common in those with head trauma.
- The inferior oblique muscle originates at the medial aspect of the maxillary bone. Here it travels so that it inserts on the posterior lateral sclera, lying inferior to the inferior rectus muscle. It is supplied by the oculomotor nerve. It acts primarily to extort the eye but its oblique insertion gives it elevation and abduction as its secondary actions.

Note that the primary muscle action relates to the main movement when the eye is in the primary position, while the secondary action relates to any additional movements the muscle makes to the eye.

Muscle	Origin	Insertion	Nerve supply	Primary action	Secondary action
Superior rectus	Annulus of Zinn	Superior sclera 7.5 mm from limbus	Oculomotor nerve	To elevate the eye	Adduction and intortion
Inferior rectus	Annulus of Zinn	Inferior sclera 6.5 mm from the limbus	Oculomotor nerve	To depress the eye	Adduction and intortion
Medial rectus	Annulus of Zinn	Medial sclera 5.5 mm from the limbus	Oculomotor nerve	To adduct the eye	None
Lateral rectus	Annulus of Zinn	Lateral sclera 7 mm from the limbus	Abducens nerve	To adduct the eye	None

Superior oblique	Annulus of Zinn	Superior outer sclera having passed through the trochlea, a small pulley situated on the medial aspect of the frontal bone; this muscle is inferior to the superior rectus	Trochlear nerve	To depress the eye	Abduction
Inferior oblique	Medial aspect of the maxillary bone	Posterior lateral sclera lying inferior to the rectus muscle	Oculomotor nerve	Extorsion of the eye	Elevation and abduction

BLOOD SUPPLY

Muscular branches of the ophthalmic artery and vein are responsible for the supply and drainage of blood.

EYE MOVEMENTS

Both eyes must move together in a coordinated manner. In order for this to occur, each extraocular muscle is paired with a muscle in the opposite eye. These pairs of muscles are known as synergistic or 'yoke' muscles. For example, to look to the right, the right eye looks outwards, i.e. abducts, while the left eye looks inwards, i.e. adducts. The right lateral rectus muscle abducts the right eye, while the left medial rectus muscle adducts the left eye. These two muscles work together to cause the eyes to look to the right. The right lateral rectus muscle and the left medial rectus muscle are therefore yoke muscles.

NINE POSITIONS OF GAZE

To look directly upward and downward, two pairs of yoke muscles are required to contract. In the other positions, only one pair of yoke muscles is needed. The nine positions of gaze and yoke muscles needed are

1. *Straight ahead* – The primary position of gaze when all the muscles are contracting to maintain the eye in this position
2. *Upward to the right (Dextro elevation)* – Right superior rectus; left inferior oblique
3. *To the right (Dextro version)* – Right lateral rectus; left medial rectus
4. *Downward to the right (Dextro depression)* – Right inferior rectus; left superior oblique
5. *Downward to the left (Laevo depression)* – Left inferior rectus; right superior oblique
6. *To the left (Laevo version)* – Left lateral rectus; right medial rectus
7. *Upward to the left (Laevo elevation)* – Left superior rectus; right inferior oblique
8. *Direct elevation* – Right superior rectus; left inferior oblique *and* left superior rectus; right inferior oblique
9. *Direct depression* – Right inferior rectus; left superior oblique *and* left inferior rectus; right superior oblique

Convergence is the position of the eyes when looking at something close by. In this case, both medial recti contract to turn the eye inwards.

ANTAGONIST MUSCLES

When each muscle in the eye contracts, in order for the eye to move, the antagonist or opposite muscle in the same eye must relax to allow the first muscle to work; for example, to look to the right, the right lateral rectus contracts and the right medial rectus must relax. In the left eye, the left medial rectus contracts while the left lateral rectus relaxes. The antagonist muscles are

- Medial rectus and lateral rectus
- Inferior rectus and superior rectus
- Inferior oblique and superior oblique

This brings us to Sherrington's law of reciprocal innervation which states that as an increase of innervational stimuli is sent to a muscle, decreased innervation is sent to the direct antagonist, helping to maintain smooth and accurate eye movement.

OCULAR MOTOR FUNCTION

The eye has five main types of eye movement that it can utilise to look at objects depending on the situation that arises. The three main types are smooth pursuit, saccades and vergence movements.

Smooth pursuit is seen as the patient follows a slow-moving object while keeping his head still. It is the movement system that is assessed during ocular motility.

Smooth pursuit movements are tested routinely during orthoptic examination but it is especially indicated that this is assessed in any patient with sudden-onset double vision, any recent history of stroke or head trauma. When investigating smooth pursuit in a patient it is recommended that you use a pen torch so that you can see the position of the corneal reflections as you get the patient to move his eyes into the nine positions of gaze. This will make it easier to see muscle under-actions.

Saccades are fast, ballistic movements of the eye that rapidly change the eyes point of fixation. They can occur voluntarily when directing ones attention towards an object or involuntarily as in when an object appears in the visual field.

Vergence movements are used to align the eyes at varying distances from the viewer. Unlike other eye movements vergence movements are disjugate, that is they move towards each other (convergence) or away from each other (divergence). It is important to note that vergence problems are common after strokes and head trauma and may cause a patient to develop double vision.

STRABISMUS OR SQUINT

Strabismus or squint is a deviation of one or either eye in an inwards, outwards, upward or downward direction (Figure 14.2). There are many types of squint. Only the most common will be described here. Orthoptists are highly trained to diagnose which muscle is involved and to treat the deviation in conjunction with ophthalmologists.

A squint causes diplopia. In younger children, this double vision can be suppressed, but older patients are unable to do this so the diplopia persists. The exact age at which this suppression is able to form is typically given as being around 78 years old; however, recent studies have shown that the neuroplacticity of the brain may well persist into a much older age. The child suppresses the vision in the squinting eye so he no longer sees double, which causes less visual confusion. In the early years, the visual process has not fully matured and if an eye is not used for any reason it may lose its ability to see. This results in reduced visual acuity, a condition

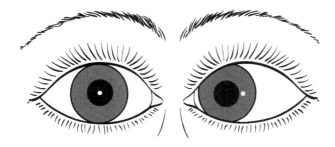

Figure 14.2 Left convergent squint.

called amblyopia. When the visual system is not mature, reduced vision can be improved with occlusion treatment up to this age. Thereafter, loss of visual acuity due to amblyopia is much harder to improve. Therefore, it is important that squint and any resulting amblyopia are diagnosed before the age of 8 years. This applies to all squints, whether manifest or latent. School eye tests are important to pick up poor vision before it is too late for treatment to be of help.

Normal vision with both eyes in use is termed binocular single vision. The images from both eyes together are seen as one visual impression by means of the fusion faculty. The aim of treatment for squint is to restore binocular single vision and prevent or reverse amblyopia.

Squints are either non-paralytic or paralytic.

NON-PARALYTIC SQUINT

Non-paralytic squint is the squint of childhood and is sometimes called a concomitant squint. It can be manifest or latent, convergent or divergent, alternating or non-alternating (unilateral):

- A manifest squint (Tropia) is where one or other eye deviates from the primary or straight-ahead position while the patient is viewing the target without interruption to either eye. It can often be an obvious squint to the observer.
- A latent squint (Phoria) is where there is a tendency for both eyes to deviate and this is not usually observed unless symptoms such as headaches or diplopia have occurred, in which case the latent squint may have become manifest. Latent squints are most easily seen when binocular vision is interrupted, i.e. when one eye is occluded. The occluded eye will usually be seen to refixate as the occlusion is removed.
- A convergent squint (esotropia/esophoria) is a squint in which one eye turns inwards.
- A divergent squint (exotropia/exophoria) is a squint in which one eye turns outwards.
- An alternating squint is a squint in which the eyes deviate alternately, whereas it is always the same eye which deviates in a non-alternating squint. In a non-paralytic squint the 'fixing eye' or the eye which is in primary position is usually the eye with the better vision; therefore alternating squints typically have a better visual prognosis as they present with near equal visual acuity and tend to remain that way.

Condition guideline: Non-paralytic squint

CAUSES

Around 5% of all children aged 5 years old have a squint. It is also common to see a brief squint in younger children, especially when tired. Children under the age of 3 months will often cross their eyes as their vision develops, this is no cause for concern. However, if the squint continues to be seen past this age or becomes constantly manifest then the patient should be referred for orthoptic assessment.

CONGENITAL SQUINTS

Congenital squints are defined as squints that are present from birth or that develop within the first 6 months. The exact cause of congenital squints is often not known. In most cases the eye will turn inwards, often called an infantile esotropia. This type of esotropia often runs in the family, so there is a genetic component to the squint but there may be no family history squints.

UNCORRECTED REFRACTIVE ERROR

Uncorrected refractive error is the most common cause of squint in childhood. Squints are most commonly convergent and are often associated with hypermetropia, which causes over-accommodation and therefore over-convergence.

In contrast to this, myopia has the opposite effect and stimulates divergence because as the eyes are already in focus to near vision without the aid of accommodation, convergence is not stimulated. Anisometropia (a different refraction in each eye) causes unequally clear images, which can also lead to a squint as the brain cannot combine the two unequal images.

The usual pattern of events to occur (if the onset of squint is under the age of 8 years) is as follows:

- Squint leads to loss of binocular single vision.
- Loss of binocular single vision results in diplopia.
- Diplopia is overcome by suppression of one image.
- Suppression leads to amblyopia (a reduction in visual acuity in one eye).
- The passage of time leads to loss of binocular function (the two eyes being no longer able to see one image together).

PROLONGED EYE INACTIVITY

Prolonged inactivity of one eye may be a dissociating factor and may enable the affected eye to deviate secondarily to the poor acuity:

- Opacities in the media, i.e. cornea, lens, vitreous humour or retina, may cause squint. A cataract or retinoblastoma may present as a squint.
- Bandaging of one eye, for example following injury to the eye, or a unilateral ptosis may also cause squint.

EXAMINATION

HISTORY

A careful history must be taken and should include

- Family history because there may be a hereditary factor.
- Age at onset, which is an important factor in prognosis for reversing amblyopia and restoring binocular single vision.
- Nature of onset – The onset of squint may occur in one or several of the following ways:
  - Suddenly the squint occurs without any previous sign.
  - Gradually the squint appears more and more frequently and possibly increasing in size over a period of time.

- Intermittently, e.g. when tired, upset or unwell; the eye may be straight at other times. Constantly the squint is present all the time.
- Changing in size at different times of day.
- When looking in a particular position of gaze or at a particular distance.
- Either eye may deviate alternately, or it may always be the same eye that deviates.

The onset may be associated with some systemic disease because the child is generally unwell.

VISUAL ACUITY

Visual acuity will be recorded using the LogMAR, Snellen, Kay picture test or other tests. Selection of test will be determined by the age, intellectual ability of the patient and his language.

DETERMINATION OF REFRACTIVE ERROR

In children, a cycloplegic drop such as G. cyclopentolate 0.5% for infants, 1% for children, by prescription or procedure guideline, is needed to prevent accommodation, which would give a false result on retinoscopy. Cycloplegia will also dilate the pupils allowing for an easier fundoscopy. A retinoscope directs a light beam onto the retina, and movement of the retinoscope produces movement of the light beam across the retina in a particular direction. A lens is selected and held in front of the eye while continuing to move the retinoscope.

A change is noted in the amount and direction of the movement of the light beam. Finally, the lens, which actually neutralises or abolishes the movement of the light beam, determines the refractive error.

PHYSICAL EXAMINATION

1. The presence of the following features is noted:
   a. Epicanthus if a child has broad epicanthic folds. It can give the appearance of a convergent squint but, if the cover test is negative, this is called a pseudosquint.
   b. Ptosis or other feature leading to asymmetry of the palpebral apertures.
   c. Nystagmus.
   d. An abnormal head posture, which could be compensating for squint.
   e. Unequal pupil sizes.
2. An inspection of the eyes is carried out:
   a. Corneal reflections.
   b. Cover test.
   c. Ocular movements.
   d. Measuring the angle of deviation.
   e. Stereoscopic vision.

CORNEAL REFLECTIONS

Method

A pen torch is held at 0.33 m directly in front of both eyes. The position of the reflection on each eye is then compared.

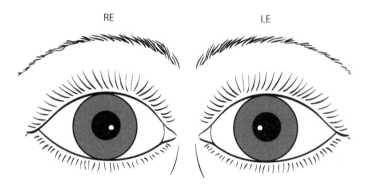

RE   LE

Figure 14.3 Normal corneal reflections. The corneal reflections are symmetrical, usually slightly nasal in each eye. *Note:* corneal reflections may not be central, but check symmetry.

RESULTS

The results may be

- Normal corneal reflections symmetrical (Figure 14.3).
- Asymmetrical corneal reflections (Figure 14.4). It is important to note that if the corneal reflection is displaced temporally, it indicates the eye is turned inwards and vice versa. An upturning eye or a downturning eye can also be detected by observing the corneal reflections (such squints are less common).

COVER TEST

The cover test is a simple, objective test carried out to detect the presence of a squint, and it should be used in conjunction with observation of the corneal reflections.

METHOD

An accommodative target is held approximately 0.33 m from the child. The child must be looking at the light while the cover test is carried out. It is important to perform the cover test using a detailed target, e.g. a small picture on a tongue depressor, because some squints are only present when looking at detailed objects. The cover test should also be carried out at 6 m, where possible, because other squints are only present when looking into the distance, i.e. intermittent squints.

To perform a cover test, ensure the patient is comfortably fixating on an adequate target for their ability and visual acuity. Then occlude one eye and look for any movement of the uncovered eye to take up fixation, repeat this for both eyes. The alternate cover test is performed by ensuring one eye is always covered by an occluder throughout the test and switching quickly between the eyes, noting the movement of the eye as it goes from being covered to fixating, again, this should be tested at both 33 cm and 6 m. The size and direction of any latent squints should be noted.

RESULTS

The results may be

- No manifest squint (Figure 14.5)
- Manifest squint right convergent squint (Figure 14.6)
- Manifest squint right divergent squint (Figure 14.7)

(a) RE LE

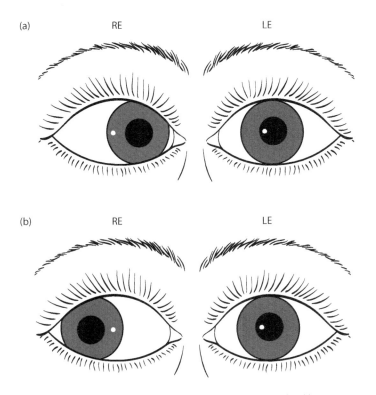

(b) RE LE

Figure 14.4 Asymmetrical corneal reflections. (a) Right convergent squint. Note asymmetry of corneal reflections. The left corneal reflection is in the normal position, i.e. slightly nasal. The right corneal reflection is displaced temporally, because the right eye is turning inwards. (b) Right divergent squint. Note asymmetry of corneal reflections. The left corneal reflection is in the normal position, i.e. slightly nasal. The right corneal reflection is displaced nasally, because the right eye is turning outwards.

An intermittent convergent squint may not be present when the child is looking at a light but becomes manifest when focussing on a detailed target. Therefore, it is important to check the corneal reflections and to carry out the cover test using a light and a detailed target.

An intermittent divergent squint may not be present for near vision, but becomes manifest in the distance. Therefore, it is important to carry out a cover test for both near and distance vision.

OCULAR MOVEMENTS

The examiner sits in front of the patient and, using a pen torch, and a toy if appropriate, observes both eyes moving in all nine positions of gaze. This will include up, down, both sides and in all four corners, always returning to the straight-ahead or primary position. The patient's head must be held still. Any muscle imbalance, over-actions and under-actions or areas of diplopia are then noted.

MEASURING THE ANGLE OF DEVIATION

The angle of deviation can be measured using objective or subjective methods. Objective methods are based on the observer neutralising the patient's deviation as it takes up

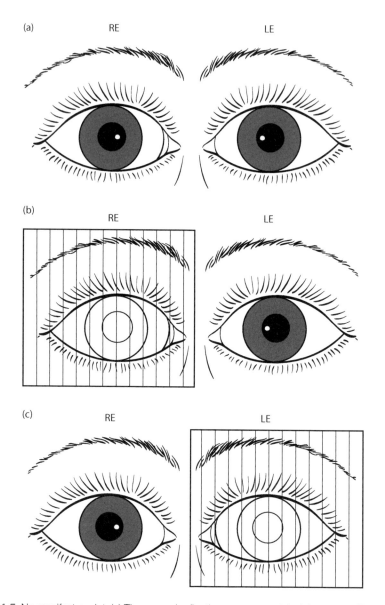

Figure 14.5 No manifest squint. (a) The corneal reflections are symmetrical, i.e. no manifest squint detected. (b) No movement of the left eye when the right eye is covered. (c) No movement of the right eye when the left eye is covered.

fixation. Subjective measurements are where the patient tells the observer the position of each image from each eye on a calibrated scale of some sort.

The following methods include both objective and subjective measurements.

The prisms cover test is the most commonly used objective method of measuring the angle of a manifest or a latent squint. The measurements are performed at near (0.33 m), distance (6 m) and occasionally beyond 6 m (far distance). Loose prisms, or a prism bar, are introduced in front of the squinting eye in a manifest squint, or in front of either eye in a latent squint, with the apex of the prism in the direction of the deviation. It can

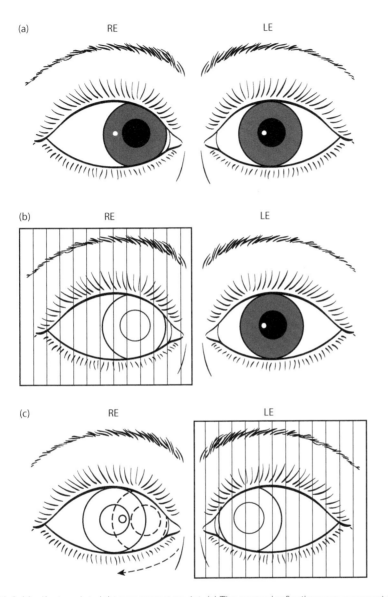

Figure 14.6 Manifest squint: right convergent squint. (a) The corneal reflections are asymmetrical, showing a right convergent squint. Confirm with cover test. (b) No movement of the left eye when the right eye is covered. (c) The right eye moves out to fix when the left eye is covered.

be performed by using an alternate cover test with a prism held in front of the eye. The strength and direction of the prism required to neutralise the deviation should be noted.

Using major amblyoscope (synoptophore), the angle of deviation can be measured both objectively and subjectively. Slides are introduced, and the measurement can be read from the scales in degrees or prism dioptres. The synoptophore has the advantage of being able to accurately reproduce measurements in different positions of gaze.

The Maddox rod is used in conjunction with a light at 6 m and measures small degrees of squint. The Maddox rod is made of a series of parallel cylinders, red in colour, which

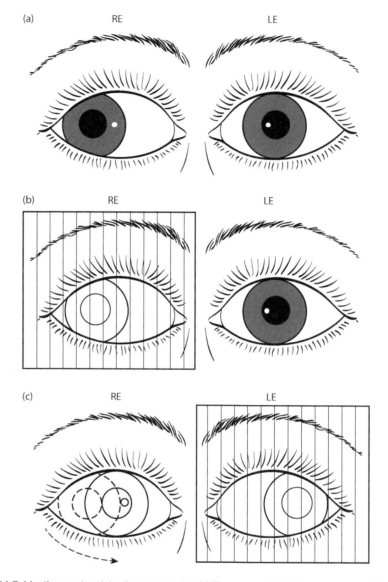

Figure 14.7 Manifest squint: right divergent squint. (a) The corneal reflections are asymmetrical, showing a right divergent squint. Confirm with cover test. (b) No movement of the left eye when the right eye is covered. (c) The right eye moves *in* to fix when the left eye is covered.

convert a light image into a red line. This is placed before one eye while the patient is fixing on a light at 6 m distance with both eyes open. The eye looking through the Maddox rod sees a red line instead of a white light, and the other eye sees the light as it really is.

These images are too dissimilar for fusion to take place, so the eyes deviate to the position of squint. Prisms are introduced until the light and the red line are superimposed. The Maddox wing enables measurements of latent and small manifest deviations to be made at a near distance. The Maddox rod and wing allow measurement of horizontal and vertical deviations. The wing also allows torsional measurements to be made. Maddox wings and rods are rarely used in practice as their measurements tend to be quite variable. Maddox wings are especially prone to falsely identifying torsional deviations depending on the patient's head posture.

STEREOSCOPIC VISION

The ability to see in 'depth' or 3D vision is the highest form of binocular sight.

The main tests measuring stereo acuity in seconds of arc (the measurement of minimum disparity that gives rise to appreciation of depth) include

- Frisby test
- Wirt fly test (Titmus test)
- TNO (red/green test)
- Lang stereo test

Frisby is considered the gold standard for testing stereopsis so it should be used where possible. However, Wirt and TNO work better with younger patients as their 3D illusion can be quite entertaining. Reduced stereopsis can be a sign of reduced visual acuity or of a decompensating phoria.

TREATMENT

There are several treatment choices for a non-paralytic squint:

- Optical treatment – Accurate refraction must be carried out and appropriate glasses ordered. This in itself might correct the squint.
- Occlusion therapy – The visual acuity must be assessed and, if amblyopia is present, it must be reversed. This is performed by occluding the 'good' eye to encourage the amblyopic eye to work harder and develops the visual cortex. In cases of very dense amblyopia, inverse occlusion may be used, i.e. occluding the good eye for a small period of time to interrupt the suppression of that eye. Occlusion therapy is carried out according to the state of amblyopia and should be administered by an orthoptist. Patients and parents should be made aware that occlusion therapy will not alter the angle of the eye and will not cure a patient of a squint.
- Orthoptic exercises are used to stimulate binocular single vision and strengthen fusion by means of binocular instruments such by using stereograms. These instruments use pairs of slides, one for each eye, which match together to form a picture; slides may include two diagrams of cats which are missing details so that a single, complete cat can be made by fusing the two images.
- Operative measures will not improve binocular vision once it has been lost. The muscles operated on in convergent and divergent squint are usually the medial and lateral recti. They may be resected (tightened) or recessed (weakened). Sometimes surgery is directed to the non-squinting eye, which worries parents and sometimes nurses. It may not matter which eye is operated on, the aim being to align one eye with the other.
  - Early surgery is performed if there is either potential binocular function present, or if there is poor cosmetic appearance with no binocular vision.
  - Surgery can be delayed if the deviation is cosmetically reasonably good.
  - Surgery is not performed if the cosmetic appearance is good in the presence of no binocular function.
- Botulinum toxin is used to correct some types of convergent and divergent squint, particularly where surgery may be contraindicated as with Graves' disease or when

the angle of the deviation is too small to warrant surgery. It is primarily used for cosmetic reasons. The botulinum toxin is injected directly into the muscle; however, the paralysis of the muscle is not instantaneous. It can take up to 48 hours to take effect and the action is relatively short lived, between 5 and 8 weeks. Because of this, the treatment needs to be repeated every 23 months. Botulinum toxin injections must be administered using Aseptic Non Touch Technique (ANTT) principles.

PARALYTIC SQUINT

A paralytic or incomitant (non-concomitant) squint is more common in adults than in children. If it occurs in a child under the age of 8 years, the child will be able to suppress the resulting double vision, and the same events that occur with a non-paralytic squint will follow.

Adults, however, have no capacity to suppress the vision in one eye to eliminate the diplopia. This can be distressing and can be associated with nausea and giddiness.

Condition guideline: Paralytic squint

CAUSES

A paralytic squint is caused by an abnormality in the extraocular muscles or their nerve supply.

MUSCLE DISORDERS

- Trauma, e.g. forceps delivery at birth
- Congenital abnormality
- Disease, e.g. exophthalmic ophthalmoplegia from
    - Thyroid eye disease
    - Myasthenia gravis
    - Neoplasm

NERVE DISORDERS

Trauma

- Bruising or severing of nerves following head injury
- Strokes; infarcts or haemorrhages
- Septic infection

Inflammation

- Mastoid disease
- Peripheral neuritis
- Encephalitis
- Multiple sclerosis
- Tertiary syphilis
- Haemorrhage
- Thrombosis
- Aneurysm
- Neoplasm, e.g. pituitary tumour

- Diabetes mellitus
- Temporarily following cataract extraction

TREATMENT

- Orthoptic assessment should be carried out to establish which muscle is affected, e.g. examination of eye movements, the Hess chart and diplopia tests.
- Give temporary Fresnel prism to join the diplopia to binocular single vision if possible.
- Teach compensatory head posture, if this is applicable. The patient is taught to hold his head in the position that relieves the diplopia.
- Occlude on eye if the diplopia cannot be fused.
- Referral is required to a neurologist or physician for investigation of the cause.
- Botulinum toxin can be used to paralyse muscles and thereby straighten the eye. It is used to treat strabismus, paralytic strabismus and diplopia post-retinal detachment surgery. Patients need to be aware that the maximum effect is not immediate, but may be felt some 25 days later. The effect is only temporary and lasts for between 2 and 3 months.
- Wait 6–9 months for recovery to occur.
- If recovery does not occur after 9 months, surgery can be performed or prisms can be permanently incorporated into glasses to restore binocular single vision.
- Correction of squint for cosmetic reasons (children are especially teased at school).
- Correction of amblyopia and restoration of binocular single vision.
- Relief of diplopia if an adult.

NURSING ACTION

1. Assist with examination in the outpatient department.
2. Instil prescribed cycloplegic drops, e.g. G. cyclopentolate hydrochloride.
3. Liaise with the orthoptic department if necessary about patching and exercises, and offer teaching and encouragement to the parents and child on the use of patching.
4. Give advice on occluding one eye, prisms in glasses or compensatory head posture to relieve the symptoms.
5. Prepare the patient for botulinum injections.
6. Admit the patient to day unit if surgery is to be performed.
7. Give pre-operative care, e.g. explain reasons for possibility of surgeon operating on the 'good' eye. Warn adult patients that they may feel unwell for about 1 week; the reason for this is not readily understood.
8. Give post-operative care:
   a. The eye is not usually padded post-operatively.
   b. There may be conjunctival injection present, including a subconjunctival haemorrhage.
   c. Instil prescribed antibiotic or steroid and antibiotic drops.
   d. Give analgesia intramuscularly if adjustable sutures have been employed prior to their being adjusted. This can occur any time from immediately coming round from the anaesthetic to 24 hours later. Adjustable sutures are suitable for any patient over the age of 10 years old. Topical anaesthetic is used immediately prior to adjustment such as G. oxybuprocaine 0.4% to facilitate adjustment.
   e. Liaise with the orthoptic department regarding the necessity of continuing with non-surgical treatment such as wearing glasses, occlusion, etc.

    f.   Avoid swimming or contact sports for 4 weeks.

    g.   Children should only need to be kept off school for a few days.

9. Ensure that the patient has a follow-up orthoptic appointment on discharge.

COMPLICATIONS

- Stitch abscess.
- The muscle slipping away from its new position because the sutures have failed.
- Failure of the operation to result in binocular single vision when this is the expected outcome.
- Failure of the operation to give good cosmesis.
- Overcorrection of the squint; a convergent squint results in a consecutive divergent squint, and vice versa.

Condition guideline: Pseudosquint

A pseudosquint is the appearance of a squint occurring in the presence of binocular single vision.

CAUSES

- Epicanthus.
- Abnormal angle alpha – a larger or smaller than normal angle between the optic axis and the visual axis; similar to that of angles kappa and gamma.
- Facial asymmetry.
- Wide or narrow inter-pupillary distance giving the appearance of divergent squint; and a narrow inter-pupillary distance, giving the appearance of convergent squint.
- Enophthalmos may result in pseudoesotropia, whereas exophthalmic eyes will appear more exotropic.
- Displacement of the orbits, either as a result of trauma or congenital defects may give the appearance of a squint when there is none.

Reflective activities

Consider a patient whom you have seen recently with a problem with the extraocular muscles:

- What were the presenting signs and symptoms?
- Was there any associated systemic disease or diseases?
- What tests and investigations were carried out and why?
- How did you arrive at a diagnosis?
- What was the treatment plan?
- Outline the care and management of the patient.
- If there were any challenges in caring for the patient, what were they?
- Was any other member of the multidisciplinary team involved in the care and what was his or her input?

- Utilising a recognised health promotion framework, how would you explain the condition and treatment to the patient in order to ensure that he or she adheres to the treatment?
- What was the clinical outcome?
- What local or national policies, guidelines or protocols influenced the care and management of this patient?
- On reflection, would you have done anything differently and, if so, what? Your completed case study can be used to contribute to your continuing professional development portfolio for Registration and your Knowledge and Skills Framework or appraisal review.

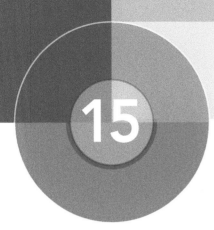

Ophthalmic trauma

This chapter examines some of the more common conditions seen in emergency settings.

The ophthalmic nurse requires special skills of observation and history taking, together with the ability to care for a patient who has received trauma to the eye or its surrounding area.

Penetrating (perforating) injury and ocular burns are considered ophthalmic emergencies. Blunt trauma can result in serious ocular damage. Therefore, the nurse must take an accurate history, examine the eye carefully and decide in what order of priority each patient presenting with ocular trauma needs to be placed.

A blow to the eyeball causes shock waves to pass through it, damaging many structures such as the cornea, iris, lens and retina. Blunt trauma may accompany a penetrating injury, and therefore any patient presenting with a history of a forceful blow to the eye must have all ocular structures examined carefully. The importance of accurate history taking and accurate measurement of visual acuity cannot be overemphasised.

Children presenting with ocular trauma, and whose history is not appropriate for the injury sustained, must be carefully screened for any sign of child abuse, and appropriate action taken if found.

Minims drops, which are sterile and preservative free, must be used in all eye examinations for ocular trauma.

Patients presenting with ocular trauma must have their visual acuity checked to establish baseline reading.

It is assumed in the following text that all patients will be treated for accompanying shock if present and that this may be a priority. Where appropriate analgesia and antiemetic, and also a tetanus toxoid injection, must be given if the skin or ocular tissue has been cut.

Condition guideline: Intraocular foreign body

An intraocular foreign body (IOFB) results when something enters the eye under force, such as fragments generated when using a hammer and chisel or a lathe. The foreign body may lodge itself in any of the structures of the eye, and examination may not reveal its presence, highlighting the importance of history taking. History taking should include whether appropriate eye protection has been worn at time of injury.

PATIENT'S NEEDS

- Thorough ocular examination to determine the extent of the injuries
- Explanation of the extent of the injuries and the required treatment
- Admission to hospital for removal of the IOFB
- Post-operative and discharge care

NURSING ACTION

1. Obtain accurate history.
2. Inform medical staff.
3. Prepare the patient for an x-ray or computed tomography (CT) scan to locate the IOFB.
4. Prepare the patient for removal of the foreign body if one is present. If it is metallic, it may be removed with a specialised magnet in the operating theatre.
5. Give post-operative care, clean the eye and instil drops. Give any necessary information including advice on appropriate eye protection to prevent future injuries.
6. Plan discharge.

Condition guideline: Fracture of the orbit

Fractures of the orbit occur as a result of trauma. Usually they are easily recognised by the irregularity of the outline of the orbit. A 'blowout' fracture of the orbit occurs following trauma to the maxillary bone which fractures, and the eye tends to sink down into the gap created in the bone. Patients with suspected 'blow-out' fracture should be told not to blow their nose to minimise emphysema and consider oral antibiotics and steroids. Emphysema (the skin crackles when pressed) may be present due to a fractured maxillary sinus. All patients with suspected orbital fracture will need an evaluation of optic nerve function and an orthoptic assessment and a full eye examination (McMullen 2013). Orbital fractures are generally managed by the maxillofacial department and referral to them is mandatory. Children with 'white-eyed blowout' fractures may well be toxic with a fever and tachycardia due to muscle entrapment.

SIGNS AND SYMPTOMS

- Enophthalmos
- Inability to move the eye in all fields of gaze because the extraocular muscles have become trapped in the fractured bone
- Jerky eye movement in the upward gaze because the inferior oblique and inferior rectus muscle have been trapped
- Diplopia
- Areas of facial paraesthesia, which may suggest damage of the infraorbital or supraorbital nerve

PATIENT'S NEEDS

- Diagnosis of the presence of a fracture
- Relief of symptoms of
  - Decreased sensation of the skin over the maxilla
  - Diplopia

- Repair of skin laceration if present
- Repair of fracture if severe (may not be performed for up to 6 months)
- Cleaning of any wounds present

NURSING ACTION

1. Explain to the patient the extent of the injuries and the treatment to be carried out.
2. Preparation for x-ray examination to confirm and isolate the fracture.
3. Clean wound if present.
4. Admit the patient to the ward if surgery is to be performed.
5. Prepare the patient for the operation to free the trapped muscles and repair the fracture. A Teflon plate or orbital implant may be inserted.
6. Give post-operative care:
   a. Clean the wound.
   b. Instil antibiotic drops.
   c. Give prescribed systemic antibiotics.
7. Plan discharge.
8. Remove sutures, usually as an outpatient procedure, 5–7 days post-operatively.

Condition guideline: Trauma to the eyelids

Trauma to the eyelids is a common occurrence as their function is to protect the globe. The following may occur:

- Bruising
- Laceration
- Burns

PATIENT'S NEEDS

- Exploration of the extent of the injuries.
- Relief of symptoms – if a sub-tarsal foreign body is present, there will be profuse lacrimation and blepharospasm.
- Treatment of injuries.

NURSING PRIORITIES

- Inform medical staff.
- Commence irrigation if a burn has occurred.

NURSING ACTION

1. Explain to the patient the extent of the injuries received and the necessary treatment.
2. Assist the doctor in examining the eye.
3. Treat the injuries:
   a. Bruising: apply cold compress and instruct the patient how to do this.
   b. Laceration:
      i. Clean wound.
      ii. Prepare the patient and equipment for suturing of the laceration or apply Steri-Strip if superficial. The two edges of the lacerated lid must be aligned very carefully to prevent trichiasis occurring.

    c. Burns:
       i.   Clean area.
      ii.   Irrigate eye.
     iii.   Admit patient if necessary.
     iv.   Do not pad an eye with an ocular burn.
      v.   Prepare the patient for skin grafting, which may need to be carried out before scar tissue forms.
    d. Sub-tarsal foreign body – remove the foreign body.

Condition guideline: Trauma to the lacrimal system

Laceration of the lacrimal drainage apparatus is fairly common. If the canaliculus is torn, accurate apposition of the tear ducts must be performed to prevent permanent epiphora. In children, the injury is often caused by the claws of a dog as it jumps up to greet the child.

PATIENT'S NEEDS

- Cleaning of the wound
- Admission to hospital if necessary
- Repair of the laceration
- Prophylactic antibiotic cover
- Analgesia as required

NURSING PRIORITIES

The nursing priority is to inform medical staff of the extent of the injuries.

NURSING ACTION

Clean the wound

1. Assist the doctor to examine the wound.
2. Admit the patient to the ward if necessary.
3. Prepare the patient for surgery to repair the laceration.
4. Give post-operative care:
    a. Clean the wound.
    b. Instil antibiotic drops.
    c. Administer analgesia as required.
    d. Give oral antibiotics if prescribed.
    e. Remove sutures 5–7 days post-operatively.

Condition guideline: Trauma to the conjunctiva

SUBCONJUNCTIVAL HAEMORRHAGE

Subconjunctival haemorrhage can result from a penetrating or blunt trauma which causes the conjunctival blood vessels to bleed.

PATIENT'S NEEDS

Investigations into the extent of the injuries need to be carried out.

NURSING ACTION

1. Obtain accurate history.
2. Examine the patient or assist the doctor. It is important to be able to visualise the scleral margin posterior to the bleed. If it is absent, the bleeding may have tracked from elsewhere, typically the anterior cranial fossa, and is more serious.
3. Reassure the patient that the haemorrhage will not cover the cornea and so will not affect vision.
4. Inform the patient that the blood may spread before it resolves and that it may take 2–3 weeks to clear completely, similar to a bruise. There is no specific treatment for the haemorrhage.

LACERATION OF THE CONJUNCTIVA

Laceration of the conjunctiva may occur as a result of trauma to the eye. The eye must be examined to see if the underlying sclera has been involved. If there is a possibility of a foreign body having entered the eye, an x-ray must be taken to exclude or confirm this.

PATIENT'S NEEDS

- Cleaning and examination of the wound and eye to discover the extent of the injuries
- Suturing of the wound if necessary, although this is not always performed
- Prophylactic antibiotic cover

NURSING ACTION

1. Inform the doctor of the patient's condition.
2. Assist the doctor in the examination.
3. Prepare the patient and equipment for cleaning and suturing of the laceration under local anaesthetic, unless the patient is a child, when a general anaesthetic will usually be administered. Small lacerations may be left to heal without suturing.
4. Apply pad following the procedure.

Condition guideline: Ocular burns

Ocular burns can result in patients losing their sight.

Acid substances entering the eye coagulate with the protein of the ocular surface and cease to act, although damage is caused by the initial impact. Alkaline substances, such as lime found in cement and brick dust, continue to be active in the eye, destroying the superficial layers and penetrating the anterior segment of the eye. Collagenase is released by the cornea following an alkali burn, and this destroys the cornea. It is therefore vitally important that the eye(s) are thoroughly cleaned of all particles of lime. Immediate washing of the eye with whatever harmless liquid is at hand is the best first-aid measure that can be employed. The patient should then be transferred to an ophthalmic unit. The eye must never be padded following chemical injury.

PATIENT'S NEEDS

- Irrigation of eye(s).
- Treatment of burns to the lids and skin around the eye that may have occurred.
- Reassurance and information on the extent of the injuries and treatment; patients can be very worried about the threat of sight loss following a chemical burn.
- Pain relief.

NURSING PRIORITIES

- If a severe alkali burn has occurred, inform the doctor immediately of the patient's arrival.
- Check the pH of the conjunctival sac (normally 7.3–7.7).
- Commence irrigation of the eye(s) after instillation of local anaesthetic drop. If working single-handed, commence the irrigation before informing the doctor.

NURSING ACTION

1. Irrigate the eye(s). Ensure all particles have been removed. It may be necessary to double-evert the lid.
2. Allay anxiety.
3. Test visual acuity once the patient's condition allows this.
4. Instigate the following treatment, which will be prescribed after the eye has been examined, to establish the extent of the damage to the conjunctiva and the cornea.

MILD BURNS

1. Instil G. mydrilate 1% to 'rest' the eye and prevent uveitis.
2. Instil G. or Oc. chloramphenicol to prevent infection and provide lubrication.
3. Give prescribed analgesia.

MODERATE TO SEVERE BURNS

- Instil:
  - G. potassium ascorbate to aid healing, intensively (such as hourly) initially, reducing to 2-hourly after 3 days; advise the patient that these drops sting.
  - G. chloramphenicol to prevent infection.
  - A steroid such as G. dexamethasone (Maxidex) to prevent/treat inflammation.
  - G. homatropine 2% to 'rest' the eye and prevent/treat uveitis. Drugs that inhibit collagenase, such as metaloproteinase inhibitors, may be used.
- Apply a bandage contact lens to prevent symblepharon forming. Rodding of the fornices may be employed. Apply steroid ointment to the skin around the eye if prescribed.

OTHER TREATMENTS

The excimer laser has been used to treat chemical burns. Keratoepithelioplasty or cadaveric limbal cell transplantation has also been successfully employed.

COMPLICATIONS

SYMBLEPHARON

Symblepharon is the adhesion of the bulbar conjunctiva to the palpebral conjunctiva. It occurs following alkaline burns to the eye when the epithelial layer of the conjunctiva is stripped off and the two areas of the conjunctiva stick together. When this occurs, the fornices are lost and the eye is immobile. The lids may not be able to cover and protect the eyeball. It is therefore important to keep the fornices well lubricated and to apply a bandage contact lens to separate the two conjunctival surfaces or to rod them to break up any adhesions that might occur. This latter procedure can be painful. Nasal mucosal grafts can be performed.

CORNEAL OPACITIES

Corneal opacities occur from destruction of the layers of the cornea from the burns. Blindness may result.

Condition guideline: Welder's flash

Welder's flash or exposure to light from a sun lamp or snow blindness burns the cornea if protective goggles have not been worn. Both eyes are affected and become very red and sore, typically after 6 hours.

PATIENT'S NEEDS

The patient requires relief of symptoms of acute pain, watering, photophobia and reduced vision. These symptoms do not become evident until about 8 hours after the incident has occurred.

NURSING ACTION

1. Instil local anaesthetic drops. Local anaesthetic drops must never be given to patient to take home as these drops inhibit epithelial healing.
2. Commence the prescribed treatment once the eye that has been examined with G. fluorescein shows punctate staining over most of the cornea, especially within a central band. The treatment is with Oc. chloramphenicol immediately – once only.

Condition guideline: Trauma to the cornea

CORNEAL FOREIGN BODIES

Many different kinds of foreign bodies can adhere to the cornea: dirt specks, sawdust, pieces of metal or rust (Figure 15.1). Anyone working in an environment, whether at work or at home, where particles can fly into the eye, or working with a hammer and chisel, should wear protective goggles. However, these do not always afford complete protection.

The eye with a corneal foreign body present may or may not be red, depending on what the foreign body is, how long it has been in the eye and how much the patient has rubbed it.

PATIENT'S NEEDS

- Removal of the foreign body to relieve pain and discomfort
- Treatment of any corneal abrasion

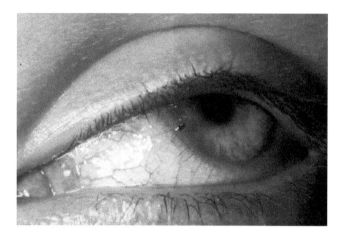

Figure 15.1 Metallic corneal foreign body. (From Marsden, J., *Ophthalmic Care*. Wiley, Chichester, 2006, reproduced with permission.)

NURSING ACTION

1. Record the visual acuity before removal of the foreign body. This is particularly important if the accident has occurred at work. It may be necessary to instil a drop of local anaesthetic into the eye before the patient can read the Snellen chart.
2. Assist the doctor or nurse practitioner to remove the foreign body.
3. Apply antibiotic ointment.
4. Apply a pad, if necessary, for patient comfort, but bear in mind the evidence indicating that the corneal epithelium is slower to heal under a pad.
5. If the foreign body is a piece of metal, a rust ring may be left around the abrasion resulting from the foreign body. This rust ring will need to be removed either at the first visit or the following one.
6. Instil G. mydrilate 1% to prevent the complication of uveitis occurring.
7. Ensure the patient is not driving if he has an eye pad on. Although it is not illegal to drive with one eye padded, it is not safe to do so and the patient's insurance will not be valid. Stereoscopic vision is lost and the field of vision reduced, especially if the right eye is covered. If the patient has arrived by car and there is no one to take him home, he can be given a pad to apply at home following instructions on how to do so.
8. Ensure the patient understands the need for any follow-up visit(s) required to check on healing.

COMPLICATIONS

- Corneal ulceration
- Corneal scarring

CORNEAL ABRASION

Corneal abrasions can result from a foreign body as seen above. Other common causes are babies' fingernails, twigs, flower stalks, pens and pencils. In fact a great variety of items can cause abrasion.

PATIENT'S NEEDS

- Relief of symptoms, which can vary in severity: pain; lacrimation, photophobia, blepharospasm and reduced vision
- Treatment of the abrasion

NURSING ACTION

1. Record visual acuity. It may be necessary to instil a local anaesthetic drop first.
2. Examine/assist the doctor to examine the eye. The abraded area will show up with the instillation of G. fluorescein and illumination with a blue light.
3. Instigate prescribed treatment:
   a. If large, G. mydrilate 1% will be instilled to prevent uveitis and afford some pain relief as the pupil will dilate and prevent ciliary spasm.
   b. Apply Oc. chloramphenicol.
   c. Apply a pad or pad and bandage if the abrasion is large.
4. Warn the patient that this condition will be painful and ensure that he has adequate analgesia to take.
5. A short-term non-steroidal anti-inflammatory, such as Voltarol, may be prescribed as a topical analgesia for pain management. Long-term use of Voltarol is not advocated due to the likelihood of corneal melt. Caution should be exercised when prescribing any non-steroidal anti-inflammatory in the presence of any underlying corneal pathology, such as a history of herpes virus infection or keratoconus.
6. Ensure that the patient understands the need for any follow-up visit(s) required to monitor healing. A large abrasion may take several days to heal.

COMPLICATIONS

- Corneal ulceration is a potential complication.
- Recurrent corneal abrasion/erosion – these can recur up to 1 year or longer after the initial incident. The patient, on waking, finds that he has difficulty opening the eye and that it is painful. On examination, the epithelium will have debrided again. This occurs because the epithelium is loosely adherent to Bowman's membrane. There may be a hereditary tendency to recurrent erosions. The treatment is as above. The excimer laser has been used to treat these erosions. Application of eye ointment, such as simple eye ointment at night, can prevent this recurring condition.

PERFORATION OF THE CORNEA

Usually when the cornea perforates from injury, the iris herniates into the perforation, blocking it and causing the anterior chamber to collapse.

PATIENT'S NEEDS

- Immediate attention
- Relief of anxiety about possible loss of the eye
- Admission to hospital

NURSING PRIORITIES

The nursing priority is to inform medical staff of the patient's injuries.

NURSING ACTION

1. Allay anxiety.
2. Record visual acuity if possible.
3. Assist the doctor to examine the eye.
4. Clean any wounds around the eye.
5. Admit the patient to hospital for
   a. Rest and recovery from the accident.
   b. Pre-operative care prior to excision of prolapsed iris, repair of corneal wound and restoration of anterior chamber; if the prolapsed iris shows no signs of deterioration and has not been prolapsed for long, it may be repositioned under intensive antibiotic cover.
6. Post-operative care. Observe the eye for
   a. Hyphaema.
   b. Depth of anterior chamber.

COMPLICATIONS

IMMEDIATE COMPLICATIONS

- Loss of anterior chamber
- Disorganisation of ocular contents
- Endophthalmitis

LONG-TERM COMPLICATIONS

- Corneal scarring
- Astigmatism due to scarring
- Glaucoma
- Recurrent uveitis
- Phthisis bulbi

Condition guideline: Trauma of the uveal tract

HYPHAEMA

Following blunt or penetrating injury to the uveal tract, the iris or ciliary body may bleed into the anterior chamber causing a hyphaema (see Figure 15.2). If, by looking through a slit lamp, the blood cells are seen floating in the anterior chamber, prior to settling inferiorally, this is termed a microscopic hyphaema.

A blackball hyphaema is one which fills the whole of the anterior chamber. Sometimes the blood clots in the anterior chamber and may be attached to the iris.

PATIENT'S NEEDS

Treatment of the hyphaema by

- Rest at home
- More rarely, admission to hospital

NURSING ACTION

1. Inform medical staff of the patient's condition and history of trauma.
2. Admit the patient if necessary.

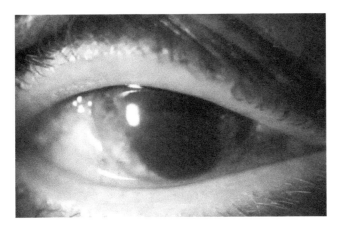

Figure 15.2 Hyphaema.

3. Inform the patient of the importance of rest. A severe bleed may occur 48 hours later in a minority of patients, especially if the large ciliary body vessels have bled. The intraocular pressure may rise acutely and a prolonged rise in intraocular pressure can cause damage to the optic nerve.
4. Prepare the patient for an anterior chamber washout in the case of a blackball hyphaema, or if the hyphaema has not resolved after four to five days.
5. Give post-operative care. Eye care should be as follows:
   a. Instil prescribed drops, e.g. G. chloramphenicol and G. maxidex (dexamethasone).
   b. Observe the anterior chamber for depth and recurrence of hyphaema.
6. Following a blow to the eye, the fundus needs to be examined. There is differing opinion as to whether this should be carried out immediately. Some authorities believe immediate dilation will induce further bleeding (Ragge and Easty 1990).

COMPLICATIONS

- Secondary bleed 24–48 hours after the initial injury.
- Secondary glaucoma:
  - The blood cells, or blood clot, in the anterior chamber block the drainage angle.
  - Following trauma, angle recession may not become evident for some years, so the patient must have annual eye examinations.
- In long-standing hyphaema, the cornea may become blood stained.

TRAUMATIC MYDRIASIS

Following trauma (usually blunt) to the iris, the pupil may become fixed and dilated. This is due to paralysis of the sphincter muscle in the iris. It may resolve itself after a few days. If it is permanent, the patient will experience photophobia.

TRAUMA TO THE LENS: TRAUMATIC CATARACT

Cataract formation can result from a direct or indirect assault on the lens; for example a penetrating injury, such as a hammer and chisel injury, or a blunt injury, such as from a squash ball. An IOFB may lodge on the lens causing a surrounding opacity. This may be the only indication of the IOFB. Trauma to the lens during intraocular surgery falls into this category. When the capsule of the lens is injured, aqueous humour enters the lens substance, causing it to swell and become cloudy. Opacities are most often found in the posterior cortex and sometimes appear like a flower with several petals. They gradually enlarge to cover the whole lens. Lens matter may leak out of the injured capsule into the anterior chamber, where it may cause uveitis or a secondary (phacolytic) glaucoma by blocking the drainage angle. Leaked lens matter can be absorbed by the aqueous humour, in which case it will not cause any complications.

The development of a traumatic cataract can occur from within a few hours after the incident to several months later.

Treatment of a traumatic cataract is similar to that of other causes.

Condition guideline: Trauma to the retina, vitreous choroid and optic nerve

Trauma to the posterior segment of the eye may result in a vitreous haemorrhage, retinal tear, retinal detachment, choroidal haemorrhage, choroidal tear, macular tear, optic nerve contusion, or commotio retinae (oedema of the retina).

PATIENT'S NEEDS

- Accurate diagnosis and prognosis
- Preparation for repair of damaged structures
- Post-operative care and discharge planning

NURSING ACTION

1. Take an accurate history.
2. Report to medical staff.
3. Assist in examination.
4. Allay the patient's anxiety.
5. Prepare the patient for surgery as appropriate.
6. Give post-operative care.
7. Plan discharge.
8. Commotio retinae is managed by rest.

PREVENTION OF OCULAR TRAUMA AND EYE PROTECTION

Nurses working in the ophthalmic casualty area are ideally suited to advise patients on how to prevent ocular trauma. Posters can be displayed in the waiting area and public places outside the hospital that highlight the danger to eyes from certain activities and what protection is available. Eye protection should be worn for racquet sports, and for some contact sports, as well as in industry. The incidence of ocular trauma has risen with the increase in DIY activities. Suppliers of DIY equipment do not always emphasise the need for eye protection, although hire firms are obliged to. There are many types of eye protectors on the market, although some scratch easily or become steamed up. The most effective protectors are more expensive to purchase.

Reflective activity

Consider a patient whom you have seen recently with an ophthalmic emergency:

- What were the presenting signs and symptoms?
- Was there any associated systemic disease or diseases?
- What tests and investigations were carried out and why?
- How did you arrive at a diagnosis?
- What was the treatment plan?
- Outline the care and management of the patient.
- If there were any challenges in caring for the patient, what were they?
- Was any other member of the multidisciplinary team involved in the care and what was his or her input?
- Utilising a recognised health-promotion framework, how would you explain the condition and treatment to the patient in order to ensure that he or she adheres to the treatment?
- What was the clinical outcome?
- What local or national policies, guidelines or protocols influenced the care and management of this patient?
- On reflection, would you have done anything differently and, if so, what?

Your completed case study can be used to contribute to your continuing professional development portfolio for Registration and your Knowledge and Skills Framework review or appraisal.

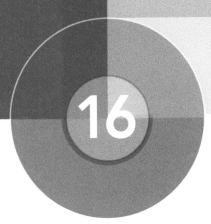

Ocular manifestations of systemic disease

16

This chapter summarises the effects of systemic disease on the eye. Most of the detailed information has already been discussed and can be found in the chapters on the diseases of the specific ocular structures.

DIABETES MELLITUS

Diabetes mellitus can cause the following ocular conditions:

- Lids
  - Styes
  - Chalazions
- Cornea
  - Keratitis
- Iris
  - Rubeosis iridis from neovascularisation
  - Atrophy of the iris
  - Spontaneous hyphaema from rubeosis iridis
- Chronic open-angle glaucoma
- Secondary glaucoma from rubeosis iridis and peripheral anterior synaechiae
- Lens
  - Cataract
  - Intermittent refractive errors due to changes in blood glucose levels and therefore changes in the glucose levels in the lens
- Uveal tract
  - Uveitis
- Retina
  - Retinal vein occlusion
  - Retinopathy
  - Retinal detachment
- Vitreous humour
  - Haemorrhage

- Optic nerve
  - Retrobulbar neuritis
  - Optic atrophy
- Nerve palsies (occur, rarely, due to inflammation of the third, fourth and sixth cranial nerves causing paralysis of the extraocular muscles)

ACQUIRED IMMUNE DEFICIENCY SYNDROME

Acquired immune deficiency syndrome (AIDS) can cause the following conditions:

- Microvascular disease
  - Retina – usually asymptomatic
    - Cotton wool spots
    - Haemorrhages
    - Microaneurysms
  - Conjunctiva (vessels have altered appearance)
- Opportunistic infections affecting the retina
  - Cytomegalovirus
  - Herpes simplex and zoster
  - Toxoplasmosis
  - *Candida*
  - Tuberculosis
  - Syphilis
  - *Molluscum contagiosum*
  - *Pneumocystis*
- Neoplasms
  - Kaposi's sarcoma
    - Eyelid
    - Conjunctiva
    - Nose
    - Orbit
  - Burkitt's lymphoma
    - Orbit
- Neuro-ophthalmic
  - Cranial nerve palsies
  - Visual field defects
  - Papilloedema
  - Optic atrophy

THYROID DISEASE

Thyrotoxicosis affects the eye in the following ways:

- Lid lag
- Lid retraction
- Exophthalmos
- Conjunctival chemosis

- Exposure keratitis
- Ophthalmoplegia

COMPLICATIONS OF THYROID DISEASE

- Corneal ulceration leading to perforation
- Optic nerve compression
- Glaucoma
- Central retinal artery and vein occlusion
- Cataract

HYPERTENSION

Hypertension causes a retinopathy. Changes to the walls of the retinal vasculature result in the presence of exudates, wool spots, flame haemorrhage and retinal oedema.

GIANT CELL ARTERITIS

Giant cell arteritis, or temporal arteritis, is a condition affecting those from the over-60s age group, affecting all arteries, and having an effect especially on the heart and kidneys. It is also associated with polymyalgia rheumatica. In the eye, it causes a sudden loss of vision in one or both eyes. This is caused by infarctions in the ciliary arteries which supply the optic nerve head, causing ischaemia and swelling of the optic disc. The temporal artery is often prominent, hard and tender to touch.

Condition guideline: Giant cell arteritis

PATIENT'S NEEDS

- Relief of symptoms
  - Sudden loss of vision
  - General malaise
  - Temporal headaches
  - Pain on chewing
  - Tenderness on scalp when combing hair
- Instigation of treatment

NURSING PRIORITY

Inform the doctor of the patient's history of sudden loss of vision.

NURSING ACTION

1. Instil prescribed mydriatic drops to facilitate ophthalmoscopy.
2. Take blood for erythrocyte sedimentation rate estimation. A high reading is indicative of giant cell arteritis. It can be as high as 100 mmHg in 1 hour.

3. Prepare patient and equipment and assist the doctor in performing a temporal artery biopsy. This is not always performed as a false-negative result can occur.
4. Admit the patient to hospital if the condition is severe enough to warrant high-dose systemic steroids, possibly via the intravenous route.
5. If the patient is not admitted, explain the treatment by oral steroids and the importance of carrying a steroid card.
6. Ensure the patient has an outpatient follow-up appointment.
7. High doses of oral steroids are given to prevent further visual loss in the presenting eye if unilateral and to prevent the disease affecting the other eye. These steroids will be gradually reduced and the disease monitored by regular erythrocyte sedimentation rate estimations. A maintenance dose of steroids may need to be continued for several years. Patients with severe visual loss resulting from this disease may need to be registered as blind or partially sighted.

HERPES SIMPLEX VIRUS

Herpes simplex virus causes a conjunctivitis and keratitis resulting in a dendritic corneal ulcer.

HERPES ZOSTER VIRUS

In the eye, the herpes zoster virus affects the trigeminal nerve. Usually only the ophthalmic branch is involved, but the maxillary branch may be affected too. It causes

- Vesicular eruptions on the forehead, eyelids and nose of the affected side of the face, which crust over
- Keratitis
- Conjunctivitis

COMPLICATIONS OF HERPES ZOSTER VIRUS

- Uveitis
- Cataract
- Glaucoma
- Ophthalmoplegia
- Persistent pain
- Ptosis
- Corneal scarring
- Anaesthetic cornea

TUBERCULOSIS

Tuberculosis can cause a uveitis. Rarely, miliary tuberculosis causes discrete yellow nodules in the choroid. A retinitis may develop. Phlyctenular conjunctivitis can be caused by tuberculosis.

SARCOID

Sarcoid can cause a bilateral uveitis with mutton fat keratic precipitates present on the corneal endothelium. Dry eyes result from sarcoid involvement of the lacrimal gland.

BEHÇET'S DISEASE

Behçet's disease is a chronic idiopathic multisystem condition causing inflammation to different systems of the body. Presentation is usually in the second and third decade of life, and the disease is seen in Mediterranean countries, the Middle East, Japan and South-East Asia. The disease is characterised by oral and genital ulceration. Lesions can also develop on the skin of the face or back, and vascular lesions can give rise to occlusions of blood vessels, in turn giving rise to major internal venous occlusions. Ocular involvement includes acute recurrent iridocyclitis, retinitis and occlusive retinal periphlebitis.

SYPHILIS

Congenital syphilis can cause interstitial keratitis. It may, rarely, cause a dacryoadenitis. Acquired syphilis can cause a uveitis and chorioretinitis.

TOXOPLASMOSIS

Toxoplasmosis is shown in Figure 16.1.

Toxoplasma can be transmitted in utero if the mother has been infected by ingesting infected meat. It also spreads in the excreta of cats. The parasite causes choroiditis and chorioretinitis.

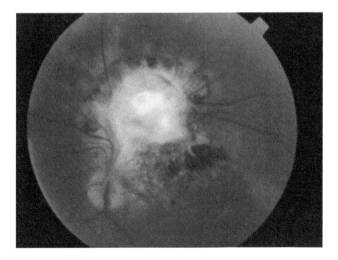

Figure 16.1 Toxoplasmosis.

TOXOCARA

Toxocara is transmitted via the faeces of puppies and kittens and can cause a unilateral uveitis and choroiditis, affecting children under the age of 10 years. A chronic endophthalmitis can occur, resulting in severe loss of vision. The parasite can be treated with pyrimethamine and steroids.

RHEUMATOID ARTHRITIS

Rheumatoid arthritis can cause

- Episcleritis
- Scleritis
- Uveitis
- Dry eyes

STILL'S DISEASE

Still's disease, or juvenile rheumatoid arthritis, can cause uveitis.

ANKYLOSING SPONDYLITIS

Ankylosing spondylitis is the main known cause of uveitis and scleritis.

ULCERATIVE COLITIS AND CROHN'S DISEASE

Ulcerative colitis and Crohn's disease can cause uveitis, scleritis and episcleritis.

NEUROFIBROMATOSIS

Neurofibromatosis is a genetic disorder affecting mainly the nervous system. There are two different types of neurofibromatosis – Nf1 and Nf2. Nf1 is also known as Von Recklinghausen's Peripheral Nf, and Nf2 is known as Von Recklinghausen's bilateral Nf. Nf1 is more common, but Nf2 is generally more serious. Neurofibromatosis causes non-cancerous growths on nerves throughout the body. The ocular manifestations of neurofibromatosis are as follows:

- Tumours of the optic nerve occur in children of less than 5 years and may not be clinically apparent.
- Optic nerve gliomas result in asymmetrical visual field defects, colour defects, optic nerve pallor or proptosis.
- Lisch nodules occur on the iris and congenital ectropion uvea.
- Patchy choroidal abnormalities and corkscrew retinal vessels are sometimes seen in patients with Nf1.

- In Nf2, posterior subcapsular or juvenile cataracts can precede central nervous system symptoms.
- Congenital glaucoma is a rare manifestation of neurofibromatosis.

MIGRAINE

Migraine is a severe headache giving rise to a number of symptoms including nausea and visual problems. Migraine can be triggered by certain factors such as drinking alcohol and coffee, a lack of sleep, high stress levels and eating cheese. There are two different types of migraine – classical migraine when a patient experiences a headache follows a series of symptoms known as aura and common migraine with no aura symptoms. Patients suffering from classical migraine may present themselves to the Emergency Eye Centre with visual problems such as flashing lights, visual distortions and seeing zigzag patterns. They may also be complaining of neck stiffness, nausea, problems with coordination and speech difficulty. General measures include eliminating other causes of symptoms and establishing the diagnosis of migraine. Once the diagnosis has been established, treatment such as simple analgesia and anti-emetic can be given if appropriate. Advice including elimination of known conditions that may precipitate an attack should be provided.

Reflective activity

Consider a patient whom you have seen recently with a systemic disease with an associated ocular problem:

- What were the presenting ocular signs and symptoms?
- Was there any associated systemic disease or diseases?
- What tests and investigations were carried out and why?
- How did you arrive at a diagnosis?
- What was the treatment plan?
- Outline the care and management of the patient.
- If there were any challenges in caring for the patient, what were they?
- Was any other member of the multidisciplinary team involved in the care and what was his or her input?
- Utilising a recognised health-promotion framework, how would you explain the condition and treatment to the patient in order to ensure that he or she adheres to the treatment?
- What was the clinical outcome?
- What local or national policies, guidelines or protocols influenced the care and management of this patient?
- On reflection, would you have done anything differently and, if so, what?

Your completed case study can be used to contribute to your continuing professional development portfolio for Registration and your Knowledge and Skills Framework or appraisal review.

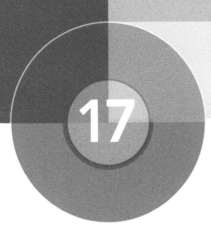

Ophthalmic drugs

This chapter gives brief details of drugs commonly used in ophthalmic practice.

MYDRIATICS

Mydriatic drugs are used to dilate the pupil for the following purposes:

- To examine the retina
- To maintain dilation of the pupil in uveitis, with corneal ulcers, severe corneal abrasions and after surgery
- To break down posterior synaechiae which may be present in uveitis
- To allow a cataract to be extracted
- To enable retinal surgery to take place
- To improve vision when a nuclear cataract is present
- To perform refraction in children

There are two groups of mydriatics:

1. Parasympatholytics, which cause pupillary dilation – mydriasis and cycloplegia – paralysis of the ciliary muscle
2. Sympathomimetics, which cause only mydriasis

PARASYMPATHOLYTICS

G. ATROPINE SULPHATE 0.5% OR 1%; OC. ATROPINE SULPHATE 1%

Derived from the belladonna plant.

- *Onset* – 30 minutes
- *Duration* – 7–14 days
- *Dosage* – Usually once or twice a day – may be up to four times
- *Side effects* – Can be local or as a result of systemic absorption
    - May cause an allergic reaction
    - Toxic effects, especially in the elderly, including tachycardia, confusion, drowsiness, hallucinations and thirst
- *Single use* – Available in minims, which are preservative free

- *Disadvantages*:
  - Not readily reversed by miotics
  - Prolonged duration
  - May provoke acute glaucoma in eyes with narrow angles

G. HOMATROPINE HYDROBROMIDE 1% OR 2%

This is a man-made derivative of atropine.

- *Onset* – 30 minutes
- *Duration* – 24–48 hours
- *Dosage* – Two, three or four times a day
- *Advantages*:
  - Can be reversed by pilocarpine
  - Shorter duration than atropine
- *Side effects* – Similar to those for atropine

G. CYCLOPENTOLATE HYDROCHLORIDE 0.5% OR 1% (MYDRILATE)

- *Onset* – 30 minutes
- *Duration* – 24 hours
- *Dosage* – Two, three or four times a day
- *Uses* – Often used in refraction of children; pre- and post-operatively
- *Side effects* – Similar to those for atropine
- *Single use* – Available in minims, which are preservative free

G. TROPICAMIDE 0.5% OR 1% (MYDRIACYL)

- *Onset* – 20 minutes
- *Duration* – 6 hours
- *Dosage* – Usually only once before examination because of its short-lived effect
- *Advantage* – Short duration makes it suitable for ophthalmoscopy in outpatient or casualty patients
- *Side effects* – Similar to those for atropine
- *Single use* – Available in minims, which are preservative free

SYMPATHOMIMETICS

G. PHENYLEPHRINE 2.5%

- *Onset* – 20 minutes
- *Duration* – 3 hours
- *Dosage* – Two, three or four times daily, or up to 4-hourly to break down posterior synaechiae
- *Use* – Effective in combination with parasympatholytics, especially in the breaking down of posterior synaechiae
- *Disadvantages*:
  - Does not cause cycloplegia

- Can cause corneal epithelial damage
- May cause cardiovascular reactions that may be severe
- *Single use* – Available in minims, which are preservative free

Some ophthalmologists may still prescribe G. phenylephrine 10% but, because of side effects, including confusion, it is rarely used.

NOTES ON MYDRIATICS

Mydriatics must be used with care in patients who have shallow anterior chambers, as dilating the pupils may provoke an attack of closed-angle glaucoma. Some ophthalmologists would argue that if such an episode occurred while the patient was in an ophthalmic unit, they could treat the patient easily and prevent a problem from occurring later on in the patient's life.

All mydriatic drops sting on instillation to some degree. Phenylephrine usually causes the most discomfort.

MIOTICS

Miotic drugs constrict the pupil and the ciliary muscle, which opens up the drainage channel for aqueous flow. Therefore their main use is in the treatment of glaucoma.

G. PILOCARPINE 0.5%, 1%, 3%, 4% (MAY BE UP TO 10% IN OTHER PARTS OF THE WORLD); ALSO AVAILABLE AS A LONG ACTING GEL ONLY IN 4% STRENGTH

This is a natural compound from the *Pilocarpus* tree found in South America. It is a parasympathomimetic.

- *Onset* – 30 minutes.
- *Duration* – 10–12 hours.
- *Dosage* – Two, three or four times a day, or intensively for acute glaucoma.
- *Disadvantages*:
  - G. pilocarpine can cause headaches.
  - The eye is fixed at accommodation.
  - The pupil remains permanently miosed, increasing the risk of accidents especially at night as light adaptation is restricted.
  - Care must be taken when used intensively as overdose can cause vomiting.
  - G. pilocarpine may cause an allergic reaction.
  - G. pilocarpine can sting on instillation.
- *Single use* – Available in minims, which are preservative free, only in 2% strength.

ACETYLCHOLINE CHLORIDE 1% (MIOCHOL)

A freshly prepared solution of acetylcholine is injected into the anterior chamber after a cataract extraction to constrict the pupil rapidly to prevent vitreous humour loss, or to retain a posterior chamber or iris clip intraocular lens in position.

DRUGS OF CHOICE USED IN THE TREATMENT OF GLAUCOMA

PROSTAGLANDIN ANALOGUES

- *Actions* – Prostaglandin analogues reduce the intraocular pressure by increasing the uveoscleral outflow. They are used to treat open-angle glaucoma and ocular hypertension.
- *Disadvantages* – The patient needs to be warned that this drug may change the colour of his iris. Caution should be taken if the patient has asthma.
- *Side effects* – Brown pigment on the iris, irritation, lengthening of the eyelashes, periorbital oedema, cystoid macular oedema, iritis, uveitis.

G. LATANOPROST (XALATAN) 50 MCG/ML

- *Use* – Once per day, ideally in the evening

G. TRAVAPROST (TRAVATAN) 40 MCG/ML

- *Use* – Once per day, ideally in the evening

G. BIMATOPROST (LUMIGAN) 300 MCG/ML

- *Use* – Once per day, ideally in the evening

G. BRIMONIDINE TARTRATE (ALPHAGAN) 0.2%

- *Use* – Twice per day

G. BRIMONIDINE TARTRATE 0.2%; TIMOLOL MALEATE 10.5% (COMBIGAN)

- *Use* – Twice per day

G. TAFLUPROST (SAFLUTAN) 15 MCG/ML, PRESERVATIVE FREE

- *Use* – Once per day

CARBONIC ANHYDRASE INHIBITORS

Carbonic anhydrase is an enzyme necessary for the production of aqueous humour. These drugs therefore cause a reduction in the amount of aqueous humour produced.

ACETAZOLAMIDE (DIAMOX)

- *Dosage*:
  - 500 mg intravenously stat. in acute glaucoma.
  - 500 mg orally stat.

- 250 mg orally as maintenance, four times a day, reducing to three or two doses a day, or slow-release capsules 250 mg given once or twice a day.
- *Uses* – In acute, chronic and secondary glaucoma.
- *Side effects* – Drowsiness, gastrointestinal upset, nausea and potassium loss resulting in tingling of extremities. Potassium supplements such as potassium chloride are sometimes given. It is a weak diuretic.

G. DORZOLAMIDE 2% (TRUSOPT)

- *Dosage* – Three times a day, or twice a day if given with a beta-blocker
- *Uses* – In chronic and secondary glaucoma as an adjuvant therapy to beta-blockers or as a single therapy to non-responders or in those who are unable to tolerate beta-blockers
- *Side effects* – Conjunctivitis, eyelid irritation

G. DORZOLOMIDE HYDROCHLORIDE 2% AND TIMOLOL MALEATE 0.5% (COSOPT)

- *Dosage* – Twice per day; timolol maleate is a beta-blocker
- *Use* – To reduce intraocular pressure in open-angle glaucoma

G. BRINZOLAMIDE 10 MG/1 ML AND TIMOLOL MALEATE 5 MG/1 ML (AZARGA SUSPENSION)

- *Dosage* – Twice per day. Timolol maleate is a beta-blocker
- *Use* – To reduce intraocular pressure in open-angle glaucoma

BETA-BLOCKERS

G. timolol maleate 0.25% or 0.5% (Timoptol)
G. betaxolol hydrochloride 0.5% (Betoptic)
G. carteolol hydrochloride 1% or 2% (Teoptic)
G. levobunolol hydrochloride 0.5% (Betagan)

- *Actions* – Reduce the production of aqueous humour and, after several weeks of use, increase the outflow of aqueous humour
- *Dosage* – 12-hourly, strictly (Betagan may be used daily)
- *Advantages* – Do not cause miosis or accommodation spasm
- *Disadvantages* – Cannot be used in patients with a history of asthma or congestive cardiac failure

Timolol and levobunolol are available in single-dose presentations.

OTHER DRUGS

MANNITOL 20%

- *Use* – Given intravenously in acute glaucoma when acetazolamide has failed to reduce the intraocular pressure. It can be given pre-operatively. Usually 1.5–2 g/kg body weight is given over a 1-hour period.

GLYCEROL

- *Action* – An osmotic.
- *Use* – Oral dose given in acute glaucoma when acetazolamide has failed to reduce the intraocular pressure.
- *Dosage* – 1.5 g/kg body weight in fruit juice to disguise the taste. It must be drunk within 20 minutes to affect the intraocular pressure. Topical glycerol 50% can be used to clear corneal oedema temporarily for ophthalmoscopy to take place.

ANTIBIOTICS

G. CHLORAMPHENICOL 0.5%, OC. 1%

- *Action* – Bacteriostatic, broad spectrum.
- *Uses* – In ocular infections; can penetrate the corneal epithelium; prophylactic use.
- *Dosage* – 2-hourly or two, three or four times a day.
- *Advantage* – Resistance is slow to develop.
- *Single use* – G. chloramphenicol is available in minims, which are preservative free.
- *Storage* – Guttae should be stored in a refrigerator.

GENTAMICIN 0.3% (GENTICIN) (DROPS AND OINTMENT) 1.5% FORTIFIED

- *Action* – Bactericidal, broad spectrum
- *Uses* – Ocular infections resistant to chloramphenicol; for *Pseudomonas aeruginosa* infections
- *Dosage* – 2-hourly or two, three or four times a day; subconjunctival injection: 10–20 mg

NEOMYCIN SULPHATE 0.5% (DROPS AND OINTMENT)

- *Action* – Bactericidal, broad spectrum
- *Uses* – In conjunctivitis, blepharitis, superficial infections
- *Dosage* – 2-hourly or two or four times a day
- *Disadvantages*:
  - Does not penetrate corneal tissue
  - May cause an allergic reaction

G. CIPROFLOXACIN 0.3%

- *Action* – Broad-spectrum antibiotic
- *Dosage* – Intensively for severe infections or two, three or four times a day
- *Uses* – Corneal ulcers, especially caused by *Pseudomonas*
- *Side effects* – Local burning and itching, lid-margin crusting
- Also available as ointment 0.3%

G. FUCIDIC ACID 1% (FUCITHALMIC)

- *Action* – Broad-spectrum antibiotic
- *Dosage* – Usually twice a day
- *Uses* – Superficial infections
- *Advantages* – A viscous substance that is not absorbed as readily as drops and therefore need not be administered as frequently; useful in children

G. OFLOXACIN 0.3%

- *Action* – Broad-spectrum antibiotic
- *Dosage* – Two to four times per day, but may be used more frequently if required

G. PROPAMIDINE ISETHIONATE 0.1% (BROLENE)

- *Use* – In *Acanthamoeba* keratitis
- *Dosage* – Four times a day
- *Disadvantage* – Little value in bacterial conjunctivitis

ANTIVIRAL AGENTS

OC. ACYCLOVIR (ZOVIRAX) 3%

- *Dosage* – Five times a day
- *Uses* – In herpes simplex virus and herpes zoster ophthalmicus; cream preparation 5% is available for use on skin lesions
- Also available as tablets or injection

CORTICOSTEROIDS

Corticosteroid drops are used for

- Allergic conditions
- With an antibiotic in bacterial inflammatory conditions, e.g. chronic conjunctivitis
- Inflammatory conditions such as uveitis, sympathetic ophthalmia, episcleritis

G. PREDNISOLONE (PREDSOL) 0.001%–0.5% (1% PRED FORTE)

- *Dosage* – Four times a day
- *Single use* – Available in minims, which are preservative free as 0.5%

METHYLPREDNISOLONE (DEPO-MEDRONE) 20 MG

- *Dosage* – One dose injected onto the orbital floor; must not be mixed with other drugs in the same syringe

BETAMETHASONE (BETNESOL) G. AND OC. 0.1%

- *Dosage* – 2-hourly, two, three or four times a day, ointment at night; 2–4 mg subconjunctivally

G. HYDROCORTISONE 1% (OINTMENT 0.5%, 1%, 2.5%)

- *Dosage* – Four times a day, ointment at night

G. DEXAMETHASONE (MAXIDEX) 0.1%

- *Dosage* – Hourly, or 2-hourly if needed intensively, with frequency gradually reducing, or two or four times a day; must be shaken before instillation

NEOMYCIN-STEROID COMBINATION

Neomycin can be combined with a steroid:

- Predsol-*N* (prednisolone 0.5% and neomycin 0.5%)
- Betnesol-*N* (betamethasone 0.1% and neomycin 0.5%) drops and ointment
- Maxitrol (dexamethasone 0.1%, neomycin 0.5% and polymyxin B)

DISADVANTAGES OF CORTICOSTEROID USE

- Lowers the resistance to micro-organisms.
- Masks signs of infection.
- Increases the activity of herpes simplex virus.
- May cause herpes simplex viral infection if prescribed for conjunctivitis.
- May cause secondary glaucoma.
- Cataract formation may be caused with prolonged use.

LOCAL ANAESTHETICS

All are single use: Available in minims, which are preservative free.

G. OXYBUPROCAINE HYDROCHLORIDE 0.4% (BENOXINATE)

- *Dosage* – Usually once only is sufficient
- *Use* – Prior to minor ophthalmic procedures

G. PROXYMETACAINE 0.5% (OPHTHAINE)

- *Dosage* – Usually once only is sufficient
- *Use* – Minor ophthalmic procedures; often used in children due to reduced stinging on instillation

G. TETRACAINE HYDROCHLORIDE 0.5% AND 1%

- *Dosage* – Usually once only is sufficient
- *Use* – Prior to minor ophthalmic procedures

DIAGNOSTIC DROPS

FLUORESCEIN

- *Drops* – 2%.
- *Uses*:
  - Stains conjunctival and corneal epithelial damage; i.e. corneal ulcers, erosions and conjunctival or corneal abrasions.
  - Assessment of the tear film.
  - Tonometry.
  - Seidel's test shows fluorescein-stained aqueous humour leaking from a wound on the cornea/limbus.
  - Contact lens fitting.
- *Single use* – Available as minims, which are preservative free.

Fluorescein is also available in paper strips. Fluorescein should not be dispensed in a multiple container as it is a good medium for *Pseudomonas* bacterial growth.

INTRAVENOUS INJECTION: USUALLY 2.5 ML OF 25%

- *Use* – For fundal fluorescein angiography, which demonstrates the condition of the retinal blood vessels, the condition of the macula and optic disc and the presence of choroidal tumours
- *Disadvantage* – Discolours the skin and urine

INDOCYANINE GREEN

Intravenous injection 25 mg in 5 mL of aqueous solvent followed by a bolus dose of normal saline.
- *Use* – To highlight retinal and choroidal blood vessels

TEAR REPLACEMENT

The following are used for dry eyes and must be used as often as is necessary to keep the eyes feeling comfortable. This may be as often as every hour. Once dry eyes have been diagnosed, the patient may need to continue to use tear-replacement drops for life:

- G. hypromellose
- G. tears naturale
- G. liquifilm tears
- G. acetylcystein

- G. viscotears (long-acting gel formulation)
- G. celuvisc
- Oc. lacri-lube
- G. polyvinyl alcohol (Liquifilm Tears) (Sno Tears)
- G. povidone (Oculotec)

MISCELLANEOUS

G. ANTAZOLINE SULPHATE 0.5% AND XYLOMETAZOLINE HYDROCHLORIDE 0.05% (G. OTRIVINE-ANTISTIN)

- *Use* – In allergic conjunctivitis, especially caused by hay fever; for short-term use only
- *Dosage* – Two or three times a day

G. SODIUM CROMOGLYCATE (OPTICROM) 2%

- *Use* – In allergic conjunctivitis, especially vernal catarrh
- *Dosage* – Four times a day

G. LODOXAMIDE (ALOMIDE) 0.1%

- *Use* – In allergic conjunctivitis, as an alternative to Opticrom
- *Dosage* – Four times daily

G. OLOPATADINE (OPATANOL)

- *Use* – Seasonal allergic conjunctivitis
- *Dose* – Twice daily

AFLIBERCEPT (EYLEA)

- *Use* – Wet, age-related macular degeneration (AMD); diabetic macular oedema (DMO).
- *Dose*:
  - AMD – One intravitreal injection monthly for three doses, then one intra-injection every 2 months for the first year. Treatment may be extended based on vision and anatomical outcomes.
  - DMO – One intravitreal injection per month for five doses, then one intra-injection every 2 months for the first year. Treatment may be extended based on vision and anatomical outcomes

VERTEPORFIN (VISUDYNE)

- *Use* – To treat subfoveal choroidal neovascularisation in wet, age-related macular degeneration.

- *Dose* – Intravenous infusion based on body mass index; each eye will require more than one treatment.
- *Disadvantages* – Photosensitivity for up to 48 hours; sunlight, halogen lights or sun beds should be avoided.
- *Side effects* – Blurred vision, flashing lights, field defects, nausea, vomiting, fever, back pain, hypertension.

RANIBIZUMAB (LUCENTIS)

- *Use* – To treat subfoveal choroidal neovascularisation in wet, age-related macular degeneration.
- *Dose* – Intravitreal injection 500 micrograms into affected eye once a month for 3 months.
- *Side effects* – Headache, back pain, nausea, anaemia, eye pain, vitreous floaters.
- *Dose* – Intravenous infusion based on body mass index. Each eye will require more than one treatment.
- *Disadvantages* – Photosensitivity for up to 48 hours; sunlight, halogen lights and sun beds should be avoided.
- *Side effects* – Blurred vision, flashing lights, field defects, nausea, vomiting, fever, back pain, hypertension.

SODIUM HYALURONATE (HEALONID)

This is a viscoelastic polymer normally present in aqueous humour.

- *Use* – During surgical procedures to protect internal structures and maintain depth of anterior chamber
- *Side effects* – Occasional hypersensitivity, transient rise in intraocular pressure

BOTULINUM TOXIN (CLOSTRIDIUM BOTULINUM TYPE A; DYSPORT, BOTOX)

- *Action* – Paralysis of muscles.
- *Uses* – To treat blepharospasm and strabismus and to induce ptosis to protect the cornea.
- *Dosage* – Varies depending on use and which product is used.
- *Side effects* – As it is a biological product, anaphylaxis may occur.

G. DICLOFENAC SODIUM 0.1% (VOLTEROL OPHTHA)

- *Uses* – Inhibits intraoperative miosis, reduces post-cataract surgery inflammation
- *Dosage*:
  - Pre-operative: half-hourly four times
  - Post-operative: four times a day
- *Advantage* – Preservative-free preparation

GENERAL NOTE

As indicated, many ophthalmic drugs are prepared in single-dose containers that contain no preservative. Therefore they are useful for those patients who may be allergic to the preservative used in ophthalmic preparations.

As with any medication, for more detailed prescribing information, it is essential to consult the British National Formulary (medicines complete).

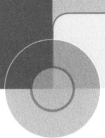

Appendix 1: Correction of refractive errors

Light travels in rays that are reflected from objects into the eyes. Light rays travel in straight lines from a distance of 6 m or more. At a shorter distance, they diverge as they enter the eye. When light rays meet a transparent object at an angle, they bend. This is called 'refraction'. Light rays entering the eye meet the curved cornea and bend inwards or converge. They continue to converge as they pass through each of the refractive media of the eye, the cornea, the aqueous humour, the lens and the vitreous humour, so that they are brought to a focal point on the retina (American Academy of Ophthalmology 2009/2010).

The 'refractive power' of the eye is the degree to which the eye is able to refract the light rays. This power is expressed in dioptres. One dioptre brings rays of light to a focus over 1 m. Ten dioptres bring rays of light to a focus over 0.1 m, or 10 cm. The refractive power of the eye is 60 dioptres (that of the lens is 20 dioptres and of the cornea 40 dioptres).

LONG SIGHT OR HYPERMETROPIA

A long-sighted person has a short eyeball. The light rays therefore come to a focus behind the retina, causing blurred vision. A long-sighted person consequently has to accommodate for their distant vision to be clear. No further accommodation is possible for near vision, so this is blurred. If a convex lens is placed in front of the eye, the light rays will converge more sharply and come to a focus on the retina. A convex lens is a spherical lens because its shape is equal in all meridians. It is known as a 'plus' lens.

SHORT SIGHT OR MYOPIA

A short-sighted person has a long eyeball. The light rays therefore come to a focus in front of the retina. The vision is usually more blurred for distant vision than near vision as the lens can accommodate for near vision. If a concave lens is placed in front of the eye, the light rays will diverge before converging through the cornea and lens and will come to a focus at the retina. A concave lens is also spherical and is known as a 'minus' lens.

PRESBYOPIA

From the age of about 45 years, the lens in the eye no longer has the ability to accommodate for near vision. The light rays therefore fall behind the retina before coming to a focus. This is known as presbyopia. Convex or plus lenses are needed to bring the image into focus on the retina. An increasingly powerful lens is required until the age of 70 years, when no further deterioration in focussing occurs.

ASTIGMATISM

The astigmatic cornea has an uneven curvature, so that there is no point of focus of the light rays on the retina. A cylindrical lens placed in front of the eye with its axis corresponding to the abnormal plane on the cornea will focus the light rays. The cylindrical lens can either be concave or convex.

Most spectacles combine both spherical (plus or minus) lenses with cylindrical lenses to provide a compound lens to correct myopia/hypermetropia and astigmatism. Full information on optics is beyond the scope of this book.

TECHNIQUES FOR CORRECTING REFRACTIVE ERRORS

The main principle of correcting refractive errors is to modify the refractive power. Correction of refractive errors can be made in a variety of ways as listed below.

SPECTACLES

Spectacles are still the most widely used correction technique and are universally the safest devices. However, for various reasons, some people find spectacles unacceptable and they are not necessarily the answer to their vision problems. For example, wearing spectacles in some working environments can be hazardous, while others find glasses impractical for certain sports such as rugby or football and, for the rest, spectacles are cosmetically unacceptable.

CONTACT LENSES

Contact lenses are more popular as they provide convenience and are reasonably safe, but they are not risk free. Usually contact lenses can either be gas permeable or soft lenses. Soft lenses can be daily or monthly disposables, or extended wear. Users of contact lenses can encounter problems such as eye infections, abrasions, chemical injury (as a result of inadvertently using contact lens cleaner instead of the wetting solution), corneal ulcers and problems of over-wearing their lenses. People should be informed that they should not shower or swim in contact lenses. Wearers of contact lenses must visit their opticians for regular eye checks if problems are to be avoided. Cleaning guidelines must be strictly adhered to, both the lenses and the carrying case. Handwashing before and after insertion or removal must be undertaken to prevent infection. However, some people cannot tolerate contact lenses, either because of dry eyes or because of an allergy to the solution or to the lenses themselves. Certain environments, such as very dusty or smoky surroundings, make the wearing of contact lenses intolerable.

REFRACTIVE SURGERY

In recent years, there has been an increased interest in refractive surgery. Initially, this was performed for myopia, but recent advances have enabled patients with hypermetropia and astigmatism also to be treated. While there is an increase in popularity for refractive surgery, it is not without its long- and short-term complications, including pain, photophobia, epithelial defects and over- or under-correction (Bashour and Benchimol 2014).

RADIAL KERATOTOMY

Radial keratotomy consists of radial incisions involving 90% of the corneal thickness near the limbus. Radial keratotomy is more successful in individuals who are within the myopic range of −2 to −4. Side effects, such as fluctuations of vision and glare, have been reported. Corneal infections as a result of delayed healing of the corneal incisions are another complication. This procedure is rarely used now but is included here as you may come across patients who have had it.

LASER-ASSISTED SUB-EPITHELIAL KERATOMILEUSIS

Laser-assisted sub-epithelial keratomileusis (LASEK) has largely replaced radial keratotomy. In LASEK, the cornea is subjected to light energy from the excimer laser to excise tissue from the cornea. A computer estimates the depth and position of the corneal tissue to be removed, which will vary depending on the refractive error being treated. The energy from the laser beam is subjected to the central cornea with resultant flattening of the cornea. The corneal epithelium is removed during LASEK. The shortcomings of the procedure are

- Visual results are better predicted in patients whose refractive error is less than −6 dioptres than in higher myopes (−6 to −10). However, higher myopes can obtain a reduction in their myopia.
- Severe pain can be experienced for approximately 48 hours while the epithelium regenerates.
- Complications include corneal haze, which is significantly more in myopes greater than −10 dioptres, regression, loss of best corrected visual acuity, night-halo effects, glare and starbursts, wound infection, delayed healing and perforation.

LASER *IN SITU* KERATOMILEUSIS

Laser *in situ* keratomileusis is a surgical procedure used to correct myopia, hypermetropia and astigmatism. The current method is to use a femtosecond laser to create a corneal 'flap' of approximately 110 or 120 microns. The thickness of the flap is dependent on the degree of myopia to be corrected and the individual's corneal thickness. The flap is lifted towards the hinge. The excimer laser is focussed and centred on the exposed middle layer of the cornea. When laser treatment is completed, the flap is placed back into position.

The patient is seen the day following surgery to measure the visual acuity, to inspect the flap position and to ensure that no signs of infection or inflammation are present. A broad-spectrum antibiotic such as chloramphenicol is prescribed. However, a consensus on the use of steroids does not exist.

PATIENT'S NEEDS

- The patient must have detailed explanations given of the procedure itself, and of any complications.
- Topography and pachymetry investigations are measurements of the cornea presented in detailed maps that show the curvature and thickness of the cornea.
- Schirmer's test is used to exclude dry eyes.
- Pre- and post-operative care is required.
- Follow-up information should be given.

NURSING ACTION

- Assist/perform topography and pachymetry.
- Ensure the patient has a full understanding of the procedure and that the patient does not have unrealistic expectations.
- Give pre-operative care. Local anaesthetic drops will be instilled. The eye area will be cleaned with betadine.
- Assist in the laser surgery.
- Give post-operative care:
  - A bandage contact lens may be used for LASEK.
  - Ensure the patient has adequate oral and topical analgesia.
  - Ensure the patient has follow-up information and eye drops as prescribed.

PARALYTIC SQUINT

When a paralytic squint occurs, the image to each eye is not focussing on the same area of each retina. If a prism is placed in front of the squinting eye, the light rays bend towards the base of the triangular-shaped prismatic lens and will cause the image to focus in the area of the retina of that eye corresponding to the area of retina in the other eye. This results in a single image being seen or binocular single vision.

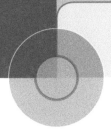

Appendix 2: Contact lenses

USES OF CONTACT LENSES

- Refractive errors. People may wear contact lenses for cosmetic reasons instead of glasses. High myopes benefit from wearing contact lenses because they would need to wear glasses with thick lenses, which cause visual distortion. Contact lenses afford much improved vision involving the whole visual field.
- Wearing contact lenses can be helpful for patients with aphakia.
- The effect of corneal abnormalities, such as keratoconus, can be minimised through the use of contact lenses.
- Protection. A bandage lens can protect the eye from perforating or becoming too dry. Painted contact lenses are worn by people who are albinos or people with aniridia to prevent too much light entering the eye.
- Some people seek to have myopia corrected by the insertion of an intraocular lens surgically so they do not have to wear glasses or contact lenses.

TYPES OF LENS

- Hard or rigid lens
- Gas-permeable lens
- Soft lens
- Extended-wear lens
- Bandage lens
- Disposable – monthly/weekly/daily
- Toric and bi-toric for astigmatism
- Bifocal
- Varifocal

HARD AND GAS-PERMEABLE LENSES

Hard and gas-permeable lenses must be removed before sleep, or if the eye is irritable. If they are kept in the eye under these circumstances, corneal damage is likely to occur. Artificial tear-drops may be required to prevent the cornea from drying out. Gas-permeable lenses should cause less corneal dryness.

SOFT LENSES

Soft lenses are slightly larger than hard lenses. They tend to be used if the wearer finds hard lenses intolerable. They should also be removed at night and if the eye is irritable. More scru-pulous care is required for soft lenses as they are more likely to cause corneal damage; because they are made of a softer material than hard lenses, a scratch on the cornea or a small foreign body underneath the lens is not so likely to be felt until damage has been done.

Fluorescein drops should never be put into an eye with a soft contact lens in, as the dye will be taken up by the lens and is extremely difficult, if not impossible, to remove. Only eye drops without preservative should be used with soft contact lenses, as the preservative can be absorbed by the lens, which may provoke an allergic reaction. Soft lenses should be stored in normal saline if no soaking solution is available; water, whether sterile or not, will cause them to dry out.

EXTENDED-WEAR LENSES AND BANDAGE LENSES

Extended-wear lenses and bandage lenses are essentially similar to soft lenses but are larger in size. They can be worn for up to 3 months without being removed so are therefore useful for the young and the elderly. The optician removes the lens and replaces it with a new one. Artificial teardrops will be required to prevent the cornea from drying out. Bandage lenses do not have a prescription incorporated.

DISPOSABLE MONTHLY/WEEKLY/DAILY LENSES

Disposable lenses are becoming more popular. Initially, the lenses were designed to be worn day and night for 6 days and then discarded. The eyes were rested on the seventh day. Some contact lens wearers now use disposable lenses, but as daily wear, removing them at night to reduce the complications.

CARE OF CONTACT LENSES

Contact lenses require great care to prevent corneal damage and eye infection. There are several different brands of products on the market for use with contact lenses. Two important steps in the care of the lenses are handwashing before and after handling the lenses, and cleaning the contact lens case. There are different solutions for hard and soft lenses. Care of non-disposable lenses involves the following:

- Meticulous attention should be paid to hand hygiene and cleaning of the contact lens case.
- Lenses should be cleaned with a cleansing solution rubbed on the lens with the finger and washed off with sterile water or saline. It has been suggested that solutions containing hydrogen peroxide are better in that they destroy *Acanthamoeba*.
- Wetting solution is dropped onto the corneal surface of the lens before it is inserted into the eye.
- When the lens is not in the eye, i.e. overnight, it is placed in a contact lens case filled with soaking solution. This fluid should be changed each time the container is used. The container should be washed out with warm water and rinsed with the soaking solution.
- There are now 'all-in-one' solutions available that reduce the number of processes involved in the care process. By doing so, it is hoped that the wearer will better comply with a simple regimen.

Lenses should be cleaned well and checked by an optician before being reinserted following corneal damage.

COMPLICATIONS OF CONTACT LENS WEAR

- Intolerance. Some people find wearing contact lenses intolerable. Hard lenses are usually prescribed initially as they cause fewer problems. If these are difficult to wear, gas-permeable or soft contact lenses are prescribed. Some people have to abandon contact lens wearing and resort to spectacles.
- Corneal abrasion is a potential complication of contact lens wear.
- Dry eyes. The lens prevents the tear film from adequately covering the cornea. Artificial teardrops can be prescribed for people who do experience dry eyes.
- Giant papillary conjunctivitis or contact lens-associated papillary conjunctivitis. This is more common in wearers of soft contact lenses. It may not manifest itself for months or years after starting to wear lenses. Symptoms include
  - Itching
  - Mucus discharge
  - Increasing intolerance to lens wear
  - Large conjunctival papillae (Kanski 2007)
- Hypoxia. The cornea is deprived of oxygen from the tear film by the presence of the contact lens. The cornea becomes oedematous, and new vessels may develop in the limbal area. This usually occurs after years of contact lens wear.
- Sensitivity. This may develop in response to the preservative in the cleaning and soaking solutions.
- Keratitis. People wearing extended-wear soft contact lenses are 21 times more likely to get microbial keratitis than gas-permeable lens wearers, and daily soft contact lens wearers are four times more likely to suffer from keratitis at some point. *Acanthamoeba* is the most dangerous organism requiring intensive antibiotic application (Kanski 2007). This may be chlorhexidine and polyhexamethylene biguanide. The contact lens should not be reinserted into the eye until the infection has cleared and the lens itself has been cleaned or replaced.

It is advisable for all contact lens wearers to have a spare pair of spectacles to wear in case they are unable to use their contact lenses for a while.

NURSE'S ROLE

Although nurses do not prescribe or fit contact lenses, they are in an ideal position to educate people on the care of contact lenses, whether the person has a problem or in a more informal advisory capacity.

Nurses must stress the importance of the following:

- Complying with scrupulous and effective care regimes of their contact lenses (American Academy of Ophthalmologists 2009/2010) is essential. However, wearers of extended-wear soft contact lenses have an increased risk of keratitis despite complying with hygiene instructions.
- It is important to discard any remaining solution after 28 days of use. Saliva and tap water must not be used as wetting or cleaning solutions.
- Other people's contact lens cases, which may not be clean, must not be 'borrowed' for their lenses.
- It is important to allow time for the cornea to 'breathe', by removing the lenses for a period of time each day.

- Removal of lenses, except extended-wear lenses, at night is essential.
- Washing of hands prior to handling lenses, avoiding creamy soft soaps and ensuring that all traces of hand cream are removed from fingertips are important.
- Avoiding swimming/Jacuzzis while wearing contact lenses is essential.
- Remove the lenses if the eye becomes sore, and seek medical advice.
- Remove contact lenses before going to sleep.

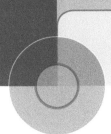

Appendix 3: Competency assessment tools

COMMUNICATING WITH THE VISUALLY IMPAIRED COMPETENCY TOOL

PERFORMANCE CRITERIA AND ASSESSMENT DOCUMENT FOR COMMUNICATIING WITH THE VISUALLY IMPAIRED

You need to be able to demonstrate your knowledge, understanding and skill of communication with a patient who is visually impaired. The individual staff member must be able to demonstrate the following:

1. Communicating effectively with a patient with visual impairment using a range of strategies
2. What action to take in order to maintain effective communication

The staff member is able to perform the following competently	Evidence	Yes	No	Further practice required/ Action plan
Is able to demonstrate effective communicating skills and strategies	Discussion and direct observation Reflective account			
Is able to demonstrate how to communicate effectively with someone with a visual impairment	Discussion and direct observation Reflective account			
Is able to demonstrate alternative strategy of communicating with someone with a visual impairment	Discussion and direct observation Reflective account			
Is able to demonstrate the importance of good positioning to communicate with the patient needs with a visual impairment	Discussion and direct observation Reflective account			
Is able to demonstrate communication in an appropriate place	Discussion and direct observation Reflective account			
Is able to demonstrate that the individual need of the patient is taken into account	Discussion and direct observation Reflective account			
Is able to demonstrate through discussion or direct observation how to communicate effectively	Discussion and direct observation Reflective account			

Is able to demonstrate through discussion or direct observation how to communicate effectively	Discussion and direct observation Reflective account			
Where communication issues are identified, is able to seek alternative strategies of communication	Discussion and direct observation Reflective account			
Is able to demonstrate the ability to communicate effectively with a patient needs with visual impairment	Discussion and direct observation Reflective account			
Ensures patient's understanding	Discussion and direct observation Reflective account			
Is able to demonstrate through discussion or direct observation how to communicate effectively	Discussion and direct observation Reflective account			
Is able to seek assistance as appropriate	Direct observation Reflective account			

Staff signature:………………………………...............

Mentor/coach signature:………………………….…..

Date of assessment:…………………………...............

GUIDING A PATIENT WITH VISUAL IMPAIRMENT COMPETENCY TOOL

PERFORMANCE CRITERIA AND ASSESSMENT DOCUMENT FOR GUIDING THE VISION IMPAIRED

You need to be able to demonstrate your knowledge, understanding and skill of communication with a patient who is visually impaired. The individual staff member must be able to demonstrate the following:

- To be able to safely guide a person with visual impairment

The staff member is able to perform the following competently	Evidence	Yes	No	Further practice required/ Action plan
Is able to demonstrate the most appropriate way to approach a patient taking into account the patient's visual impairment	Discussion and direct observation Reflective account			
Is able to accurately assess and take into account the individual need of the patient	Discussion and direct observation Reflective account			
Is able to demonstrate if assistance is required and the type of assistance needed	Discussion and direct observation Reflective account			

Is able to demonstrate the correct procedure for guiding a patient with visual impairment	Discussion and direct observation Reflective account			
Is able to demonstrate how to guide a patient through a doorway, upstairs and downstairs and safely to a chair	Discussion and direct observation Reflective account			

Staff signature:..

Mentor/coach signature:..................................

Date of assessment:..

VISUAL ACUITY COMPETENCY TOOL

PERFORMANCE CRITERIA AND ASSESSMENT DOCUMENT FOR TESTING VISUAL ACUITY

You need to be able to demonstrate your knowledge, understanding and skill of assessing a patient's visual acuity. The individual staff member must be able to demonstrate the following:

1. Underpinning knowledge of why visual acuities are recorded
2. An understanding of what the recorded visual acuity means in relation to the patient's vision and the care and management of the patient with that amount of vision
3. Ability to measure visual acuity on a wide range of patients with special needs such as learning difficulties, hard of hearing, different age group
4. Ability to accurately record and document visual acuity

The staff member is able to perform the following competently	Evidence	Yes	No	Further practice required/ Action plan
Ascertain that the correct patient is identified using the Trust ID policy	Discussion and direct observation			
Assess the patient's ability to perform the test without appropriate support	Discussion and direct observation			
Ensure that privacy and dignity are maintained throughout the test	Discussion and direct observation			
Ensure that the patient's learning needs and any other barriers are taken into account such as language barrier, hard of hearing, etc. and appropriate action taken	Discussion and direct observation			
Ensure the patient is at a correct distance from the test chart	Discussion and direct observation			
Ensure the room and Snellen/ LogMAR box is adequately illuminated for the task	Discussion and direct observation			

Confirm that the patient has brought the most appropriate optical correction with him and that the appropriate optical correction is utilized during the test	Discussion and direct observation			
Give clear and concise instructions to the patient to allow accurate measurement of visual acuity	Discussion and direct observation			
Encourage patient at all stages of the visual acuity testing to obtain the most accurate reading possible	Discussion and direct observation			
Where appropriate, demonstrate the measurement of visual acuity using a different visual acuity format chart, e.g. E chart	Discussion and direct observation			
Where appropriate, record a patient's visual acuity using a pinhole	Discussion and direct observation			
Demonstrate when to use a pinhole	Discussion and direct observation			
Give clear and concise instructions on the use of a pinhole	Discussion and direct observation			
Know what action to take if a patient is unable to perform visual acuity at a stated distance using a pinhole	Discussion and direct observation			
Produce accurate, legible and complete documentation of a patient's visual acuity taking into account the following: • Was visual acuity aided or unaided or with a pinhole • Reasons why patient is unable to complete the test • The use of alternative format of visual acuity testing, e.g. E chart • Any eccentric viewing by the patient	Discussion and direct observation			
Record any adverse event or critical incident	Discussion and direct observation			

Staff signature:..…....

Mentor/coach signature:...................................

Date of assessment: ....….............

INSTILLING TOPICAL EYE MEDICATION COMPETENCY TOOL

PERFORMANCE CRITERIA AND ASSESSMENT DOCUMENT FOR INSTILLING TOPICAL EYE MEDICATION

You need to be able to demonstrate your knowledge, understanding and skill in the instillation of eye medication.

The staff member is able to perform the following competently	Evidence	Yes	No	Further practice required/ Action plan
Ascertain that the correct patient is identified using the Trust ID policy	Discussion and direct observation Reflective account			
Correct handwashing technique Questioning on the spread of infection and the importance of handwashing	Discussion and direct observation Reflective account			
Discuss the pharmacology of the prescribed medication including side effects	Discussion and direct observation Reflective account			
Ensure correct procedure is followed in relation to checking eye against prescription	Discussion and direct observation Reflective account			
Follow correct procedure in relation to checking drops against prescription	Discussion and direct observation Reflective account			
Follow the correct procedure in relation to checking for expiry dates and clarity of drops	Discussion and direct observation Reflective account			
Correct procedure followed for checking sterility of eye medication	Discussion and direct observation Reflective account			
Ensure verbal consent was given	Discussion and direct observation Reflective account			
Give explanation to patient in relation to side effects and effects of drops	Discussion and direct observation Reflective account			
Confirm the patient's allergy status	Discussion and direct observation Reflective account			
Accurately assess patient and take appropriate action before drop instillation	Direct observation Reflective account			
Accurately assess the eye and take action where appropriate before drop instillation	Direct observation			

Observe the administration of eye medication in a safe and competent manner and take appropriate action	Direct observation			
Observe the correct procedure for disposal of waste	Direct observation			
Observe the correct documentation has taken place	Direct observation			
Staff signature:... Mentor/coach signature:.................................... Date of assessment:...				

TAKING A CONJUNCTIVAL SWAB COMPETENCY TOOL

PERFORMANCE CRITERIA AND ASSESSMENT DOCUMENT FOR TAKING A CONJUNCTIVAL SWAB				
You need to be able to demonstrate your knowledge, understanding and skill in the taking of a conjunctival swab.				
The staff member is able to perform the following competently	**Evidence**	**Yes**	**No**	**Further practice required/ Action plan**
Ascertain that the correct patient is identified using the Trust ID policy	Discussion and direct observation Reflective account			
Ensure verbal consent was given by the patient	Discussion and direct observation Reflective account			
Use correct handwashing technique	Discussion and direct observation Reflective account			
Discuss the rationale for taking eye swab	Discussion and direct observation Reflective account			
Answer questioning on the spread of infection and the importance of handwashing	Discussion and direct observation Reflective account			
The patient will have the following outcomes: • Understand and be able to cooperate with the investigation • Be comfortable and able to maintain position during the procedure • Will not be exposed to the risk of cross-infection	Discussion and direct observation Reflective account			

Demonstrate the correct procedure for swab taking so that sufficient cells are taken	Discussion and direct observation Reflective account			
Demonstrate the recording of correct patient's details on specimen	Discussion and direct observation Reflective account			
Transport specimen in a timely way so that cells will reach labs in optimum condition for identification of microorganisms	Discussion and direct observation Reflective account			
Demonstrate that patient is not exposed to unnecessary anxiety	Direct observation Reflective account			
Washes hands after procedure				
Accurately document swabs taken				

Staff signature:...

Mentor/coach signature:...................................

Date of assessment:...

FLUORESCEIN ANGIOGRAPHY COMPETENCY (FFA) TOOL

PERFORMANCE CRITERIA AND ASSESSMENT DOCUMENT FOR PERFORMING INTRAVENOUS FLUORESCEIN ANGIOGRAM

You need to be able to demonstrate your knowledge, understanding and skill in performing intravenous fluorescein angiogram. The individual staff member must be able to demonstrate the following:

A factual awareness and working understanding of the current policies and protocols which affect your work practice in relation to

- Health and safety and infection control
- The handling of equipment required for intravenous fluorescein angiogram and other resources
- Accountability and responsibility for checking equipment (including emergency resuscitation drugs and equipment) and other resources, including vicarious liability

A working understanding and factual knowledge of the importance of the following:

- Your role and the importance of working within your own sphere of competence
- The roles and responsibilities of other team members
- Standard precautions in relation to intravenous fluorescein angiogram
- Understanding of the potential consequences of poor practice in relation to the application of standard precautions
- Preparing and setting out correctly essential resources safely and efficiently
- Having all the resources including equipment ready before starting the procedure
- Selecting and preparing resources according to the individual's care plan
- How to set up and prepare equipment including any adjustments which are specific to an individual's needs, the nature and function of equipment used and how to check whether or not it is functioning correctly

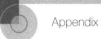

- What procedures you are permitted to undertake when problems arise with equipment or resources and when you must refer the problems to others
- The correct procedure to follow for reporting problems or faults with resources without delay to the relevant member of the senior staff
- The types of records and documentation required for the clinical activity and how they should be documented

The staff member must be able to perform competently	Evidence	Yes	No
Demonstrates the importance of establishing patient's identity in accordance with Trust guideline	Discussion and direct observation Reflective account		
Demonstrates the ability to take into account patient's privacy and dignity during FFA	Discussion and direct observation Reflective account		
Attends the Trust venipuncture and cannulation course	Discussion and direct observation Reflective account		
Demonstrates underpinning knowledge of the following: • Anatomy and physiology of the veins • Theory and principles of FFA • Reasons for performing FFA • Review of the literature on FFA • Pharmacological knowledge of FFA including side effects • Dealing with any emergencies as a result of FFA • The principles of good history • Taking a consent	Discussion and direct observation Reflective account		
Establishes rapport with patient, e.g. showing respect, concern and interest in patient during FFA	Discussion and direct observation Reflective account		
Through observation, demonstrates how the operator's and patient's comfort and safety are maintained during FFA	Discussion and direct observation Reflective account		
During FFA, demonstrates patient comfort and safety on the more challenging patient, i.e. patient with learning disability, lack of mental capacity, physical disability, etc.	Discussion and direct observation Reflective account		
Demonstrates how to accurately position patient during FFA	Discussion and direct observation Reflective account		
Demonstrates the use of good interpersonal and communication techniques to minimise patient anxiety during the patient's time in the ophthalmic unit	Discussion and direct observation Reflective account		

Demonstrates competence to carry out a FFA pre-assessment	Discussion and direct observation Reflective account		
Demonstrates the ability to obtain a valid consent from the patient	Discussion and direct observation Reflective account		
Demonstrates effective handwashing technique	Discussion and direct observation Reflective account		
Demonstrates the use of good interpersonal and communication techniques to minimize patient anxiety before, during and after the procedure	Discussion and direct observation Reflective account		
Checks for patient's allergy before instillation of drops	Discussion and direct observation Reflective account		
Demonstrates correct ANTT with the instillation of dilating drops pre FFA	Discussion and direct observation Reflective account		
Demonstrates the ability to cannulate patients using ANTT and complete appropriate documentation in relation to the administration of fluorescein and cannulation	Discussion and direct observation Reflective account		
Demonstrates the ability to competently manage any emergencies	Discussion and direct observation Reflective account		
Demonstrates the ability to care for patients and relatives before, during and after FFA	Discussion and direct observation Reflective account		
Demonstrates the ability to complete all appropriate paperwork and ensure the patient's awareness of any after-care management	Discussion and direct observation Reflective account		

Staff signature:..

Mentor/coach signature:....................................

Assessment date:...

ASSESSING RELATIVE AFFERENT PAPILLARY DEFECT COMPETENCY TOOL

PERFORMANCE CRITERIA AND ASSESSMENT DOCUMENT FOR ASSESSING RELATIVE AFFERENT PUPIL DEFECT
You need to be able to demonstrate your knowledge, understanding and skill in assessing the pupils for relative afferent papillary defect. The individual staff member must be able to demonstrate the following: 1. Underpinning knowledge of pupillary pathway 2. Knowledge and understanding of different papillary abnormalities

3. Ability to assess pupillary reaction of a wide range of patients with special needs such as learning difficulties, hard of hearing, different age group 4. Demonstrate accurate recording and documentation of pupil reaction				
The staff member is able to perform the following competently	**Evidence**	**Yes**	**No**	**Further practice required/ Action plan**
Ascertain that the correct patient is identified using the Trust ID policy	Discussion and direct observation Reflective account			
Ensure verbal consent given by patient	Discussion and direct observation Reflective account			
The patient will have the following outcomes: • Will understand and consent to procedure • Will be comfortable and able to maintain position during the procedure • Gaze will be in correct position to carry out procedure • Will have accurate assessment made of results • Will have any consensual defect identified • Will have any defect identified	Discussion and direct observation Reflective account			
Accurate record is maintained in patient's record	Discussion and direct observation Reflective account			

Staff signature:..

Mentor/coach signature:...................................

Date of assessment:..

MEASURING INTRAOCULAR PRESSURE USING THE TONO-PEN COMPETENCY TOOL

PERFORMANCE CRITERIA AND ASSESSMENT DOCUMENT FOR MEASURING INTROCULAR PRESSURE USING THE TONO-PEN

You need to be able to demonstrate your knowledge, understanding and skill in measuring intraocular pressure using the Tono-Pen. The individual staff member must be able to demonstrate the following:

1. Underpinning knowledge of ability to demonstrate a factual awareness and working understanding of the current policies and protocols which affect your work practice in relation to
   a. Health and safety and infection control
   b. The handling of equipment required for Tono-Pen applanation tonometry and other resources
   c. Accountability and responsibility for checking equipment (including emergency resuscitation drugs and equipment) and other resources, including vicarious liability
2. Ability to demonstrate a working understanding and factual knowledge of the importance of the following:
   a. Your role and the importance of working within your own sphere of competence.
   b. The roles and responsibilities of other team members
   c. Standard precautions in relation to Tono-Pen applanation tonometry
   d. Understanding of the potential consequences of poor practice in relation to the application of standard precautions
   e. Preparing and setting out correctly essential resources safely and efficiently
   f. Having all the resources including equipment ready before starting the procedure
   g. Selecting and preparing resources according to the individual's care plan
   h. How to set up and prepare equipment including any adjustments which are specific to an individual's needs, the nature and function of equipment used and how to check whether or not it is functioning correctly
   i. What procedures you are permitted to undertake when problems arise with equipment or resources and when you must refer the problems to others
   j. The correct procedure to follow for reporting problems or faults with resources without delay to the relevant member of the senior staff
   k. The types of records and documentation required for the clinical activity and how they should be documented

The staff member is able to perform the following competently	Evidence	Yes	No
Demonstrates the importance of establishing the patient's identity in accordance with Trust guideline	Discussion and direct observation Reflective account		
Ensure verbal consent is given by patient	Discussion and direct observation Reflective account		

Demonstrates the ability to take into account the patient's privacy and dignity during IOP measurement	Discussion and direct observation Reflective account		
Demonstrates effective health and safety issues before, during and after IOP measurement including correct handwashing technique	Discussion and direct observation Reflective account		
Demonstrates the correct procedure of calibrating the Tono-Pen and takes appropriate action to address calibration errors	Discussion and direct observation Reflective account		
Checks patient for any allergies to latex and demonstrates the correct technique for applying the protective cover over probe	Discussion and direct observation Reflective account		
Demonstrates the correct checking of drug allergies prior to instillation of topical analgesia	Discussion and direct observation Reflective account		
Demonstrates the instillation of appropriate analgesia prior to IOP procedure	Discussion and direct observation Reflective account		
Demonstrates correct technique of intraocular pressure measurement using Tono-Pen	Discussion and direct observation Reflective account		
Demonstrates methodical and accurate documentation of IOP readings	Discussion and direct observation Reflective account		
Demonstrates the use of good interpersonal and communication techniques to minimize patient anxiety during IOP measurements	Discussion and direct observation Reflective account		
Demonstrates the ability to recognize incorrect IOP measurement and uses solutions to address	Discussion and direct observation Reflective account		
Demonstrates and discusses the probability value in relation to IOP measurement and takes appropriate action if values are outside normal limits	Discussion and direct observation Reflective account		
Demonstrates a deeper understanding of IOP readings to pathophysiology in relation to abnormal IOP readings			

Staff signature:……………………………...............

Mentor/coach signature:………………………………

Date of assessment:………………………...............

OPTICAL COHERENCE TOMOGRAM COMPETENCY TOOL

PERFORMANCE CRITERIA AND ASSESSMENT DOCUMENT FOR RECORDING OPTICAL COHERENCE (OCT)

You need to be able to demonstrate your knowledge, understanding and skill in recording OCT. The individual staff member must be able to demonstrate the following:

A factual awareness and working understanding of the current policies and protocols which affect your work practice in relation to

- Health and safety and infection control
- The handling of equipment required for OCT and other resources
- Accountability and responsibility for checking equipment (including emergency resuscitation drugs and equipment) and other resources, including vicarious liability

A working understanding and factual knowledge of the importance of the following:

- Your role and the importance of working within your own sphere of competence
- The roles and responsibilities of other team members
- Standard precautions in relation to OCT
- Understanding of the potential consequences of poor practice in relation to the application of standard precautions
- Preparing and setting out correctly essential resources safely and efficiently
- Having all the resources including equipment ready before starting the procedure
- Selecting and preparing resources according to the individual's care plan
- How to set up and prepare equipment including any adjustments which are specific to an individual's needs, the nature and function of equipment used and how to check whether or not it is functioning correctly
- What procedures you are permitted to undertake when problems arise with equipment or resources and when you must refer the problems to others
- The correct procedure to follow for reporting problems or faults with resources without delay to the relevant member of the senior staff
- The types of records and documentation required for the clinical activity and how they should be documented

The staff member is able to perform the following competently	Evidence	Yes	No
Demonstrates the importance of establishing patient's identity in accordance with Trust guideline	Discussion and direct observation Reflective account		
Demonstrates the ability to take into account the patient's privacy and dignity during OCT	Discussion and direct observation Reflective account		
Demonstrates effective health and safety issues before, during and after OCT	Discussion and direct observation Reflective account		

Demonstrates underpinning knowledge of the following: • Anatomy and physiology of the macroscopic and microscopic of the retina • Theory and principles of OCT • A review of the literature on OCT • General workings of the OCT including troubleshooting • Understanding of optical principles • Common diseases requiring referral for an OCT	Discussion and direct observation Reflective account		
Demonstrates ability to establish rapport with patient, e.g. showing respect, concern and interest in patient during OCT	Discussion and direct observation Reflective account		
Demonstrate how the operator's and patient's comfort and safety are maintained during OCT	Discussion and direct observation Reflective account		
During OCT, demonstrates patient's comfort and safety on the more challenging patient, i.e. patients with learning disability, lack of mental capacity, physical disability, etc.	Discussion and direct observation Reflective account		
Demonstrates how to accurately position patient during OCT	Discussion and direct observation Reflective account		
Demonstrates the use of good interpersonal and communication techniques to minimize patient anxiety during OCT	Discussion and direct observation Reflective account		
Demonstrates the ability to give accurate information to patient regarding fixation of the patient's gaze during OCT	Discussion and direct observation Reflective account		
Demonstrates knowledge, skills and understanding on the following aspects of OCT: • Switching the machine • Accurate positioning of the patient • Recording and aligning the patient and chin rest • Assessing the suitability of an image • Repeating the procedure when necessary • Printing and documenting appropriate information • Describing and demonstrating the correct OCT procedures for troubleshooting • Demonstrating and discussing infection control measures	Discussion and direct observation Reflective account		
Demonstrates an understanding of OCT printout to pathophysiology in relation to abnormal OCT	Discussion and direct observation Reflective account		

Staff signature:..

Mentor/coach signature:...................................

Date of assessment:...

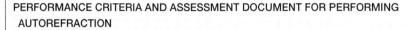

PERFORMANCE CRITERIA AND ASSESSMENT DOCUMENT FOR PERFORMING AUTOREFRACTION

You need to be able to demonstrate your knowledge, understanding and skill in performing autorefraction. The individual staff member must be able to demonstrate the following:

A factual awareness and working understanding of the current policies and protocols which affect your work practice in relation to

- Health and safety and infection control
- The handling of equipment required for autorefraction and other resources
- Accountability and responsibility for checking equipment (including emergency resuscitation drugs and equipment) and other resources, including vicarious liability

A working understanding and factual knowledge of the importance of following

- Your role and the importance of working within your own sphere of competence
- The roles and responsibilities of other team members
- Standard precautions in relation to autorefraction
- Understanding of the potential consequences of poor practice in relation to the application of standard precautions
- Preparing and setting out correctly essential resources safely and efficiently
- Having all the resources including equipment ready before starting the procedure
- Selecting and preparing resources according to the individual's care plan
- How to set up and prepare equipment including any adjustments which are specific to an individual's needs, the nature and function of equipment used and how to check whether or not it is functioning correctly
- What procedures you are permitted to undertake when problems arise with equipment or resources and when you must refer the problems to others
- The correct procedure to follow for reporting problems or faults with resources without delay to the relevant member of the senior staff
- The types of records and documentation required for the clinical activity and how they should be documented

The staff member is able to perform the following competently	Evidence	Yes	No
Demonstrates the importance of establishing the patient's identity in accordance with Trust guideline	Discussion and direct observation Reflective account		
Demonstrates the ability to take into account the patient's privacy and dignity during autorefraction	Discussion and direct observation Reflective account		
Demonstrates effective health and safety issues before, during and after autorefraction	Discussion and direct observation Reflective account		
Demonstrates underpinning knowledge of the following • Anatomy and physiology of the eye including an in-depth knowledge of the cornea and lens • In-depth knowledge and understanding of the autorefractor	Discussion and direct observation Reflective account		

Demonstrates patient's comfort by moving autorefractor close to patient and adjusting height and chin rest position to promote comfort and full movement of joystick	Discussion and direct observation Reflective account		
Demonstrates the use of good interpersonal and communication techniques to minimize patient anxiety during autorefraction	Discussion and direct observation Reflective account		
Demonstrates the ability to give accurate information to patient regarding positioning of patient by asking patient to place his chin on the chin rest and fixate his gaze onto the red sail of the boat in the picture ahead	Discussion and direct observation Reflective account		
Demonstrates the ability to use the joystick to locate the patient's cornea on the relevant eye and focus the circle until it is in crisp focus and it has a cross in the centre of the circle	Discussion and direct observation Reflective account		
Has a deeper understanding of autorefractor readings to pathophysiology in relation to abnormal autorefractor readings	Discussion and direct observation Reflective account		
Demonstrates how to press print to print off readout and instruct patient to sit back	Discussion and direct observation Reflective account		

Staff signature:……………………………............

Mentor/coach signature:……………………………

Date of assessment:……………………….............

SPECULAR MICROSCOPY COMPETENCY TOOL

PERFORMANCE CRITERIA AND ASSESSMENT DOCUMENT FOR PERFORMING SPECULAR MICROSCOPY

You need to be able to demonstrate your knowledge, understanding and skill in performing specular microscopy. The individual staff member must be able to demonstrate the following:

A factual awareness and working understanding of the current policies and protocols which affect your work practice in relation to

- Health and safety and infection control
- The handling of equipment required for specular microscopy and other resources
- Accountability and responsibility for checking equipment (including emergency resuscitation drugs and equipment) and other resources, including vicarious liability

A working understanding and factual knowledge of the importance of the following:

- Your role and the importance of working within your own sphere of competence
- The roles and responsibilities of other team members
- Standard precautions in relation to specular microscopy
- Understanding of the potential consequences of poor practice in relation to the application of standard precautions

- Preparing and setting out correctly essential resources safely and efficiently
- Having all the resources including equipment ready before starting the procedure
- Selecting and preparing resources according to the individual's care plan
- How to set up and prepare equipment including any adjustments which are specific to an individual's needs, the nature and function of equipment used and how to check whether or not it is functioning correctly
- What procedures you are permitted to undertake when problems arise with equipment or resources and when you must refer the problems to others
- The correct procedure to follow for reporting problems or faults with resources without delay to the relevant member of the senior staff
- The types of records and documentation required for the clinical activity and how they should be documented

The staff member is able to perform the following competently	Evidence	Yes	No
Demonstrates the importance of establishing the patient's identity in accordance with Trust guideline	Discussion and direct observation Reflective account		
Demonstrates the ability to take into account the patient's privacy and dignity during specular microscopy	Discussion and direct observation Reflective account		
Demonstrates effective health and safety issues before, during and after specular microscopy	Discussion and direct observation Reflective account		
Demonstrates underpinning knowledge of the following: • Anatomy and physiology of the macroscopic and microscopic of the cornea • Anatomy of the tear film and tear film stability • Theory and principles of specular microscope • A review of the literature on specular microscopy • General workings of the specular microscope including troubleshooting • Understanding of optical principles • Common diseases and trauma of the eye and cornea affecting specular microscopy findings • The impact of contact lenses on specular microscopy	Discussion and direct observation Reflective account		
Demonstrates ability to establish rapport with patient, e.g. showing respect, concern and interest in patient during specular microscopy	Discussion and direct observation Reflective account		
Through observation, demonstrates how the operator's and patient's comfort and safety are maintained during specular microscopy	Discussion and direct observation Reflective account		
During specular microscopy, demonstrates patient's comfort and safety on the more challenging patient, i.e. patients with learning disability, lack of mental capacity, physical disability, etc.	Discussion and direct observation Reflective account		

Demonstrates how to accurately position the patient during specular microscopy	Discussion and direct observation Reflective account		
Demonstrates the use of good interpersonal and communication techniques to minimise patient anxiety during specular microscopy	Discussion and direct observation Reflective account		
Demonstrates the ability to give accurate information to patient regarding fixation of the patient's gaze during specular microscopy	Direct observation		
Has a deeper understanding of specular microscopy readings to pathophysiology in relation to abnormal specular microscopy readings	Discussion and reflective account		

Staff signature:………………………………..............

Mentor/coach signature:……………………………..

Date of assessment:………………………...............

PERFORMANCE CRITERIA AND ASSESSMENT DOCUMENT FOR PERFORMING PACHYMETRY

You need to be able to demonstrate your knowledge, understanding and skill in performing pachymetry. The individual staff member must be able to demonstrate the following:

A factual awareness and working understanding of the current policies and protocols which affect your work practice in relation to

- Health and safety and infection control
- The handling of equipment required for pachymetry and other resources
- Accountability and responsibility for checking equipment (including emergency resuscitation drugs and equipment) and other resources, including vicarious liability

A working understanding and factual knowledge of the importance of the following:

- Your role and the importance of working within your own sphere of competence
- The roles and responsibilities of other team members
- Standard precautions in relation to pachymetry
- Understanding of the potential consequences of poor practice in relation to the application of standard precautions
- Preparing and setting out correctly essential resources safely and efficiently
- Having all the resources including equipment ready before starting the procedure
- Selecting and preparing resources according to the individual's care plan
- How to set up and prepare equipment including any adjustments which are specific to an individual's needs, the nature and function of equipment used and how to check whether or not it is functioning correctly
- What procedures you are permitted to undertake when problems arise with equipment or resources and when you must refer the problems to others
- The correct procedure to follow for reporting problems or faults with resources without delay to the relevant member of the senior staff
- The types of records and documentation required for the clinical activity and how they should be documented

The staff member is able to perform the following competently	Evidence	Yes	No
Demonstrates the importance of establishing the patient's identity in accordance with Trust guideline	Discussion and direct observation Reflective account		
Demonstrates the importance of establishing patient's identity in accordance with Trust guideline	Discussion and direct observation Reflective account		
Demonstrates the ability to take into account the patient's privacy and dignity during pachymetry	Discussion and direct observation Reflective account		
Demonstrates effective health and safety issues before, during and after a pachymetry	Discussion and direct observation Reflective account		
Demonstrates underpinning knowledge of the following: • Anatomy and physiology of the macroscopic and microscopic of the cornea • Anatomy of the tear film and tear film stability • Theory and principles of pachymetry • Importance of performing pachymetry • Literature review of pachymetry • General workings of the pachymeter including troubleshooting • Understanding of optical principles • Common diseases of the cornea affecting pachymetry measurement • Normal corneal thickness • Correct storage and maintenance of the pachymeter microscope	Discussion and direct observation Reflective account		
Demonstrates ability to establish rapport with patient, e.g. showing respect, concern and interest in patient during pachymetry	Discussion and direct observation Reflective account		
Through observation, demonstrates how the operator's and patient's comfort and safety are maintained during pachymetry	Discussion and direct observation Reflective account		
During pachymetry, demonstrates patient's comfort and safety on the more challenging patient, i.e. patients with learning disability, lack of mental capacity, patients with physical disability, etc.	Discussion and direct observation Reflective account		
Demonstrates the importance of good explanation to patient to relieve anxiety and fear during pachymetry including the small risk of a corneal abrasion	Discussion and direct observation Reflective account		
Demonstrates how to accurately position patient during pachymetry	Discussion and direct observation Reflective account		

Demonstrates effective handwashing technique	Discussion and direct observation Reflective account		
Demonstrates the use of good interpersonal and communication techniques to minimise patient anxiety during the procedure	Discussion and direct observation Reflective account		
Checks for patient's allergy before instillation of drops	Discussion and direct observation Reflective account		
Demonstrates correct ANTT with the instillation of local anesthetic	Discussion and direct observation Reflective account		
Demonstrates the ability to give accurate information to patient regarding fixation of their gaze during pachymetry	Discussion and direct observation Reflective account		
Demonstrates the ability to take accurate pachymetry readings	Discussion and direct observation Reflective account		
Demonstrates knowledge and understanding of how to interpret pachymetry readings and the implications of the care and management of patient with abnormal readings	Discussion and direct observation Reflective account		
Has a deeper understanding of pachymetry readings to pathophysiology in relation to abnormal pachymetry readings	Discussion and direct observation Reflective account		
Demonstrates ability to accurately document pachymetry readings	Discussion and direct observation Reflective account		

Staff signature:..

Mentor/coach signature:..................................

Assessment date:..

APPLANATION CONTACT BIOMETRY COMPETENCY TOOL

PERFORMANCE CRITERIA AND ASSESSMENT DOCUMENT FOR PERFORMING APPLANATION CONTACT BIOMETRY COMPETENCY

You need to be able to demonstrate your knowledge, understanding and skill in the following:
A factual awareness and working understanding of the current policies and protocols which affect your work practice in relation to

- Health and safety and infection control
- The handling of equipment required for applanation contact biometry and other resources
- Accountability and responsibility for checking equipment (including emergency resuscitation drugs and equipment) and other resources, including vicarious liability

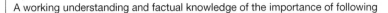

A working understanding and factual knowledge of the importance of following

- Your role and the importance of working within your own sphere of competence
- The roles and responsibilities of other team members
- Standard precautions in relation to applanation contact biometry
- Understanding of the potential consequences of poor practice in relation to the application of standard precautions
- Preparing and setting out correctly essential resources safely and efficiently
- Having all the resources including equipment ready before starting the procedure
- Selecting and preparing resources according to the individual's care plan
- How to set up and prepare equipment including any adjustments which are specific to an individual's needs, the nature and function of equipment used and how to check whether or not it is functioning correctly
- What procedures you are permitted to undertake when problems arise with equipment or resources and when you must refer the problems to others
- The correct procedure to follow for reporting problems or faults with resources without delay to the relevant member of the senior staff
- The types of records and documentation required for the clinical activity and how they should be documented

The staff member is able to perform the following competently	Evidence	Yes	No
Demonstrates the importance of establishing the patient's identity in accordance with Trust guideline	Discussion and direct observation Reflective account		
Demonstrates the ability to take into account the patient's privacy and dignity during biometry	Discussion and direct observation Reflective account		
Demonstrates effective health and safety issues before, during and after biometry measurement	Discussion and direct observation Reflective account		
Demonstrates underpinning knowledge of the following: • Anatomy and physiology of the eye including an in-depth knowledge of the cornea and lens • In-depth knowledge and understanding of IOL Master biometry machine • In-depth knowledge and understanding of the test eye machine	Discussion and direct observation Reflective account		
Demonstrates ability to establish rapport with the patient, e.g. showing respect, concern and interest in patient during biometry measurement	Discussion and direct observation Reflective account		
Through observation, demonstrates how the operator's and patient's comfort and safety are maintained during biometry measurement	Discussion and direct observation Reflective account		
During biometry measurement, demonstrates the patient's comfort and safety on the more challenging patient, i.e. patients with learning disability, lack of mental capacity, physical disability, etc.	Discussion and direct observation Reflective account		

Demonstrates the importance of a good explanation to the patient to relieve anxiety and fear during biometry measurement, including the small risk of a corneal abrasion	Discussion and direct observation Reflective account		
Checks for patient's allergy before instillation of drops	Discussion and direct observation Reflective account		
Demonstrates how to accurately position patient during biometry measurement	Discussion and direct observation Reflective account		
Demonstrates correct procedure for entering patient's demographic and other details in the machine	Discussion and direct observation Reflective account		
Demonstrates effective handwashing technique	Discussion and direct observation Reflective account		
Demonstrates correct ANTT with the instillation of local anesthetic	Discussion and direct observation Reflective account		
Demonstrates health and safety issues when performing applanation contact biometry	Discussion and direct observation Reflective account		
Gives clear instruction for patient to look straight ahead	Discussion and direct observation Reflective account		
Demonstrates the use of good interpersonal and communication techniques to minimize patient anxiety during the patient's time in the ophthalmic unit	Discussion and direct observation Reflective account		
Ensures scan settings are correct. Dense/normal cataracts are taken into consideration, as is aphakia. Automatic or manual modes are identified.	Discussion and direct observation Reflective account		
Demonstrates correct application of probe to corneal surface perpendicular to the visual axis. (Poor perpendicularity will produce inaccurate scans and may misalign along the optic nerve causing a longer axial length without a scleral spike.)	Discussion and direct observation Reflective account		
Demonstrates a working knowledge that scan produced will freeze automatically on auto mode. (Press pedal to unfreeze screen. The next scan may be obtained.)	Discussion and direct observation Reflective account		
Demonstrates a working knowledge that if difficulty is experienced gaining scans, instill one drop of G. hypromellose to provide a better contact medium as dry eyes will not have sufficient to obtain scans	Discussion and direct observation Reflective account		
Demonstrates ability to repeat procedure until five consecutive scans are produced as five scans will allow evaluation to ensure accuracy of scans	Discussion and direct observation Reflective account		

Demonstrates ability to measure glasses using the focimetry and establish current refraction using autorefractor and/or current O.O. prescription	Discussion and direct observation Reflective account		
Has an understanding that degree of myopia or hypermetropia should be mirrored in axial length measurements to evaluate validity of measurements (i.e. R eye – 2.5, L eye – 1.25; right axial length is expected to be longer than the left). (Degree of astigmatism should be mirrored in keratometry (K) readings obtained on IOL Master. *Note*: Index-linked myopia in cataract must be taken into consideration, i.e. an eye may be expected on focimetry to be longer than it really is.)	Discussion and direct observation Reflective account		
Demonstrates ability to print the best scan and fix in patient's case notes, showing documented evidence of axial length and scan quality	Discussion and direct observation Reflective account		
Has a deeper understanding of biometry measurement pathophysiology in relation to abnormal biometry readings	Discussion and direct observation Reflective account		
Demonstrates ability to evaluate scans by ensuring five clear spikes (cornea, anterior capsule, posterior capsule, retina and sclera) and retinal spike are steeply rising at 90 degrees, with perpendicularity indicated by all five spikes being equal in height	Discussion and direct observation Reflective account		
Knows how to promote accuracy by deleting any scans which do not meet the above requirements and re-scan to achieve five consistent scans	Discussion and direct observation Reflective account		

Assessor/coach signature:...................................

Staff nurse signature:...

Assessment date:...

NON-CONTACT BIOMETRY USING IOL MASTER COMPETENCY TOOL

PERFORMANCE CRITERIA AND ASSESSMENT DOCUMENT FOR PERFORMING NON-CONTACT BIOMETRY USING IOL MASTER

You need to be able to demonstrate your knowledge, understanding and skill to demonstrate the following:

A factual awareness and working understanding of the current policies and protocols which affect your work practice in relation to

- Health and safety and infection control
- The handling of equipment required for non-contact biometry and other resources
- Accountability and responsibility for checking equipment (including emergency resuscitation drugs and equipment) and other resources, including vicarious liability

A working understanding and factual knowledge of the importance of the following:

- Your role and the importance of working within your own sphere of competence
- The roles and responsibilities of other team members
- Standard precautions in relation to non-contact biometry
- Understanding of the potential consequences of poor practice in relation to the application of standard precautions
- Preparing and setting out correctly essential resources safely and efficiently
- Having all the resources including equipment ready before starting the procedure
- Selecting and preparing resources according to the individual's care plan
- How to set up and prepare equipment including any adjustments which are specific to an individual's needs, the nature and function of equipment used and how to check whether or not it is functioning correctly
- What procedures you are permitted to undertake when problems arise with equipment or resources and when you must refer the problems to others
- The correct procedure to follow for reporting problems or faults with resources without delay to the relevant member of the senior staff
- The types of records and documentation required for the clinical activity and how they should be documented

The staff member must be able to perform the following competently:	Evidence	Yes	No
Demonstrates the importance of establishing the patient's identity in accordance with Trust guideline	Discussion and direct observation Reflective account		
Demonstrates the ability to take into account the patient's privacy and dignity during biometry	Discussion and direct observation Reflective account		
Demonstrates effective health and safety issues before, during and after biometry measurement	Discussion and direct observation Reflective account		
Demonstrates underpinning knowledge of the following: • Anatomy and physiology of the eye including an in-depth knowledge of the cornea and lens • In-depth knowledge and understanding of IOL Master biometry machine • In-depth knowledge and understanding of the test eye machine	Discussion and direct observation Reflective account		
Demonstrates the correct procedure of calibrating the IOL Master through the use of the test eye machine and take appropriate action to address calibration errors	Discussion and direct observation Reflective account		
Demonstrates ability to establish rapport with the patient, e.g. showing respect, concern and interest in patient during biometry measurement	Discussion and direct observation Reflective account		
Through observation, demonstrates how the operator's and patient's comfort and safety are maintained during biometry measurement	Discussion and direct observation Reflective account		

During biometry measurement, demonstrates the patient's comfort and safety on the more challenging patient, i.e. patients with learning disability, lack of mental capacity, physical disability, etc.	Discussion and direct observation Reflective account		
Demonstrates the importance of good explanation to patient to relieve anxiety and fear during biometry measurement	Discussion and direct observation Reflective account		
Demonstrates how to accurately position patient during biometry measurement	Discussion and direct observation Reflective account		
Demonstrates correct procedure for entering patient's demographic and other details in the machine	Discussion and direct observation Reflective account		
Demonstrates ability to accurately position the patient on the machine and ensure alignment to the red indicator	Discussion and direct observation Reflective account		
Demonstrates the ability to instruct the patient accurately by asking the patient to focus the testing eye on the light and placing the circular guiding display over the pupil	Discussion and direct observation Reflective account		
Demonstrates how to firmly press the button on the top of the control stick for axial length and focus the pinpoint and line by moving the stick backwards or forwards slowly	Discussion and direct observation Reflective account		
Demonstrates ability to instruct patient not to blink or move eye while measurements are being taken and that up to five measurements of axial length (AL) are taken. (Click button on top of control stick, move machine to left eye (OS) and repeat procedure. Always measure both eyes.)	Discussion and direct observation Reflective account		
Demonstrates the ability to know what to do in the event of differing readings in each eye, e.g. the following steps address differing readings: • Keep pinpoint over centre of pupil at all times • IOL Master will identify 'error' if AL markedly different or if lens opacity too thick for sound wave to penetrate • If different check with surgeon • If too thick proceed to contact/immersion biometry	Discussion and direct observation Reflective account		
Demonstrates the ability to take accurate K readings by pressing the button on top of the control stick for keratometry readings and focussing the circular guidance by moving the stick backwards or forwards slowly; also asks patient to blink to improve clarity	Discussion and direct observation Reflective account		
Demonstrates the ability to proceed to IOL calculations section of biometry procedure	Discussion and direct observation Reflective account		

Demonstrates the ability to take second readings by clicking button on top of control stick	Discussion and direct observation Reflective account		
Demonstrates the ability to know what to do in the event of differing K readings in each eye	Discussion and direct observation Reflective account		
Demonstrates thoroughness by checking AL & K readings once more until confident with procedure and accuracy of measurements	Discussion and direct observation Reflective account		
Demonstrates the ability to choose appropriate surgeon's name from list and click on IOL calculations for three formulae: • Hoffer Q • Halliday • SRK T II (These are found at the top of the screen. Move the cursor to highlight the appropriate formula.)	Discussion and direct observation Reflective account		
Demonstrates the capability to print IOL print-out for each formula when calculations appear	Discussion and direct observation Reflective account		
Demonstrates the ability to place printed biometry measurements and calculation into the patient's medical record and escort patient to wait outside the clinic room for the appropriate surgeon	Discussion and direct observation Reflective account		
Demonstrates the use of good interpersonal and communication techniques to minimise patient anxiety during the patient's time in the ophthalmic unit	Discussion and direct observation Reflective account		
Has a deeper understanding of biometry measurement pathophysiology in relation to abnormal biometry readings	Discussion and direct observation Reflective account		
Demonstrates accurate documentation of findings	Discussion and direct observation Reflective account		

Assessor signature:..

Staff nurse signature:..

Assessment date:...

DIRECT OBSERVATION OF PROCEDURAL SKILLS

Name of student:

Name of assessor:

Date of assessment:

Name of skill assessed:

Competency Statement	Yes	No	Comments
Through direct observation and discussion, is able to demonstrate indications, relevant anatomy and physiology and technique of procedure			
Uses Trust's policy for correct identification of patient			
Obtains informed consent			
Gives appropriate explanation of procedure to patient			
Demonstrates appropriate preparation pre-procedure			
Demonstrates technical ability			
Uses aseptic technique			
Seeks help where appropriate			
Demonstrates post-procedure management			
Uses communication skills			
Shows consideration of patient/professionalism			
Demonstrates overall ability to perform procedure			
Provides documentation			

PLEASE USE THIS SPACE TO RECORD AREAS OF STRENGTH OR ANY SUGGESTIONS FOR DEVELOPMENT

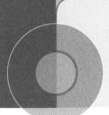

Appendix 4: Competency frameworks*

HISTORY-TAKING COMPETENCY TOOL

Competent	Proficient	Experienced
Able to demonstrate a factual awareness and working understanding of the current policies and protocols which affect your work practice in relation to • Health and safety and infection control Able to demonstrate a working understanding and factual knowledge of the importance of the following: • Your role and the importance of working within your own sphere of competence • The roles and responsibilities of other team members • Understanding the potential consequences of poor practice in relation to the application of standard precautions • The importance of preparing and setting out correctly essential resources safely and efficiently • The importance of selecting and preparing resources according to the individual's care plan	Able to problem solve around the history-taking consultation in complex situations Consistently demonstrates techniques of effective communication and effectively employs a range of communication skills to meet challenging situations Able to use complex strategies to deal with communication issues such as breaking bad news Able to maximise the use of integrated care pathways in fast-tracking patients requiring urgent ophthalmic care after history taking and slit lamp examination Initiates appropriate investigations after history taking and slit lamp examination and after consultation with the ophthalmologist Takes responsibility for initiating immediate care or follow-up care of patients after deciding on priorities of care by using advanced history taking, ocular examination and diagnostic reasoning skills in conjunction with other members of the multidisciplinary team and within protocols	Uses expert knowledge and experience to develop others, using history-taking skill to full potential Able to lead multiprofessional team within the department Uses knowledge to communicate effectively with patients and their families in challenging situations Uses methods of communication to include body language, spoken and written communications during history taking Demonstrates expertise in diagnostic skills after history taking and slit lamp examination Independently organises nursing care delivery after history taking and slit lamp examination Takes responsibility for initiating treatment and after consultation with ophthalmologist (if appropriate), deciding on priorities of care based on advanced history taking, ocular examination and diagnostic reasoning skills Takes responsibility for the whole episode of care for some patients with complex problems

* RCN 2012. *Ophthalmic Nursing: An Integrated Career and Competence Framework*. Royal College of Nursing, London.

Competent	Proficient	Experienced
• What procedures you are permitted to undertake when problems arise with equipment or resources and when you must refer the problem to others • The types of records and documentation required for the clinical activity and how they should be documented Able to demonstrate the ability to take into account patient's privacy and dignity during patient's consultation Able to demonstrate the importance of establishing patient's identity in accordance with Trust guideline Demonstrate ability to establish rapport with patient, e.g. showing respect, concern and interest in patient during consultation Able to demonstrate knowledge and understanding of the importance of good history taking Demonstrates excellent communication skills (both verbal and non-verbal) during the process of history taking Demonstrates the ability to ask relevant questions through open- and closed-ended questions	Discharges patients with a range of conditions within protocols after history taking and slit lamp examination Able to manage follow-up provision after history taking and slit lamp examination Refers patients to other members of the multidisciplinary team appropriately Provides/prescribes medication for patients under protocol or by independent or supplementary prescribing after slit lamp examination Demonstrates and teaches from a basis of wide knowledge and experience on effective history taking Relates knowledge of specific ophthalmic drugs to the treatment of specific conditions Has a deeper understanding of pathophysioloy in relation to systemic and topical medications Works autonomously, managing the episodes of care including consultation, investigations and treatment within protocols Demonstrates the ability to evaluate information gained through ophthalmic examination and assessment in relation to normal and abnormal patient presentations to prioritise patients needing specialist investigations and treatments	Uses theoretical knowledge and professional experience to plan the consultation effectively and adapts systems to meet the needs of the more challenging patients and carers Uses expertise to prescribe, initiate, interpret and monitor diagnostic tests, interventions and treatment regimens independently and without supervision Uses expertise to coordinate and contribute towards a multidisciplinary approach to patient care delivery including expert knowledge to inform the development and delivery of local ophthalmic provision Develops protocols and guidelines to support the competent and experienced nurse in the delivery of patient care in an ophthalmic setting Researches, develops and promotes the use of new ophthalmic pain management strategies Has a good working knowledge of pharmacological developments in pain management and ophthalmic disorders Draws on a wide range of ophthalmic experience during consultation of patient and carer and provides contemporary advice and management plan

Competent	Proficient	Experienced
Able to demonstrate the ability to summarise effectively patient's history		Uses a wide range of ophthalmic experience, and advises on unusual or unexpected ophthalmic findings
Able to demonstrate the ability to use appropriate language and avoid medical jargon		Acts in advisory capacity in usual situations
Able to demonstrate knowledge of anatomy and physiology of the eye		Advises in unfamiliar or unexpected situations
Demonstrates knowledge of ophthalmic disorders		Explores/researches the rationale/evidence base for ophthalmic care interventions
Demonstrates knowledge of medical management associated with ophthalmic disorders		Actively seeks to develop a sound evidence for care in practice
Demonstrates knowledge of nursing care and management of patients with ophthalmic disorders		Prioritises care needs in response to changes
Demonstrates skill, knowledge and systematic history taking of the following aspects:		Supports the development of a learning environment for staff and patients

1. Mode of referral
2. Presenting complaint including length of problem
3. Relevant medical history that potentially might impact on presenting ophthalmic problems
4. Surgical history
5. Ophthalmic history (past and present)
6. Any ophthalmic pain – pain assessment must take into account the following:
   - Type, site and spread
   - Severity using the verbal pain score

Competent	Proficient	Experienced
• Consistency • Relieving factors • Exacerbating factors • Associated factors Demonstrates the ability to deal with the more challenging group of patients such as learning disabilities and difficulties, visual impairment and mental health issues Able to demonstrate skill, knowledge and understanding of the following: 1. Current proprietary medication and duration of use 2. Non-proprietary medications and alternative therapies 3. Is aware that taking a history of allergies Demonstrates where appropriate to take an occupational history, to include 1. Type of work 2. Industrial hazards Demonstrates (where appropriate) skills in taking a social history which may have an impact of management and compliance Able to demonstrate the ability to assess patient's visual assessment and the impact that will have on the activities of daily living		

Competent	Proficient	Experienced
Demonstrates the ability to document history taking systematically, accurately and succinctly		
Demonstrates the ability to impart good explanation to the patient and carer on findings		
Assessor Sig:.....................	Assessor Sig:.....................	Assessor Sig:.......................
Staff nurse Sig:.................	Staff nurse Sig:...................	Staff nurse Sig:....................
Completion Date: /	Completion Date: /	Completion Date: /

SLIT LAMP COMPETENCY

Competent	Proficient	Experienced
Able to demonstrate a factual awareness and working understanding of the current policies and protocols which affect your work practice in relation to • Health and safety and infection control • The handling of equipment required for slit lamp and other resources • Accountability and responsibility for checking equipment (including emergency resuscitation drugs and equipment) and other resources, including vicarious liability	Able to problem solve around the performance of skill in complex situations Demonstrate a range of technical assessment skills including slit lamp examination Able to use communication skills in complex situation during slit lamp examination Able to use complex strategies to deal with communication issues such as breaking bad news Able to maximise the use of integrated care pathways in fast-tracking patients requiring urgent ophthalmic care after slit lamp examination Initiates appropriate investigations after slit lamp examination	Uses expert knowledge and experience to develop others, using technical skills to full potential Able to lead multiprofessional team within the department Demonstrates expertise in diagnostic skills after slit lamp examination Independently organises nursing care delivery after slit lamp examination Takes responsibility for initiating treatment and after consultation with ophthalmologist (if appropriate) on deciding on priorities of care based on advanced history taking, ocular examination and diagnostic reasoning skills Takes responsibility for the whole episode of care for some patients with complex problems

Competent	Proficient	Experienced
Able to demonstrate a working understanding and factual knowledge of the importance of the following: • Your role and the importance of working within your own sphere of competence • The roles and responsibilities of other team members • Standard precautions in relation to slit lamp examination • Understanding of the potential consequences of poor practice in relation to the application of standard precautions • The importance of preparing and setting out correctly essential resources safely and efficiently • The importance of having all the resources including equipment ready before starting the procedure • The importance of selecting and preparing resources according to the individual's care plan	Able to assess the anterior and posterior segment of the eye using slit lamp to coordinate complex admission and discharge processes Takes responsibility for initiating immediate care of patients after deciding on priorities of care by using advanced history taking, ocular examination and diagnostic reasoning skills in conjunction with other members of the multidisciplinary team and within protocols Discharges patients with a range of conditions within protocols after slit lamp examination Able to manage follow-up provision after slit lamp examination Refers patients to other members of the multidisciplinary team appropriately Provides/prescribes medication for patients under protocol or by independent or supplementary prescribing after slit lamp examination	Uses expertise to prescribe, initiate, interpret and monitor diagnostic tests, interventions and treatment regimens independently and without supervision Uses expertise to coordinate and contribute toward a multidisciplinary approach to patient care delivery including expert knowledge to inform the development and delivery of local ophthalmic provision Develops protocols and guidelines to support the competent and experienced nurse in the delivery of patient care in an ophthalmic setting Where appropriate, investigates critical incidents/complaints and offers expert advice and opinion to internal and external peer group Audits risk assessment practice and evaluates effectiveness of quality assurance activities in relation to service provision Explores/researches the rationale/evidence base for ophthalmic care interventions Actively seeks to develop a sound evidence for care in practice Prioritises care needs in response to changes Supports the development of a learning environment for staff and patients

Competent	Proficient	Experienced
• How to set up and prepare equipment including any adjustments which are specific to an individual's needs, the nature and function of equipment used and how to check whether or not it is functioning correctly • What procedures you are permitted to undertake when problems arise with equipment or resources and when you must refer the problem to others • The correct procedure to follow for reporting problems or faults with resources without delay to the relevant member of the senior staff • The types of records and documentation required for the clinical activity and how they should be documented Demonstrates the ability to take into account patient's privacy and dignity during patient's consultation Demonstrates the importance of establishing patient's identity in accordance with Trust guideline	Demonstrates the ability to evaluate information gained through ophthalmic examination and assessment in relation to normal and abnormal patient presentations to prioritise patients needing specialist investigations and treatments	

Competent	Proficient	Experienced
Demonstrates ability to establish rapport with patient, e.g. showing respect, concern and interest in patient during consultation		
Demonstrates knowledge and understanding in health and safety issues such as safety features on the slit lamp and the importance of infection control		
Able to demonstrate your understanding of the principle of the slit lamp		
Through discussion, demonstrate the uses of the slit lamp		
Through discussion be able to describe the components of the slit lamp and the function of each of the components		
Through discussion, demonstrates knowledge and understanding of the workings of the slit lamp		
Able to demonstrate how to adjust the slit lamp oculars to take into account individual operator's refractive error (if appropriate) and also take into account the correct adjustment of the pupillary aperture		
If appropriate, demonstrate the correct way to adjust for any refractive error through the use of the focussing rod		

Competent	Proficient	Experienced

Through observation, demonstrate how the operator's and patient's comfort and safety are maintained during slit lamp examination including the more challenging patient, i.e. patients with learning disability, lack of mental capacity, patients with physical disability, etc.

Demonstrates the importance of good explanation to patient to relieve anxiety and fear during slit lamp examination

Able to demonstrate how to accurately position patient on the slit lamp

Through discussion and observation, is able to demonstrate the various illumination techniques to examine the structures of the eye

Demonstrates systematic and methodical slit lamp examination of the anterior and posterior segments of the eye

Able to demonstrate methodical and accurate documentation of slit lamp findings

Demonstrates the use of good interpersonal and communication techniques to minimise patient anxiety during the patient's time in the ophthalmic unit

Competent	Proficient	Experienced
Has the ability to organise post-consultation investigations and treatment after slit lamp examination		
Is able to plan where appropriate, the provision of care in the community following discharge from the hospital, including patient education for self-care and ocular health promotion		
Assessor Sig:...............	Assessor Sig:.................	Assessor Sig:.................
Staff nurse Sig:............	Staff nurse Sig:..............	Staff nurse Sig:..............
Completion Date: /	Completion Date: /	Completion Date: /

GOLDMAN'S TONOMETRY COMPETENCY TOOL

Competent	Proficient	Experienced
Able to demonstrate a factual awareness and working understanding of the current policies and protocols which affect your work practice in relation to • Health and safety and infection control • The handling of equipment required for Goldmann's applanation tonometry and other resources • Accountability and responsibility for checking equipment (including emergency resuscitation drugs and equipment) and other resources, including vicarious liability	Demonstrates a fluid, highly proficient performance in undertaking a range of core ophthalmic examinations and assessments Demonstrates highly proficient performance in undertaking expanded skills Able to problem solve around complex intraocular pressure (IOP) measurements Consistently demonstrates techniques of effective communication and effectively employs a range of communication skills to meet challenging situations during IOP measurements	Uses expert knowledge and experience to develop others, using the measurement of IOP skills to full potential Able to lead multiprofessional team within the department Uses knowledge to communicate effectively with patients and their families in challenging situations Demonstrates expertise in diagnostic skills after history taking and slit lamp examination Independently organises nursing care delivery after history taking and slit lamp findings

Competent	Proficient	Experienced
Able to demonstrate a working understanding and factual knowledge of the importance of following: • Your role and the importance of working within your own sphere of competence. • The roles and responsibilities of other team members • Standard precautions in relation to Goldmann's applanation tonometry • Understanding of the potential consequences of poor practice in relation to the application of standard precautions • The importance of preparing and setting out correctly essential resources safely and efficiently • The importance of having all the resources including equipment ready before starting the procedure • The importance of selecting and preparing resources according to the individual's care plan	Initiates appropriate investigations after slit lamp examination and IOP measurement and after consultation with the ophthalmologist Evaluates the salient aspects of the patient's ophthalmic, medical and psychosocial history and presentation to formulate diagnosis and care plans within agreed protocols/guidelines Demonstrates the ability to solve problems and make decisions about the patient care episode based on information gained through ophthalmic examination/assessment and with reference to previous practice experience Provides/prescribes medication for patients under protocol or by independent or supplementary prescribing after slit lamp examination Demonstrates the use of highly developed communication skills to manage complex situations with both ophthalmic patients, and carers and the multidisciplinary team. Able to use complex strategies to deal with communication issues such as breaking bad news Demonstrates and teaches from a basis of wide knowledge and experience on accurate IOP measurement Relates knowledge of abnormal IOP readings to the treatment and management of raised IOP	Takes responsibility for initiating treatment and after consultation with ophthalmologist (if appropriate) for deciding on priorities of care based on advanced history taking, ocular examination and diagnostic reasoning skills Works independently to manage the patient episode of consultation, investigation and treatment through the application of theoretical and advanced practice experience and technical expertise Uses theoretical knowledge and professional experience to plan the consultation effectively and adapts systems to meet the needs of the more challenging patients and carers Uses expertise to prescribe, initiate, interpret and monitor diagnostic tests, interventions and treatment regimens independently and without supervision Uses expertise to coordinate and contribute toward a multidisciplinary approach to patient care delivery including expert knowledge to inform the development and delivery of local ophthalmic provision

Competent	Proficient	Experienced
• How to set up and prepare equipment including any adjustments which are specific to an individual's needs, the nature and function of equipment used and how to check whether or not it is functioning correctly	Has a deeper understanding of pathophysioloy in relation to abnormal IOP	Develops protocols and guidelines to support the competent and experienced nurse in the delivery of patient care in an ophthalmic setting
• What procedures you are permitted to undertake when problems arise with equipment or resources and when you must refer the problem to others	Works autonomously, managing the episodes of care including consultation, investigations and treatment within protocols	Draws on a wide range of ophthalmic experience during consultation of patient and carer and provides contemporary advice and management plan
• The correct procedure to follow for reporting problems or faults with resources without delay to the relevant member of the senior staff	Demonstrates the ability to evaluate information gained through ophthalmic examination and assessment in relation to normal and abnormal patient presentations to prioritise patients needing specialist investigations and treatments	Uses a wide range of ophthalmic experience, and advises on unusual or unexpected ophthalmic findings
• The types of records and documentation required for the clinical activity and how they should be documented		Acts in advisory capacity in usual situations
Demonstrates underpinning skills and knowledge in slit lamp examination Demonstrates the importance of establishing patient's identity in accordance with Trust guideline		Advises in unfamiliar or unexpected situations

Competent	Proficient	Experienced
Demonstrates the ability to take into account patient's privacy and dignity during IOP measurement		Where appropriate, investigates critical incidents/complaints and offers expert advice and opinion to internal and external peer group
Demonstrates effective health and safety issues before, during and after IOP measurement		Audits risk assessment practice and evaluates effectiveness of quality assurance activities in relation to service provision
Demonstrates underpinning knowledge of the following:		Explores/researches the rationale/evidence base for ophthalmic care interventions
1. Principles behind applanation tonometry		Actively seeks to develop a sound evidence for care in practice
2. Anatomy and physiology of aqueous production and outflow		Prioritises care needs in response to changes
3. Imbert-Fick principle		Supports the development of a learning environment for staff and patients
Able to demonstrate the correct procedure of calibrating the Goldman's tonometer and take appropriate action to address calibration errors		
Able to discuss the potential errors of IOP measurements		
Demonstrates ability to establish rapport with patient, e.g. showing respect, concern and interest in patient during IOP measurement		
Through observation, demonstrate how the operator's and patient's comfort and safety are maintained during IOP measurement		

Competent	Proficient	Experienced
Demonstrates patient's comfort and safety on the more challenging patient, i.e. patients with learning disability, lack of mental capacity, patients with physical disability, etc. during IOP measurement		
Demonstrates the importance of good explanation to patient to relieve anxiety and fear during IOP measurement		
Demonstrates how to accurately position patient during IOP measurement		
Able to demonstrate the correct way to mount the tonometer on the mounting plate		
Able to demonstrate the correct technique of the insertion of the prism onto the holder		
Able to demonstrate the correct technique of positioning the slit lamp and illumination arm for IOP measurement		
Able to demonstrate the setup procedure for IOP measurement such as correct illumination including width of light beam, correct magnification and colour		
Able to demonstrate the correct tonometer calibration and the rationale for this prior to IOP measurement		

Competent	Proficient	Experienced
Demonstrates the correct checking of drug allergies prior to instillation of topical analgesia		
Demonstrates the instillation of appropriate analgesia prior to IOP procedure		
Demonstrates correct technique of intraocular pressure measurement		
Demonstrates methodical and accurate documentation of IOP readings		
Demonstrates the ability to recognise incorrect IOP measurement and uses solutions to address		
Able to demonstrate accurate documentation of findings		

Assessor Sig:.................... Assessor Sig:.................... Assessor Sig:....................

Staff nurse Sig:................. Staff nurse Sig:................. Staff nurse Sig:.................

Completion Date: / Completion Date: / Completion Date: /

Glossary

Abduction Turning the eye outwards.

Acanthamoeba A genus of free-living amoeba.

Accommodation The ability of the lens to change shape to allow near objects to be focussed on the retina.

Acne rosacea Disease of the skin, characterised by bullous nose and erythema of the cheeks, forehead and nose.

Adduction Turning the eye inwards.

Afferent pupil defect A defect of the pupillary reflex, in which shining a light in the affected eye will result in a dilatation of the pupil. This condition is due to an optic nerve lesion.

Amaurosis fugax Short-lived loss of vision.

Amblyopia Reduced vision, usually due to interference with the eye's development.

Angles Alpha, Kappa and Gamma Different angles in the eye measured between the optic axis and the visual axis.

Aniridia Absence of the iris.

Aniscoria Unequal pupils.

Anterior chamber The space between the cornea and the iris that is filled with aqueous humour.

Aphakia Absence of the crystalline lens.

Applanation tonometry Measurement of the intraocular pressure by flattening the cornea.

Arcus senilis Degenerative change in the cornea, resulting in a white ring around the corneal circumference.

Argon laser Laser that uses photocoagulation.

Astigmatism Uneven curvature of the cornea.

Binocular vision Coordinated use of both eyes, resulting in a single vision.

Biometry Measurement of the axial length of the eye (A-scan).

Blepharitis Inflammation of the lid margin.

Blepharospasm Painful involuntary spasm of the eyelids.

Blind spot Optic disc where there are no nerve endings, only nerve fibres.

Bullous keratopathy Oedema of the cornea, causing 'blister' formation in the epithelium.

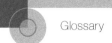

Buphthalmos Congenital glaucoma.

Burkitt's lymphoma A malignant tumour of the lympathetic system affecting mainly children.

Canthus Outer and inner areas where the upper and lower lids meet.

Capsulotomy Opening of the capsule of the lens.

Cartella shield Plastic shield to protect the eye and/or surrounding structures.

Caruncle Small fleshy area in inner corner of the eye.

Cataract Opacity of the crystalline lens.

Central field/vision Area of vision when looking straight ahead.

Chalazion Meibomian gland cyst. Internal hordeolum.

Chemosis Oedema of the conjunctiva.

Chlamydia Chronic conjunctivitis caused by serotypes D–K of *Chlamydia trachomatis*.

Commotio retinae Oedema of the retina following trauma.

Concave lens A lens which diverges light rays, used to correct myopia: a 'minus' lens.

Concretion Lipid deposit in the conjunctiva.

Convex lens A lens which converges light rays, used to correct hypermetropia: a 'plus' lens.

Cool laser Procedure similar to phacoemulsification, but uses 'cool laser' shock waves to fragment the lens.

Cover test A test for determining the presence of phoria or trophia.

Cycloplegia Paralysis of the ciliary muscles.

Cylindrical lens A lens of cylindrical shape, which refracts light rays in various directions in different meridians, used to correct astigmatism.

Dacryoadenitis Inflammation of the lacrimal gland.

Dacryocystitis Inflammation of the lacrimal sac.

Dacryocystorhinostomy An operation to make a passage from the lacrimal sac into the nose to overcome an obstruction.

Dendritic ulcer A branching ulcer of the cornea caused by the herpes simplex virus.

Descemetocele Protrusion of Descemet's membrane through the stroma and epithelium of the cornea.

Dioptre Unit of measurement of strength of the refractive power of the eye, or lenses, expressed as a fraction of a metre.

Diplopia Double vision.

Disciform keratitis Inflammation of the cornea as a complication of herpes simplex virus.

Distichiasis Double row of eyelashes.

Drusen Small yellow nodule in Bruch's membrane, or optic nerve.

Ectropion Turning out of the eyelid.

Electroretinogram A recording of electrical activity of the retina.

Emmetropia Absence of refractive error.

Endophthalmitis Inflammation/infection of inner structures of the eye.

Enophthalmos Displacement of the eyeball downward.

Entropion Turning inwards of the lid margin.

Enucleation Removal of the eyeball and length of optic nerve.

Epicanthus Broad fold of skin in inner canthus.

Epilation Removal of an eyelash.

Epiphora Watering eye.

Episcleritis Inflammation of the episcleral vessels.

Evisceration Removal of the contents of the eyeball, leaving the sclera intact.

Excimer laser Laser used for corneal surgery, e.g. for correcting refractive errors or removing corneal scars.

Exenteration Removal of the contents of the orbit, including the eyeball, the lids may or may not be conserved.

Exophthalmometer Instrument for measuring the degree of protrusion of an eye.

Exophthalmos Protrusion of one or both eyes – usually refers to that caused by thyroid eye disease.

Extracapsular lens extraction Removal of the anterior lens capsule, the cortex and nucleus but leaving the posterior lens capsule intact.

Field of vision The entire area that can be seen without moving the eye.

Fields of gaze The different areas that can be seen when moving the eye in all directions.

Fixation The eyes are fixed on an object centrally at a chosen distance.

Flare Protein in the anterior chamber, floating in the aqueous humour. Associated with anterior uveitis.

Floaters Small, dark particles in the vitreous humour.

Follicles Dome-shaped elevations on the palpebral conjunctiva containing lymphocytes. Follicles are avascular.

Fresnel prism Thin, transparent plastic disc which is attached to a pair of glasses to eliminate diplopia.

Fuch's dystrophy Disorder of Descemet's membrane of the cornea, with wart-like deposits and thickening. Defect in the endothelium is also noted.

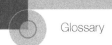

Fundus Posterior aspect of the retina including the optic disc and the macula.

Fusion Coordinating the images seen by both eyes into a single image.

Glaucoma A group of conditions characterised by an elevated intraocular pressure, optic disc changes and visual field loss.

Gonioscope A contact lens mirror used to view the anterior chamber angle.

Guttae (G.) Eye drops.

Hemianopia Half-vision – unilateral or bilateral.

Hess chart A chart for measuring and classifying strabismus.

Heterochromia Different-coloured irises in one person.

Hordeolum Internal, see Chalazion; external, see Stye.

Hydroxyapatite implant Derived material from coral used as an implant in enucleation.

Hypermetropia Long sight.

Hyphaema Blood in the anterior chamber.

Hypopyon Pus in the anterior chamber.

Imber–Fick law States that the intraocular pressure (P in mmHg) is equal to the tonometer weight (W) divided by the applanated area of the cornea. This is applicable for applanation tonometry.

Indocyanine green Newer dye than fluorescein sodium, and which gives better information on the choroidal circulation and is particularly helpful in the diagnosis of choroidal neovascular membranes.

Injection Degree of redness of the conjunctiva.

Interpupillary distance (IPD) The distance between the two pupils.

Interstitial keratitis Inflammation of the cornea due to syphilis.

Intracapsular lens extraction Removal of the entire lens including the anterior and posterior capsules.

Iridectomy Removal of a piece of the iris.

Iridodialysis Severance of the iris from the ciliary body.

Iridodonesis Quivering of iris following intracapsular cataract extraction.

Iridotomy A hole in the iris, usually performed by the laser beam.

Iris bombe Bulging forward of the iris.

Iris prolapse A section of the iris prolapsing through a wound, either surgical or traumatic.

Iritis Inflammation of the iris.

Ishihara colour plates Multicoloured charts for testing colour vision.

Kaposi's sarcoma Vascular tumour of HIV patients, appearing as multiple purple to red nodules on the skin and mucous membranes.

Keratitic precipitates Plaques of protein adhered to the corneal endothelium in uveitis.

Keratitis Inflammation of the cornea.

Keratoconus Conical-shaped deformity of the cornea.

Keratometer Instrument for measuring the curvature of the cornea.

Lacrimation Production of tears.

Lagophthalmos Incomplete closure of the eyelids.

Lamellar graft Partial thickness corneal graft.

Laser *in situ* keratomileusis (LASIK) A surgical procedure to correct myopia, hypermetropia and astigmatism by creating a corneal flap.

Laser light Amplification by stimulated emission of radiation. Energy transmitted as heat.

Lensectomy Removal of the entire crystalline lens and capsule, including an anterior segment of the vitreous humour using specialised equipment.

LogMAR A more accurate and replicable test of visual acuity.

Microphthalmos Small eyeball.

Miotic Drug that constricts the pupil.

Molluscum contagiosum Viral infection of the skin occurring on the face or eyelids manifested by a shiny, raised skin nodule.

Mydriatic Drug that dilates the pupil.

Myopia Short sight.

Needling A procedure used to remove soft lens matter on an infant or child.

Occulentum (Oc.) Eye ointment.

Operculum A semi-circular tear in the retina, covered with a flap of retina.

Ophthalmia neonatorum Severe conjunctivitis of the newborn.

Ophthalmoplegia Paralysis of the extraocular muscles.

Ophthalmoscope Instrument for examining the retina.

Optic axis The line through the centre of the optical structures of the eye.

Osteo-odonto-keraprosthesis surgery A type of surgical technique where patient's own tooth root and aveolar bone are used instead of conventional corneal graft technique.

Pachymetry A technique to measure the corneal thickness by using a pachometer.

Palpebral Pertaining to the eyelids.

Papillae Tiny elevation seen on palpebral conjunctiva with vascular cores.

Pannus Neovascularisation of the cornea.

Panophthalmitis Inflammation of the whole eyeball.

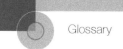

Pemphigoid An autoimmune disease of the elderly, characterised by chronic itchy blistering usually on the limbs.

Penetrating graft Full-thickness corneal graft.

Perimeter Instrument for measuring the field of vision.

Peripheral vision/field Area of vision outside central field of vision.

PGD Patient group directions.

Phacoemulsification Removal of cataract by ultrasound, breaking down lens matter prior to it being aspirated.

Phacolytic lens Lens matter leaking out, giving rise to uveitis and secondary glaucoma.

Phasing Regular frequent measurements of intraocular pressure, usually over a day.

Phlyctenule Small vesicle of allergic origin on limbal area of conjunctiva and/or cornea.

Photophobia Sensitivity to light.

Photopsia Sensation of flashing lights.

Photorefractive keratectomy (PRK) Correction of refractive errors using excimer laser.

Phthisis bulbi Shrunken eyeball.

Pinguecula A yellowish overgrowth of conjunctiva.

Placido's disc A disc with alternating black and white rings for reflecting onto the cornea to detect any irregularity in its curvature.

Presbyopia Inability to focus for near sight due to hardening of the lens nucleus after the age of 40 years.

Preseptal cellulitis Inflammation of preseptal portion of eyelids.

Prism A triangular-shaped lens used to correct diplopia.

Proptosis Protrusion of the eyeball.

Pterygium A triangular proliferation of conjunctival tissue that can invade the cornea.

Ptosis Drooping eyelid.

Radial keratotomy A surgical procedure consisting of radial incisions to the cornea used to correct myopia.

Refraction (a) Bending of light rays; (b) measurement of and correction of refractive errors of the eye.

Refractive surgery Corneal surgery to correct refractive errors.

Reiter's syndrome A condition characterised by inflammation of the conjunctiva, urethra and polyarthritis. This condition usually affects young males.

Retinal detachment Separation of the epithelial layer of the retina from its neural layers.

Retinitis pigmentosa A hereditary degeneration of the retina.

Retinoblastoma Highly malignant tumour of the retina in infancy.

Retinopathy Non-inflammatory disease of the retina.

Retinopathy of prematurity A vasoproliferative retinopathy occurring in premature infants.

Retinoscope Instrument for objective assessment of refractive errors.

Retrobulbar Behind the eyeball.

Retropunctal cautery Cautery applied behind the punctum to cause fibrosis and in-turning of the lower lid.

Rhodopsin Light-sensitive pigment of the rods in the retina – 'visual purple'.

Rodding of fornices Passing a glass rod in either fornix.

Rubeosis irides Neovascularisation of the iris.

Scleritis Inflammation of the sclera.

Scleromalacia Degeneration of the sclera.

Scotoma An area of vision loss in the visual field.

Siedel test A test to ascertain leakage of aqueous humour through a section or perforative wound using fluorescein drops.

Sjögren's syndrome Syndrome comprising arthritis, dry eyes, dysphagia and achlorhydria.

Snellen chart A chart consisting of graded letters, symbols or numbers for testing central vision.

Specular photomicroscopy Special mounted slit lamp camera which allows the corneal endothelium to be photographed and counted.

Squint Misalignment of the eyes, the eyes are not parallel.

Staphyloma A protrusion of the cornea or sclera.

Stereopsis Perception of depth with binocular vision.

Stevens–Johnson syndrome Acute mucocutaneous vesiculobullous disease.

Strabismus See Squint.

Sturge–Weber syndrome Red discolouration of the skin, often referred to as 'port wine stain', which is present at birth and which is permanent.

Stye Inflammation of one lash follicle. External hordeolum.

Superficial punctate keratitis Superficial spots of inflammation of the cornea which stain with G. fluorescein.

Symblephron Adhesion of the bulbar and palpebral conjunctiva.

Sympathetic ophthalmitis Severe uveitis in one eye following trauma involving the uvea of the other eye.

Synaechiae adhesion of the iris (a) to the lens – posterior synaechiae; (b) to the cornea – anterior synaechiae.

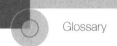

Tarsorrhaphy Suturing together of the eyelids.

Tear film The film of fluid covering the eyeball.

Tenon's capsule Membrane encircling globe from limbus to optic nerve overlying the sclera.

Tomography Computerised scan of the optic disc.

Tonometer Instrument for measuring intraocular pressure.

Topography A contour map of the curvature of the cornea.

Toric contact lens Contact lens to correct astigmatism.

Trachoma Potentially blinding infection of the conjunctiva and cornea caused by the TRIC virus.

Trichiasis Ingrowing or inturning of eyelashes.

Uveitis Inflammation of the uveal tract.

Visual acuity Detailed central vision.

Visual axis The line between a point viewed and the macula.

Visual field Area of vision.

Vitrectomy Removal of vitreous humour.

Xanthelasma Fatty deposits on the eyelids.

Xerophthalmia Lack of vitamin A, resulting in corneal and conjunctival disease.

YAG laser Laser that cuts holes in structures.

References

REFERENCES

American Academy of Ophthalmology. 2009/2010. *Clinical Optics*. AAO, San Francisco.

Bashour, M. and Benchimol, M.D. 2014. Radial keratotomy myopia. *eMedicine. Ophthalmology*. http://emedicine.medscape.com/oph/topic 669.htm.

Bettin, P. and Matteo, F. 2013. Glaucoma: Present challenges and future trends. *Ophthalmology Research*, 50(4), 197–208.

Bowling, B. 2015. *Kanski's Clinical Ophthalmology*, 8th edition, Elsevier, London, UK.

Brahma, A., Shah, S., Hiller, V., Mcleod, D., Sabala, T., Brown, A. and Marsden, J. 1996. Topical analgesia for superficial corneal injuries. *Journal of Accident and Emergency Medicine*, 1(3), 186–88.

British National Formulary. 2015. BNF 70 (British National Formulary) September 2015. British Medical Association and The Royal Pharmaceutical Society, London.

Bruce, I., McKennel, A. and Walker, E. 1991. *Blind and Partially Sighted Adults in Britain*. The Royal National Institute for the Blind Survey, HMSO, London.

Budenz, D.L., Barton, K. and Tseng, S.C. 2000. Amniotic membrane transplantation for repair of leaking glaucoma for filtering blebs. *American Journal of Ophthalmology*, 130, 580–88.

Carley, F. and Carley, S. 2001. Mydriatics in corneal abrasion. *Emergency Medicine Journal*, 18(4), 273.

Chalam K. 2007. Pilot studies suggest anti-VEGF Avastin may be effective for neovascular glaucoma. *EuroTimes*, 12(6), 42.

Collin, R. and Rose, G. 2001. *Fundamentals of Clinical Ophthalmology – Plastic and Orbital Surgery*. BMJ Books, London.

Comber, N. 2015. *Delivering Cancer Waiting Times. A Good Practice Guide*. NHS England, London.

Corbett, M.C., Rosen, E.S. and O'Bratt, D.P.S. 1999. *Corneal Topography: Principles and Applications*. BMJ Books, London.

Cordero, I. 2010. How to look after and care for a slit lamp. *Community Eye Health*, 23(73), online.

Department of Health. 2008a. *High Quality Care for All (Report by Lord Darzi)*. HMSO, London.

Department of Health. 2008b. *Releasing Time to Care*. HMSO, London.

Department of Health. 2013. *Registering Vision Impairment as a Disability*. London. https://www.gov.uk/government/publications/guidance-published-on-registering-a-vision-impairment-as-a-disability.

Dhawahir-Scala, F.E., Maino, A., Mokasht, A.A., McLauchlan, R. and Charles, S. 2008. To posture or not to posture after macular hole surgery. *Retina*, 28(1), 60–65.

Dua, H.S., Faraj, L.A., Said, D.G., Gray, T. and Lowe, J. 2013. Human corneal anatomy redefined: A novel pre-Descemet's layer (Dua's layer). *Ophthalmology*, 120, 1778–85.

Duker, J. and Tolentino, F. 1991. Retinopathy of prematurity and pediatric retina and vitreous disorders. *Current Opinion in Ophthalmology*, 2, 690–95.

Engstrom, R. and Holland, G. 1995. Local therapy for cytomegalovirus retinopathy. *American Journal of Ophthalmology*, 120(3), 376–85.

Everitt, H.A., Little, P.S. and Smith, P.W. 2006. A randomised controlled trial of management strategies for acute infective conjunctivitis in general practice. *British Medical Journal*, 333(7563), 321.

Fearnley, I. 2014. *Ophthalmia Neonatorum – Local Guidelines – Consultant Ophthalmologist*. Northampton General Hospital NHS Trust.

Fong, D.S., Ferris, F.L., Davis, M.D. and Chew, E.Y. 2000. *Early Treatment Diabetic Retinopathy Study (ETDRS)*. EDTRS study (1999). http://www.clinicaltrials.gov/ct2/show/NCT00000151.

Forrester, J.V., Dick, A.D., McMenamin, P.G. and Lee, W.R. 2002. *The Eye. Basic Sciences in Practice*, 2nd edition. W.B. Saunders, Edinburgh.

Fuchsjager-Mayrl, G. and Schmidt-Erfurth, U.M. 2007. Management of wet age-related macular degeneration. *European Ophthalmic Review*. 59–60. doi:10.17925/eor.2007.00.00.59.

Garway-Heath, D.F., Crabb, D.P. and Bunce, C. et al. 2015. Lantoprost of open-angle glaucoma (UKGTS): A randomised, multi-centre placebo control trail. *The Lancet*, 385(9975), 1295–304.

Hersch, P., Rice, B. and Baer, J. 1990. Topical non-steroidal agents and corneal wound healing. *Archives of Ophthalmology*, 108, 577–83.

James, B., Chew, C. and Bron, A. 2007. *Lecture Notes: Ophthalmology*, 10th edition. Blackwell, Oxford, UK.

Jayamanne, D., Fitt, A., Dayan, M., Andrews, R., Mitchell, K. and Griffiths, P. 1997. The effectiveness of topical diclofenac in relieving discomfort following traumatic corneal abrasions. *Eye*, 11, 79–83.

Jones, N. 2012. *Uveitis*, 2nd edition. JP Medical, Ltd., London.

Jose, R., Faria de Abreu, J.R., Silva, R. and Cunha-Vaz, J.G. 1994. The blood–retinal barrier in diabetes during pregnancy. *Archives of Ophthalmology*, 112, 1334–38.

Kanski, J. 2007. *Clinical Ophthalmology*, 6th edition. Elsevier, Oxford, UK.

Kanski, J.J., McAllister, J.A. and Salmon, J.F. 1996. *Glaucoma. A Colour Manual of Diagnosis and Treatment*, 2nd edition. Butterworth Heinemann, Oxford, UK.

Kerr A. 2014. *Local Guidelines for Herpes Simplex Keratitis and Acanthamoeba Keratitis*. Northampton General Hospital NHS Trust.

Klein, B.E., Moss, S.E., Klein, R. and Surawicz, T.S. 1991. The Wisconsin epidemiologic study of diabetic retinopathy. XIII. Relationship of serum cholesterol to retinopathy and hard exudates. *Ophthalmology*, 98, 1261–65.

Kuppens, E., Van Best, J. and Sterk, C. 1995. Is glaucoma associated with an increased risk of contact? *British Journal of Ophthalmology*, 79(7), 649–52.

Lee, S.H. and Tseng, S.C.G. 1997. Amniotic membrane transplantation for severe neurotropic ulcers. *British Journal of Ophthalmology*, 123, 302–3.

Lund-Johansen, P. 1990. The dye dilution method for measurement of cardiac output. *European Heart Journal*, 11(suppl I), 6–12.

Marsden J. 2006. *Ophthalmic Care*. Wiley, Chichester.

Marsden J., ed. 2008. *An Evidence Base for Ophthalmic Nursing Practice*. Wiley, Oxford, UK.

Martin, O., Parks, D., Mellows, S. et al. 1994. Treatment of cytomegalovirus retinitis with sustained-release ganciclovir implant. *Archives of Ophthalmology*, 112, 1531–39.

McBride, S. 2000. *Patients Talking*. RNIB, London.

McBride, S. 2002. *Patients Talking 2*. RNIB, London.

McGarey, B.E., Napalkav, J.A., Pippen, P.A. and Reaves, T.A. 1993. Corneal wound healing strength with topical anti-inflammatory drugs (ARVO abstracts). *Investigative Ophthalmology and Visual Science*, 1321.

McMullen, T. 2013. *Guide for Trainee – Orbital, Lacrimal and Adnexal Service*. Northampton General Hospital NHS Trust.

National Statistics. 2007. Health statistics quarterly, No. 33. http://www.statistics.gov.uk.

National Service Framework: Diabetes. 2002. Department of Health, London.

Nursing and Midwifery Council. 2015. *The Code*. NMC, London.

O'Conner, S. and Glasper, E.A. 1995. *Whaleyand Wong's Children's Nursing*. Mosby, London.

O'hEineachain, R. 2002. Cool laser blasts way to micro-incision cataract surgery.

Olthoff, C. and Schoutan, J. 2005. Noncompliance with ocular hypotension treatment in patients with glaucoma or ocular hypertension: An evidence based review. *Ophthalmology*, 112, 953–61.

Olver, J. and Cassidy, L. 2005. *Ophthalmology at a Glance*. Blackwell, Oxford, UK.

Public Health England. 2015. Reports of cases of tuberculosis to enhanced tuberculosis surveillance systems: United Kingdom, 2000 to 2014. Public Health England, London.

Quigley, H.A. 2006. Number of people with glaucoma worldwide. *British Journal of Ophthalmology*, 80(5), 389–93.

Quigley, H.A. and Broman, A.T. 2006. The number of people with glaucoma worldwide in 2010 and 2020. *British Journal of Ophthalmology*, 90(3), 262–7.

Ragge, N. and Easty, D. 1990. *Immediate Eye Care*. Wolfe Publications, London.

RCN 2012. *Ophthalmic Nursing: An Integrated Career and Competence Framework*. Royal College of Nursing, London.

Renouf, P. 2007. Immediate or delayed prescribing of antibiotics reduced duration of symptoms in acute infective conjunctivitis. *Evidence Based Nursing*, 10(1), 10.

Rose, P. 2007. Management strategies for acute infective conjunctivitis in primary care: A systematic review. *Expert Opinion on Pharmacotherapy*, 8(12), 1903–21.

Sabri, K., Pandit, J.C., Thaller, V.T. et al. 1998. National survey of corneal abrasion treatment. *Eye*, 12(2), 278–81.

Sheikh, A. and Hurwitz, B. 2006. Antibiotics versus placebo for acute bacterial conjunctivitis (Cochrane Review). *The Cochrane Library*, John Wiley & Sons, Ltd. http://onlinelibrary. wiley.com/doi/10.1002/14651858.CD001211.pub2/epdf/standard.

Sleat, B., Robin, A., Covert, D. et al. 2006. Patient reported behaviour, and problems in using glaucoma medication. *Ophthalmology*, 113, 431–6.

Sparrow, J.M. 2009. *The NICE Guideline. Diagnosis and Management of Chronic Open Angle Glaucoma and Ocular Hypertension*. NICE Clinical Guideline 85. (April). http://www.nice. org.uk/nicemedia/pdf/CG85NICEGuideline.pdf.

Tarlan, B. and Kiratli, H. 2013. Subconjunctival hemorrhage: Risk factors and potential indicators. *Clinical Ophthalmology*, 7, 1163–70.

Tham, Y.C., Li, X. and Wong, T.Y. 2014. Global prevalence of glaucoma and projections of glaucoma burden through 2040. *American Academy of Ophthalmology*, 121(11), 2081–90.

The Diabetes Control and Complications Trial Research Group. 1995. The effect of intensive diabetes treatment on the progression of diabetic retinopathy in insulin dependent diabetes mellitus. *Archives of Ophthalmology*, 113, 36–51.

Toma, N., Hungerford, J., Plowman, P. et al. 1995. External beam radiotherapy for retinoblastoma 2-lens-sparing technique. *British Journal of Ophthalmology*, 79(2), 112–17.

UK Prospective Diabetic Study Group. 1998. Tight blood pressure control and risk of macrovascular and microvascular complications in type 2 diabetes, UKPDS 38. *British Medical Journal*, 317, 703–13.

Waterman, H., Leatherbarrow, B.L., Waterman, C. and Hillier, V. 1998. Post-operative nausea and vomiting following hydroxyapatite orbital implant. *European Journal of Anaesthesiology*, 15, 590–94.

Wilson, S.A. and Last, A. 2004. Management of corneal abrasions. *American Family Physician*, 70(1), 123–28.

World Alliance for Patient Safety. 2008. *Forward Planning 2008–2009*. WHO, Geneva.

Wright, H.R., Turner, A., and Taylor, H.R. June 2008. Trachoma. *Lancet*, 371(9628), 1945–54.

Yanoff, M. and Duker, J.S., Eds. 2009. *Ophthalmology*, 3rd edition. Mosby Elsevier, Edinburgh.

FURTHER READING

Beare, J.D.L. 1990. Eye injuries from assault with chemicals. *British Journal of Ophthalmology*, 74, 514–18.

Bonner, E., Dowling, S. and Eustace, P. 1994. A survey of blepharitis in pre-operative cataract patients. *European Journal of Implant and Refractive Surgery*, 6, 87–92.

British Medical Association and Royal Pharmaceutical Society of Great Britain. 2009. *British National Formulary*. BMA, London.

Carson, C. and Taylor, H. 1995. Excimer laser treatment for high and extreme myopia. *Archives of Ophthalmology*, 113, 431–36.

Central Manchester Foundation Trust. 2003. *Intra-Vitreal Injection Guidelines*. CMFT, Manchester, UK.

Corbett, M.C. 2000. Corneal topography: Basic principles and applications to refractive surgery. *Optometry Today*, February, 899–905.

Damato, B. 1995. Ten FAQs on the management of uveal melanomas. *Eye News*, 1(5), 5–7.

Davies, P., Bailey, P.J., Goldeberg, M. and Ford Hutchinson, A.W. 1984. The role of arachidonic acid oxygenation products in pain and inflammation. *Annual Review of Immunology*, 2, 335–57.

De Rott, A. 1940. Plastic repair of conjunctival defects with fetal membranes. *Archives of Ophthalmology*, 23, 522–25.

Department of Health. 2003a. *Essence of Care*. HMSO, London.

Department of Health. 2003b. *Winning Ways: Working Together to Reduce Healthcare Associated Infection in England*. HMSO, London.

Department of Health. 2004. *NHS Plan*. HMSO, London.

Department of Health. 2009. *Reforming Emergency Care*. HMSO. London.

Dutton, J.J. 1991. Coralline hydroxyapatite ocular implant. *Ophthalmology*, 98(3), 370–77.

Elder, M.J. 1994. Combined trabeculotomy – Trabeculectomy compared with primary trabeculectomy for congenital glaucoma. *British Journal of Ophthalmology*, 78(10), 745–48.

Felipe, A., Medeiros, M., Pamela, A. 2002. Corneal thickness measurements and visual function abnormalities in ocular hypertensive patients. *American Journal of Ophthalmology*, 135(2), 131–137.

Field, D., Martin, D. and Witchell, L. 1999. Ophthalmic chloramphenicol: Friend or foe. *International Journal of Ophthalmic Nursing*, 2(4), 4–7.

Fishman, J. and Fishman, L. 2010. *History Taking in Medicine and Surgery*, 2nd edition. PasTest, Knutsford, UK.

Gartry, D.S. 1995. Treating myopia with the excimer laser. The present position. *British Medical Journal*, 310, 979–85.

Hawley, D.J. 1995. Psycho-educational interventions in the treatment of arthritis. *Baillieres Clinical Rheumatology*, 9, 803–23.

Hope-Ross, M., Yannuzzi, L.A., Gragoudas, E.S. et al. 1994. Adverse reactions due to indocyanine green. *Ophthalmology*, 101(3), 529–33.

Jabs, D., Grell, R., Fox, R. and Bartlett, J. 1989. Ocular manifestations of acquired immunodeficiency syndrome. *Ophthalmology*, 96(7), 1092–99.

Jones, C.A. 2001. Socket surgery. In: *Plastic and Orbital Surgery*. R. Collin and G. Rose (Eds.). BMJ Books, London.

Kalwij, S., Macintosh, M. and Baraister, P. 2010. Screening and treatment of *Chlamydia trachomatis* infections. *BMJ*, 340, c1915.

Kirkpatrick, J., Hoh, H. and Cook, S. 1993. No eye pad for corneal abrasions. *Eye*, 7(5), 468–71.

Kyngas, H., Duffy, M.E. and Kroll, T. 2000. Conceptual analysis of compliance. *Journal of Clinical Nursing*, 9, 5–12.

Laske, M., Connel, A., Schacchat, A. et al. 1994. The Barbados eye study, prevalence of open-angle glaucoma. *Archives of Ophthalmology*, 112, 821–29.

Leitman, M. 2007. *Manual for Eye Examination and Diagnosis, 7e*. Blackwell, Hoboken, NJ.

Leske, C.M., Heijl, A., Hussein, M. et al. 2003. Factors for glaucoma progression and the effect of treatment. *Archives of Ophthalmology*, 121, 48–56.

Manchester Royal Eye Hospital. 2004. *Protocol for the Management of POAG*. MREH, Manchester, UK.

McNicholl, C. 1995. Phacoemulsification. *British Journal of Nursing*, 5(2), 22–24.

Menezo, J., Cisneros, A., Hueso, J. et al. 1995. Long-term results of surgical treatment of high myopia with Worst-Fechner intraocular lenses. *Journal of Cataract and Refractive Surgery*, 21(1), 93–8.

Migdal, C. 1994. Long-term functional outcome after early surgery in open-angle glaucoma. *Ophthalmology*, 101(9), 1651–56.

Migdal, C. 1995. What is the appropriate treatment for patients with primary open-angle glaucoma: Medicine, laser or primary surgery? *Ophthalmic Surgery*, 26(2), 108–9.

National Patient Safety Agency. 2004–2009. *Seven Steps to Patient Safety. (Four Seven Steps Guides.)*. National Patient Safety Agency, London. http:// www.nrls.npsa.nhs.uk/resources/ collections/seven-steps-to-patient-safety.

NICE. 2002. Clinical effectiveness and cost utility of photodynamic therapy for wet age-related macular degeneration. http://www.nice.org.

NICE. 2007. Interventional procedure overview of corneal implants for keratonus. http://www.nice.org.

NICE. 2013. Summary of infective conjunctivitis. http://www.nice.org.

North, R. 2001. *Work and the Eye*, 2nd edition. Oxford University Press, Oxford.

Osaka, M. and Keltuer, J. 1991. Botulinum: A toxin (Oculinum) in ophthalmology. *Survey of Ophthalmology*, 36(1), 28–46.

Ottar, W., Scott, W. and Holgado, S. 1995. Photoscreening for amblyogenic factors. *Journal of Pediatric Ophthalmology and Strabismus*, 32, 289–95.

Pearce, J. 1996. Multifocal intraocular lenses. *Current Opinion in Ophthalmology*, 7(1), 2–10.

Pendleton, D., Schofield, T., Tate, P. et al. 2006. *The New Consultation: Developing Doctor–Patient Communication*. Oxford University Press, Oxford, UK.

Potter, P.A. 1994. *Pocket Guide to Health Assessment*. Mosby, London.

Pratt-Johnson, J. and Tillson, G. 1994. *Management of Strabismus and Amblyopia – A Practical Guide*. Theime Medical, New York.

Public Health England. 2004. Snapshot survey of healthcare associated infections (HCAI) reveals overall drop in infections down to 6.4 per cent. http://www.hpa.org.uk/Publications/InfectiousDiseases/AntimicrobialAndHealthcareAssociatedInfections/.

RCOph. 2014. Patient safety in ophthalmology. *Royal College of Ophthalmologists*. https://www.rcophth.ac.uk/wp-content/uploads/2014/12/2011_PROF_107_PATIENT-SAFETY-IN-OPHTHALMOLOGY.pdf.

Ricci, R. et al. 1992. Strampelli's osteo-odonto-keratoprosthesis. Clinical and histological long-term features of three prostheses. *British Journal of Ophthalmology* 76, 232–4. doi:10.1136/bjo.76.4.232. Abstract available: http://bjo.bmjjournals.com/cgi/content/abstract/76/4/232.

Richter, A., Anton, S.E., Koch, P. and Dennett, S.L. 2003. The impact of reducing dose frequency on health outcomes. *Clinical Therapeutics*, 25(8), 2307–35.

Royal College of Ophthalmologists Guidelines. 2002. Creutzfeldt-Jakob Disease (CJD) and Ophthalmology. https://www.rcophth.ac.uk/wp-content/uploads/2014/12/2010_PROF_102_MANAGING-CJD-and-vCJD-RISK-IN-OPHTHALMOLOGY.pdf.

Saude, T. 1992. *Ocular Anatomy*. Blackwell, Oxford, UK.

Schwab, I.R., Epstein, R.J., Harris, D.J. et al. 1997. *External Eye Disease and Cornea*. American Academy of Ophthalmology, San Francisco.

Shaw, M. 2001. *Principles and Protocols for Ophthalmic Medication and Instillation/Application (In-house Policy)*. Manchester Royal Eye Hospital, Manchester, UK.

Sheikh, A. and Hurwitz, B. 2001. Topical antibiotics for acute bacterial conjunctivitis: A systematic review. *British Journal of General Practice*, 51(467), 473–77.

Sorsby, A. and Symons, H.M. 1946. Amniotic membrane grafts in caustic burns of the eye. *British Journal of Ophthalmology*, 30, 337–45.

Stapleton, F. 1992. Microbial keratitis and contact lens wear. *Journal of British Contact Lens Association*, 3(1), 5–6.

Szczotka, L.B. 2002. Computerised corneal topography applications in RGP contact lens fitting. *Optometry Today*, 49, 1617–25.

Szerenyi, K., Wang, X.W., Lee, M. and McDonnell, P.J. 1993. Topical diclofenac treatment prior to eximer laser photorefractive keratometry in rabbits. *Refractive Corneal Surgery*, 9, 437–42.

Tomask, R.L. 1997. *Handbook of Treatment in Neuro-Ophthalmology*. Butterworth Heinemann, Boston.

Vaughan, D., Asbury, T. and Riordan-Eva, P. 1999. *General Ophthalmology*. Lange Medical, New York.

Visto, D. 2000. Corneal abrasion: To patch or not to patch. *Insight*, 25, 4–6, January–March.

Wakelin, S. 1995. Hygiene compliance in contact lens wearers presenting to an ophthalmic casualty department. *International Journal of Pharmacy Practice*, 3(2), 97–100.

Williams, M. 1993. Achieving patient compliance. *Nursing Times*, 89(13), 50–52.

Wilson, C.G. and O'Mahoney, B. 1999. Non-compliance in glaucoma management. *Eyenews*, 5(6), 7–9.

Wittpen, J.R. 1995. Eye scrub: Simplifying the management of blepharitis. *Journal of Ophthalmic Nursing and Technology*, 14(1), 25–28.

Wong, E.Y.H., Keefe, J.E., Rait, J.L. et al. 2004. Detection of undiagnosed glaucoma by eye health professionals. *Ophthalmology*, 111, 1508–4.

Yung, C.W., Massicotte, S. and Kuwabara, T. 1994. Argon laser treatment of trichiasis – A clinical and histopathologic evaluation. *Ophthalmic Plastic Reconstructive Surgery*, 10(2), 130–36.

WEBSITES

Aseptic Non Touch Technique (ANTT). http://www.antt.org/ANTT_Site/home.html. Provides excellent advice on infection control.

British National Formulary. http://bnf.org. The BNF is an excellent resource for sources of drug information.

British Thoracic Society. http://www.brit-thoracic.org.uk. A useful website on respiratory matters.

General Practice Notebook. http://www.gpnotebook.co.uk. Compliance with medication and other related matters.

International Glaucoma Association. http://www.glaucoma-association.com. Provides patient information on all aspects of glaucoma.

NHS Choices. How long will I have to wait to see a consultant? http://www.nhs.uk/chq/Pages/904.aspx?CategoryID = 68&SubCategoryID = 153.

Royal National Institute for the Blind (RNIB). http://www.rnib.org.uk/Pages/Home.aspx. Supporting blind and partially sighted people.

Index

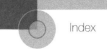

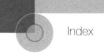

T - #1006 - 101024 - C390 - 246/189/21 - PB - 9781482249767 - Gloss Lamination